Engage more thoroughly tension in book,

4 is something anti-modern though, just b

The Grenfell Medical Mission

and American Support in

Newfoundland and Labrador, 1890s–1940s

Gillian Roberts – Reading between the Borderlines

CE Canbell – Nature, Place + Story: Rethinking Historic Sites in Canada

Mourning Nature

McGill-Queen's/Associated Medical Services Studies in the History of Medicine, Health, and Society

Series editors: J.T.H. Connor and Erika Dyck

This series presents books in the history of medicine, health studies, and social policy, exploring interactions between the institutions, ideas, and practices of medicine and those of society as a whole. To begin to understand these complex relationships and their history is a vital step to ensuring the protection of a fundamental human right: the right to health. Volumes in this series have received financial support to assist publication from Associated Medical Services, Inc. (AMS), a Canadian charitable organization with an impressive history as a catalyst for change in Canadian healthcare. For eighty years, AMS has had a profound impact through its support of the history of medicine and the education of healthcare professionals, and by making strategic investments to address critical issues in our healthcare system. AMS has funded eight chairs in the history of medicine across Canada, is a primary sponsor of many of the country's history of medicine and nursing organizations, and offers fellowships and grants through the AMS History of Medicine and Healthcare Program (www.amshealthcare.ca).

The Grenfell Medical Mission

and American Support in

Newfoundland and Labrador, 1890s–1940s

Edited by
Jennifer J. Connor and Katherine Side

McGill-Queen's University Press
Montreal & Kingston • London • Chicago

© McGill-Queen's University Press 2019

ISBN 978-0-7735-5486-3 (cloth)
ISBN 978-0-7735-5487-0 (paper)
ISBN 978-0-7735-5579-2 (ePDF)
ISBN 978-0-7735-5580-8 (ePUB)

Legal deposit first quarter 2019
Bibliothèque nationale du Québec

Printed in Canada on acid-free paper that is 100% ancient forest free
(100% post-consumer recycled), processed chlorine free

This book has been published with the help of a grant from the
Canadian Federation for the Humanities and Social Sciences, through
the Awards to Scholarly Publications Program, using funds provided
by the Social Sciences and Humanities Research Council of Canada.

Funded by the   Financé par le
Government   gouvernement   Canada   Canada Council   Conseil des arts
of Canada   du Canada   for the Arts   du Canada

We acknowledge the support of the Canada Council for the Arts,
which last year invested $153 million to bring the arts to Canadians
throughout the country. Nous remercions le Conseil des arts du
Canada de son soutien. L'an dernier, le Conseil a investi 153 millions
de dollars pour mettre de l'art dans la vie des Canadiennes et des
Canadiens de tout le pays.

Library and Archives Canada Cataloguing in Publication

The Grenfell Medical Mission and American support in Newfoundland and Labrador, 1890s–1940s / edited by Jennifer J. Connor and
Katherine Side.

(McGill-Queen's/Associated Medical Services studies in the history
of medicine, health, and society ; 49)
Includes bibliographical references and index.
Issued in print and electronic formats.
ISBN 978-0-7735-5486-3 (cloth).–ISBN 978-0-7735-5487-0 (paper).
–ISBN 978-0-7735-5579-2 (ePDF).–ISBN 978-0-7735-5580-8 (ePUB)

1. Grenfell, Wilfred Thomason, Sir, 1865–1940. 2. Grenfell Labrador
Medical Mission–History–19th century. 3. Grenfell Labrador Medical
Mission–History–20th century. 4. Missions, Medical–Newfoundland
and Labrador–History–19th century. 5. Missions, Medical–New-
foundland and Labrador–History–20th century. 6. Americans–
Newfoundland and Labrador–History–19th century. 7. Americans–
Newfoundland and Labrador–History–20th century. I. Connor,
Jennifer J. (Jennifer Jean), 1953–, editor II. Side, Katherine, 1963–,
editor III. Series: McGill-Queen's/Associated Medical Services studies
in the history of medicine, health, and society ; 49

RA390.C3G64 2018   362.109718   C2018-903634-6
                                           C2018-903635-4

Contents

Part II: The Grenfell Enterprise in Motion

Illustrations

TABLES

Acknowledgments

handwritten: property of VFLD

This collection of essays emerged from work that we editors had undertaken individually on aspects of the Grenfell mission for the period before Newfoundland became a province of Canada in 1949. Realizing that a significant gap existed in knowledge of the IGA and its history in this pre-Confederation period, we issued a call for essays on a broad range of topics addressed by the IGA beyond the organization's primary focus of health care. We therefore acknowledge first and foremost the authors of this collection who answered the call, or who were nudged to contribute, to work with us, to sustain the momentum, and to share their often deep knowledge about the IGA from years of study in Newfoundland and Labrador. We have enjoyed our collaboration with them, on studies that brought fresh and new perspectives to the subject. We are especially indebted to James K. Hiller, who helped ensure that we did not veer too close to the rocks of error, misrepresentation, and oversight in the history of Newfoundland and Labrador that might too easily undermine the best efforts of us recent CFAs (Come-from-Aways). However, we editors are responsible for any historical inaccuracies that may still be present in this volume.

Study of such an expansive enterprise as the IGA required a clear focus, and it was the research and suggestion of J.T.H. Connor that led us to emphasize the strong American connections to all the activities of Wilfred Grenfell and his mission during his lifetime. Connections of the United States to Newfoundland and Labrador had been made generally but had not been explored in relation to the IGA. This focus on American influence then invigorated the work, and we invited two other contributors – Mark Graesser and Helen Woodrow – whose research had already demonstrated important manifestations of these American ties in addition to those in essays by J.T.H. Connor, Ronald L. Numbers, and Rafico Ruiz.

No grants were specifically sought for this collective work: a testament not only to the availability of rich collections of research materials locally but also to the ability of scholars to undertake such study, as has long been the case. Nevertheless, aspects of the research and the book-making process were supported in ways that we co-editors gratefully acknowledge. Use of, and citations to, the clinical records of the IGA housed at the Charles S. Curtis Memorial Hospital in St Anthony, NL, are based on significant support from an earlier grant HOM 98740, "Interpreting Remote Medicine and Health Care in Pre-Confederation Newfoundland as 'Ecosystem,'" awarded by the Canadian Institutes for Health Research (CIHR) to principal investigators Jennifer J. Connor and J.T.H. Connor; permissions were provided to the investigators by the current owner of these records, Labrador-Grenfell Health, who aided substantially by providing in-kind support onsite towards their digital preservation and redaction by research assistant John R. Matchim. We are indebted to John Matchim, who worked on a database from these anonymized records for three years after this grant with funds provided by J.T.H. Connor, for extracting the data on patient regions that appear as table 0.2 in this volume's introduction. As culmination of the CIHR history of medicine grant, the investigators organized a public symposium to commemorate 100 years of the International Grenfell Association in 2014. Held in St John's at The Rooms – the province's combined museum, art gallery, and archives – the symposium explored the significance of Dr Wilfred Grenfell, this organization, and the delivery of health care in Newfoundland and Labrador, and it stimulated the new research in this volume. Five of the authors in this volume participated in the symposium: Ronald L. Numbers as invited guest speaker; Jennifer J. Connor, J.T.H. Connor, Heidi Coombs-Thorne, and Katherine Side as presenters. With the exception of the guest speaker, however, all four presenters wrote completely new studies for this collection of essays.

A face-to-face meeting of essay authors onsite with video link to discuss the first draft of this collection was facilitated by Katherine Side with the aid of a Seed, Bridge, and Multidisciplinary Fund grant of the Faculty of Humanities and Social Sciences at Memorial University for her work on IGA photographs. An honorarium to prepare the volume's bibliography for publication was also supported from this grant. We are particularly grateful to Helen Woodrow, who laboured above and beyond the call of duty to develop an initial draft of this bibliography with close attention to detail and timeliness.

Memorial University's Digital Archives Initiative made the magazine of the Grenfell mission, *Among the Deep Sea Fishers*, available on the internet, and without that resource much of the underlying research for the new studies in this book would have taken many years to complete. We are also grateful to Don Walsh for his help with ADSF images when this book was at proof stage. The images in this volume also come from this now-digitized magazine and from the photographic collection of The Rooms. The images are in the public domain, but efforts have been made to obtain necessary permissions for the figures in this book.

Finally, we would like to thank Kyla Madden, senior editor at McGill-Queen's University Press, who showed interest and provided necessary moral and administrative support from our first enquiry to the finished product. With her encouragement, help, and grace we met many publication and press deadlines very quickly.

Abbreviations

ORGANIZATIONS

CCNY	Carnegie Corporation of New York
CHE	Council of Higher Education (Newfoundland)
GAA	Grenfell Association of America
IGA	International Grenfell Association
MDSF	Mission to Deep Sea Fishermen
MUN	Memorial University of Newfoundland
NDBMH	Notre Dame Bay Memorial Hospital
NEGA	New England Grenfell Association
NONIA	Newfoundland Outport Nursing and Industrial Association
RNMDSF	Royal National Mission to Deep Sea Fishermen (after 1896)

ARCHIVES AND CITATIONS

ADSF	*Among the Deep Sea Fishers*
BCHL	Berea College, Hutchins Library Special Collections and Archives, Berea, KY
CBMH/BCHM	*Canadian Bulletin of Medical History/Bulletin canadien d'histoire de la médecine*
CGC	Carolyn Galbraith Correspondence (Misc. Manuscripts MS-226). Sophia Smith Archive, Smith College, Northampton, MA

CCNYR	Carnegie Corporation of New York Records. Rare Book and Manuscript Library Archives, Columbia University, NY
CMAJ	*Canadian Medical Association Journal*
DCB	*Dictionary of Canadian Biography*
DNB	*Dictionary of National Biography*
ENL	*Encyclopedia of Newfoundland and Labrador*
EPHP	Elizabeth Page Harris Papers (MS 771). Manuscripts and Archives, Yale University Library, New Haven, CT
JHA	*Journal of the House of Assembly* (Newfoundland)
LAC	Library and Archives Canada, Ottawa, ON
MU-ASC	Memorial University of Newfoundland, Archives and Special Collections, St John's, NL
MU-CNS	Memorial University of Newfoundland, Centre for Newfoundland Studies, St John's, NL
MU-FLA	Memorial University of Newfoundland, Folklore and Language Archives, St John's, NL
MU-FMA	Memorial University of Newfoundland, Faculty of Medicine Founders Archive, St John's, NL
MU-HSL	Memorial University of Newfoundland, Health Sciences Library, Historical Collection
MU-RA	Memorial University of Newfoundland Records Archives, President's Office Records and Board of Governors' Records, St John's, NL
NLS	*Newfoundland and Labrador Studies*
NQ	*Newfoundland Quarterly*
NS	*Newfoundland Studies*
PAD	The Rooms, Provincial Archives Division, St John's, NL
WGP	Wilfred Thomason Grenfell Papers (MS 254). Manuscripts and Archives, Yale University Library, New Haven, CT

TERMS

WOP	Grenfell Mission Worker "With-Out-Pay"

The Grenfell Medical Mission

and American Support in

Newfoundland and Labrador, 1890s–1940s

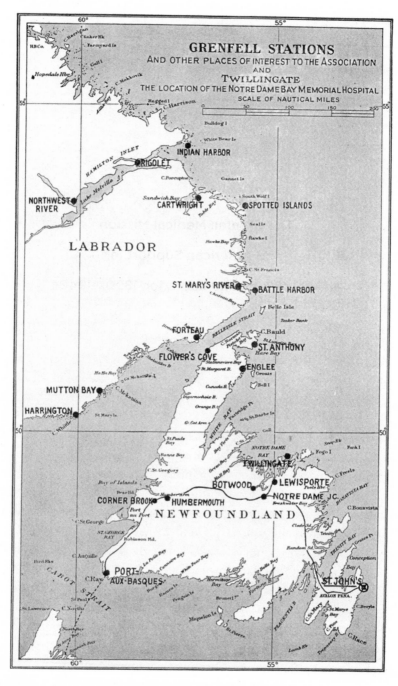

Map: International Grenfell Association stations, 1940.
ADSF (April 1940)

Editors' Introduction

"Untainted by American Ways"? Newfoundland, the United States, and the Grenfell Mission

Several decades before the creation in the 1960s of American government agencies for international aid and development, people in the United States had engaged in private aid for international health and humanitarian purposes through organized philanthropic support and volunteerism much closer to home, in North America. The beneficiaries of such generosity were not inhabitants of a foreign-language, overseas culture struggling to survive in inhospitable locales, environmental catastrophe, or war; rather, they were predominantly British descendants who eked out an existence as fishers along the cold Atlantic coast of northern Newfoundland and southern Labrador. American support for these people came through monetary donations, volunteer workers and consultants, contributions in kind (clothing, supplies, equipment, and boats), and programs for health, education, and training, all to an organization led by a single man: Wilfred T. Grenfell (1865–1940). Individual Americans donated to Grenfell's organization, as did American foundations and charities with similar aims such as the renowned Carnegie Foundation in New York and the Lend A Hand Society in Boston (which, among other things, operates a "book mission" to the American South); financial contributions specifically for hospital construction also came from the New York–based Commonwealth Fund.

Wilfred Grenfell was a British physician whose missionary life work began in 1892 with the London-based Mission to Deep Sea Fishermen (later designated Royal) in the North Atlantic British dominion that is now the Canadian province of Newfoundland and Labrador. Known widely as the Labrador, or Grenfell, Medical Mission, in 1914 the non-denominational mission incorporated as the independent International Grenfell Association (IGA). Grenfell's organization established dozens of institutions throughout the 2,400 kilometres (1,500 miles) of Labrador coast and northern Newfoundland (see map), over thirty of which were still active by his death in 1940: six hospitals, six nursing stations, five day and boarding schools, an orphanage, seven industrial centres, two agricultural and animal husbandry stations, and a sawmill. Six co-operative stores were initiated by Grenfell and often supported by him personally, though not run by his mission. Summer schools were developed in remote areas. St Anthony, at the tip of the northern peninsula of the island, was headquarters, with its hospital, orphanage, school, industrial centre, clothing store, co-operative store, and guest house; however, similarly equipped facilities were located in Cartwright and North West River, both in Labrador (table o.1).

The organization had also established a seamen's institute in St John's; libraries; and a cottage industry involving 2,000 people who created woven, knitted, and hooked goods sold in mission stores in the United States (the most well-known crafts being silk-stocking mats). In addition, it had sent over one hundred people for training in Great Britain, the United States, and Canada, to return home as skilled workers. The organization in 1937 employed over sixty permanent staff consisting of nine doctors, fourteen nurses, ten schoolteachers, six orphanage superintendents and school housekeepers, and eight industrial directors and community workers; there were also one hundred summer volunteers, including two more doctors and an assortment of "professors," dentists, laboratory technicians, more nurses, and outdoor workers. Annual operating expenses in 1937 were $120,000, but of particular interest are sources of revenue: total revenue was about $135,000 (close to $2.3 million in 2017), the majority of which came from donors to the Grenfell associations in North America, Great Britain, Ireland, and Newfoundland, with the largest amounts ($83,000) attributed to the two American associations (the equivalent of $1,431,750 in 2017) (figure o.1).[1]

Importantly, the mission had always provided medical care from Grenfell's ship that made routine visits to coastal communities in the

Table 0.1
International Grenfell Association institutions, 1937

Station/location	Hospital	Nursing station	Day and boarding school	Industrial centre	Co-operative store*	Agricultural station*	Sawmill*	Orphanage	Seamen's institute
Battle Harbour	•		•						
Brehat					•				
Cartwright	•		•	•					
Englee		•							
Flower's Cove		•			•				
Forteau		•		•	•				
Harrington Harbour	•								
Indian Harbour		•		•					
Mutton Bay		•		•					
North West River	•		•	•					
Red Bay				•	•				
Roddickton						•	•		
Spotted Islands		•							
St Anthony	•		•	•	•	•		•	
St John's									•
St Mary's River	•		•						
TOTAL	6	6	5	7	6	2	1	1	1

* Initiated by Wilfred Grenfell, not operated by the International Grenfell Association

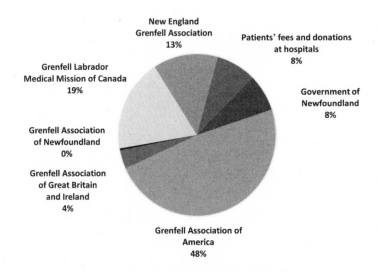

Figure 0.1 International Grenfell Association annual sources of funding, 1937. Derived from Grenfell Association of Great Britain and Ireland, *Medical Work in Labrador and Northern Newfoundland: Eleventh Annual Report* (London, [1937]); and [International Grenfell Association], *A Few Facts about the Grenfell Missions of Newfoundland and Labrador* ([1937])

summers, visits that also exchanged and distributed other provisions for residents, including clothes and reading materials. The organization's fleet by 1940 consisted of the hospital steamer *Strathcona*, motor vessels *Maraval* and *Jessie Goldthwaite*, the schooner *Geo. B. Cluett*, and other smaller vessels. Isolation thus to some extent nurtured the development of the IGA as an autonomous regional health authority, distinct from government oversight and influence. St Anthony is about 965 kilometres (600 miles) from the financial and administrative capital of St John's on the southern Avalon peninsula (an equivalent linear distance is from Bangor, Maine, to Washington, DC) – a land distance that lacks meaning during Grenfell's time, when there was neither road nor direct rail link over the mostly uninhabited terrain on the island between the two settlements. Coastal steamers instead transported people, goods, and mail along the involuted and archipelagic coastline (the main coast of Newfoundland is over 9,600 kilometres [6,000 miles] in length). A typical return trip to about fifty communities from St John's to Labrador via St Anthony took at least two weeks (much longer, if at all, in winter,

Table 0.2
Place of origin of inpatients at St Anthony Hospital, 1904–1935

Region	%*
St Anthony District, Newfoundland	38.4
White Bay District, Newfoundland	15.7
Notre Dame Bay District, Newfoundland	15.1
Straits of Belle Isle District, Newfoundland	7.5
Bonavista Bay District, Newfoundland	4.1
Conception Bay District, Newfoundland	2.9
Trinity Bay District, Newfoundland	2.1
West Coast District, Newfoundland	2.1
St John's, Newfoundland	1.0
South Coast District, Newfoundland	0.6
Labrador	4.2
Outside of Newfoundland and Labrador	0.4
Unspecified	6.0

* Derived from total number of hospital admission records (9,424), St Anthony Hospital, IGA; now housed at Charles S. Curtis Memorial Hospital, St Anthony, NL. Some records may represent the same patients who were re-admitted.

when passage could be blocked by ice until June).[2] Nevertheless, the hospital in St Anthony became the centre of health care for the whole island, attracting patients and health-care practitioners from St John's as well (table 0.2).

Hence, for several decades this was not a single-location all-purpose mission settlement; rather, its goal was to aid fishers' families along hundreds of miles of Atlantic coastline in becoming independent and self-sufficient. With Grenfell's relentless promotion in publishing and lecture tours, particularly in the United States, and his boundless enthusiasm for entrepreneurial ideas, the mission blended many of the social agendas of the period. In 1981 after most of the organization's services had increasingly been taken over by the provincial government – which by then had also become its primary funding source – the IGA sold its considerable land holdings, hospital institutions, nursing stations, and medical equipment to the government for the nominal sum of one dollar.

Since then, the IGA has operated as a private foundation providing bursaries and project grants for health, education, and wellness to benefit the region; and donation for protection and maintenance of former IGA sites such as Battle Harbour.[3] Most recently, it funded a report in 2016 that projects population figures to 2036 for Labrador and the Northern Peninsula of Newfoundland at a time of "transition" when the region is undergoing significant decline in population and associated services for the population.[4]

Historically, however, and perhaps understandably, given the broad extent of his organization, Grenfell's spirit pervades Newfoundland and Labrador. It thrives in name through the Labrador-Grenfell Regional Health Authority created in 2005 when Grenfell Regional Health Services and Health Labrador Corporation merged:[5] a Grenfell quotation on the health authority website banner reminds the community of his commitment to serve, and the health authority's fundraising arm, the Grenfell Foundation, reflects his own formidable fundraising achievements.[6] The Grenfell Interpretation Centre and the Grenfell House Museum, both in St Anthony (Grenfell's home base in Newfoundland), stand as material testaments to the man and his mission.[7] Large bronze statues of Grenfell adorn provincial sites, including the Newfoundland and Labrador government House of Assembly, and named after him are the Sir Wilfred Grenfell College (the Corner Brook campus of Memorial University of Newfoundland on the west coast of the island) and a Newfoundland-built and -based Canadian Coast Guard search and rescue vessel (equipped with a ten-bed hospital) that patrols the northeastern Atlantic Ocean. A scenic drive on the Northern Peninsula, marketed to visitors, is called "the Grenfell Loop" by the provincial government. Perhaps less obvious are the buildings that formerly belonged to his organization that serve as tourist attractions: at Battle Harbour, Labrador, now a national historic site, the Grenfell Doctors Cottage is offered for accommodations, as is the former nursing station in Forteau, Labrador.[8] Of course, Grenfell's international profile led to other tangible recognitions after his death, including postage stamps in Newfoundland (1945) and Canada (1965). And, attesting to his personal reach beyond this current Canadian province to his many supporters in the United States is a stained glass window in the National Cathedral in Washington, DC, that depicts Grenfell in parka, long boots, and gloves, holding a snowshoe and standing with Christ the Healer and Louis Pasteur.[9]

Yet despite continuing to occupy a prominent place in the area's history, and attracting significant American support, Grenfell's mission-turned-association and its evolution have yet to attract full study. This state of affairs is beginning to change, as the IGA records and other archival materials become more available, including through digitization, and scholars are investigating them initially for doctoral dissertations on aspects of the whole enterprise. For example, Heidi Coombs-Thorne used the records to analyze the class, conflict, and identity of nurses in the IGA from the 1940s to the 1980s; and Rafico Ruiz studied the organization to the 1940s as a process of social reform and, most importantly, as material re-formation of social infrastructure in the region.[10] Otherwise, rather than critical analysis, the genres of heroic biography and autobiographical narrative dominate the historical literature about the Grenfell enterprise. The contributions of individuals to both the organization and to its local communities are frequently constructed as heroic stories of adventure and risk interwoven with accounts of medical care.[11] Indeed, Wilfred Grenfell himself became an internationally storied semi-mythical figure as the "Patron Saint of Labrador"[12] with the conflation of fact with fiction – especially after his famous near-death experience in 1908 "adrift on an ice pan" when he attempted to rush across a frozen bay to attend a sick child.[13] He was the subject of many popular books[14] and featured as a fictionalized character in best-selling novels.[15] Perhaps much of his celebrity derived from his own public relations machine: Grenfell published non-stop on life in the North as well as on his own life, in countless books and magazine articles,[16] and he travelled tirelessly as lecturer and promoter for his enterprise. His narratives often described his efforts as an intrepid explorer, carving trails out of unknown terrain not traversed by coastal people in order to set up new business ventures in the interior to aid them in becoming self-reliant members of a cash economy. His presentations, illustrated with images of his mission and its people, were oriented towards church groups, middle-class social reformers – many of whom were women – and universities, to all those who could offer material and volunteer support to his mission. In these ways, Grenfell tapped into the popular – at the time insatiable – demand for missionary biographies, travels, and periodicals.[17]

In addition, Grenfell initially fostered support in these autobiographical accounts by highlighting the Indigenous population of Labrador (Inuit, Innu, and Southern Inuit) through images and narratives of individuals. In at least two instances, stories about Inuit children were used for promotion purposes. "Gabriel" Pomiuk, a Labrador Inuit who was among those exhibited at the Chicago World's Fair in 1893, was cared for at the Grenfell mission's Battle Harbour Hospital from 1895 until his death in 1897.[18] His story was often told, as was the story of Kirkina Mukko (or Mucko, and also known as Elizabeth Jeffries). After losing her lower legs to gangrene, Kirkina was briefly cared for at the mission's Indian Harbour Hospital. The cost of manufacturing and fitting prostheses was provided charitably, including by a Boston-based group, the "Cornerers," who sponsored the Gabriel Pomiuk Memorial Cot (corner cot) that Kirkina later occupied for two years in the Battle Harbour Hospital. Kirkina would then live briefly in New York, where she met many of the mission's supporters, and travel to Mexico with the doctor who provided her first prostheses before returning to Labrador. Stories about Kirkina and the assistance provided to her were recounted in the IGA's publications for many years afterward.[19]

Despite this early emphasis on Indigenous peoples and individuals in his publications, Grenfell viewed the population who received the care of his mission as akin to the British; he increasingly expressed this similarity after formation of the IGA in 1914, both in publications and in internal documents. The instructions later provided to volunteer workers informed them, for example, "It is well to remember that the people among whom you will work are of British extraction and English-speaking. Their customs and speech may differ from ours in small ways, but they are of the same stock as ourselves." A reminder, also issued in writing to volunteers, was intended to minimize the possibility of offence and distrust among these distantly related people: "It is unwise therefore, ever to talk about them, their settlement or their custom in public places ... they are sensitive to comment or criticism."[20] There were many reasons for this apparent change in priority, but it is important to know that Grenfell was not the first, or only, foreign missionary

Emphasis on shared Englishness

to work on the Labrador coast. The Protestant Moravian mission had been based on the northern Labrador coast since the late eighteenth century, working among Indigenous peoples.[21] As well, Canadian Protestant churches included Labrador among their missionary activities, often for their own denominations; as with these Canadian missionaries, Grenfell worked along the southern coast of Labrador.[22]

Perhaps paralleling his shifting priority about the beneficiaries of his enterprise, Grenfell's own life and world view, according to Ronald Rompkey, still "presents ambiguities" for people of the region: "It would be difficult to dispute the value of the medical and social benefits that followed, but not everyone tolerated Grenfell's attitude of social guardianship." This diplomatic observation about the perspective of modern-day residents obscures concerns about Grenfell's institutional legacy that arose especially in later generations, after the period of Grenfell and his mission that precedes both his death in 1940 and the political inclusion of the region within Canada in 1949.[23] As the most scholarly of Grenfell's biographers, in 1991 Rompkey wrote "not in the manner of the heroic biographies by which Grenfell has customarily been treated."[24] To the present, however, this broad interest in individuals and their heroic experiences with the mission has continued to appeal especially to book publishers and their readers.[25] At the same time, these biographical accounts, together with more recent scholarship on groups of individuals (such as nurses), point to a vitally important aspect of Grenfell's enterprise: the international connections on which it depended.[26] Staff and volunteers joined the mission from the United States, especially the New England states, the United Kingdom, and Canada. The new studies in this collection therefore spotlight the support for the organization in order to examine its operation. By describing the activities of the distributed enterprise and their historical context – for the first time – rather than the efforts of lone individuals or an occupational group, this volume also allows fuller understanding of its distinction from other missions and its place in a much larger international context.

Above all, the following chapters emphasize the critical importance of American support and influence. It was funds from the Grenfell Association of America in New York and the New England Grenfell Association in Boston that enabled the formation and incorporation of the

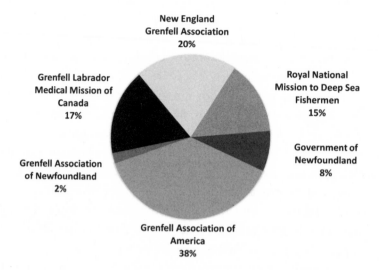

Figure 0.2 International Grenfell Association sources of funding, 1914. Derived from [International Grenfell Association], *Annual Report of the International Grenfell Association* [1915]: 17, 19

mission in 1914 as the independent International Grenfell Association: they totalled about $29,000 (about $700,000 in 2017) compared with substantially smaller contributions from the Royal National Mission to Deep Sea Fishermen in London, branch associations in Newfoundland and Canada (in Montreal, Toronto, and Ottawa), and grants from the Government of Newfoundland (figure 0.2). Although the IGA had legal charter in St John's, the first meeting of the Board of Directors was held at the Harvard Club in Boston. Furthermore, the home for the IGA was in New York, where its magazine, *Among the Deep Sea Fishers* (ADSF), then moved from Toronto. With this newly organized American base for operation, the association and its magazine shifted from British-style mission activity to American notions of systematization and philanthropy.

Moreover, published lists of the Staff Selection Committee from 1914 to 1940 show that the overwhelming majority of all 2,200 workers in the IGA was American. In fact, it is easier to count the relatively few people from Great Britain, Canada, Newfoundland, and other countries, than it is to count the thousands from the United States. A straightforward calculation of people identified each year is hindered

by repetitions of the names of full-time staff who resided at their IGA
stations and of many volunteers who returned for more than one season and who may have been assigned more than one role each time;
only the staff physicians, who often served for decades, represented
three nationalities almost equally: from England, Wilfred Grenfell and
Harry Paddon; from Scotland, John Grieve; from Canada, Donald
Hodd (Ontario) and H. Mather Hare (Nova Scotia); from Switzerland,
Herman Moret (via McGill University); and from the United States,
John Little, Charles Parsons, and Charles Curtis. Visiting physicians
who returned for years – often decades – included A.W. Wakefield from
England,[27] and Joseph Andrews and Frank Phinney from the United
States. Otherwise, over this twenty-five-year period, only about 13 per
cent of IGA workers of all kinds came from places other than the
United States: approximately 100 from the United Kingdom; 90 from
Canada; 75 from Newfoundland and Labrador; and 17 from Ireland,
France, Australia, Germany, New Zealand, Egypt, Italy, Denmark, and
Bermuda.[28] Although institutional affiliations were not listed in the
1930s in addition to place of origin, the pattern for staff and volunteers
is easily deduced for the whole period to 1940. The approximately
1,900 Americans hailed primarily from New England states and, in
addition to longstanding volunteer commitments and contributions
from post-secondary institutions like Yale, Harvard, Princeton, Johns
Hopkins, the College of Physicians and Surgeons of New York (Columbia University), the Massachusetts Institute of Technology, the
University of Pennsylvania, Vassar, Bryn Mawr, Williams, Smith, Tufts,
Amherst, Cornell, Rutgers, Wellesley, and Swarthmore, they (especially
nurses) volunteered from many hospitals: Massachusetts General Hos-
pital, Children's Hospital, Peter Bent Brigham Hospital, City Hospital,
Women's Hospital, and Charlesgate Hospital, all in Boston, along with
Lynn Hospital, Massachusetts; Johns Hopkins Hospital, Baltimore; St
Luke's Hospital, Roosevelt Hospital, and Presbyterian Hospital, all in
New York City; Hartford Hospital, Connecticut; and others in New
Hampshire, Vermont, Pennsylvania, and New York states.[29]

   While highly educated and trained Americans did not outnumber
local populations at any time, their strong presence in small, isolated
communities of tiny populations – especially in the summer seasons –

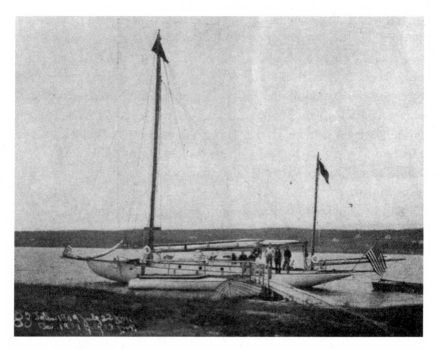

Figure 0.3 Princeton yawl, *Andrew J. McCosh*, flying US flag, 1909.
ADSF 7 (October 1909): 3

Pronounced US Presence

would have been pronounced (at times perhaps even resembling modern
college towns where the influx of students each year has great impact
on the locality). Indeed, in addition to the volunteers and staff, by the
1930s, it was routine to see the American flag at various IGA sites and
on its ships donated and staffed by Americans (figures 0.3 and 0.4).

At the very least, this sustained and significant support in finances and
personnel from people in the United States offsets a reassurance to Great
Britain in 1911 by the colonial governor that Newfoundland was "untainted by American ways,"[30] an assertion that also indicates the degree
to which Grenfell's expansive enterprise over decades was not being recognized outside the small urban centre of St John's. Just four years later,
however, his successor acknowledged to local applause the "generous
support given by Americans in the past and their guarantee of the same
in the future," as he unveiled portraits of three US presidents at the mission's Seamen's Institute in St John's.[31] That the aid and influence of

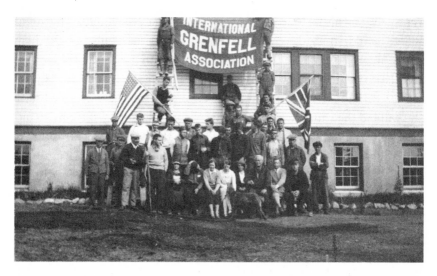

Figure 0.4 Cartwright boarding school, completion of water pipe commemoration, showing IGA banner and two flags of the United States and Great Britain, [1932]. PAD, IGA Photograph Collection, VA 92-184

Senson to Britain?

Americans was also cultural casts further doubt about any claim that Newfoundland was "untainted by American ways," in a manner that suggests the governor worried that Great Britain would react in disapproval. One cultural influence was the wide dissemination of printed publications of various kinds. To meet the need for reading material among fishers, their families, and members of his organization, Grenfell had long operated the first travelling libraries in the region as he distributed books, newspapers, and magazines from his ship, and in 1914 established the first stationary, public libraries, especially in St Anthony. Collection, organization, and distribution of books were undertaken by American volunteers, who included librarians from New York City. Grenfell's frequent appeals to donors to send this material to his mission meant that shipments routinely arrived from the United States, perhaps more than from other locales. There is some evidence that American books, expressing American values, were then destined not just for mission libraries, including that of the Seamen's Institute in St John's, but also to schools run by the mission.[32] Not just books, but also songs and games, were taught to the schoolchildren. In 1912, Theodore Greene, a volunteer teacher in St Barbe islands, northeast Newfoundland, found that the children "had a great desire to sing." He therefore "taught them a few American airs and college songs along with 'God Save the King.'" He also tried to teach them a few American games, such as "squat-tag."[33] Perhaps in light of this connection, one teacher described how she wanted the children of a community southeast of St Anthony to understand where the "States" were and took them to the map: "'What is this?' (pointing to Newfoundland)," she asked. "'Newfoundland' in a chorus. 'And what is all this?' (sweeping my hand across the map of the United States). 'White Bay, Miss Bourne.'" Knowing that "White Bay is one of the largest bays in Newfoundland," she perhaps found this response understandable, but continued her lesson: "When I asked if anyone had heard of New York, two boys had. I found out afterwards that they had two aunts in New York."[34]

By 1917, this broad American presence and support to the Grenfell enterprise was so well known that it fanned the ire of local merchants, who lodged a formal complaint to the government. In their petition they "charged the Mission with competing in the market, benefiting unfairly from customs concessions, misrepresenting Newfoundland abroad as a society of paupers, and operating with the capital of American philanthropists."[35] The subsequent government commission determined that there had been much misunderstanding about the organization's activities and that there was no connection between the IGA and co-operative stores in particular. Behind this flare-up were two decades of local criticism that Grenfell's enterprise did more than encourage self-sufficiency among fishers and that it may even be operating for profit. A complex history of trade based on the "truck" or "credit" form of payment, whereby fishers traded their harvest for clothes, food, fishing gear, and other supplies from the merchants' stores, suffused this criticism. Recent scholarship on the truck method shows not just the paternalistic impulse behind some of the merchant activity, but also the mutual benefit for merchants and fishers, with actions taken by fishers for improved credit.[36] At the time, however, Grenfell and his early supporters openly perceived this credit method as exploitation: as Dr Curwen explained in 1893, the merchants "seem determined not to allow people to make money ... they take their salmon, cod, herring & fur at a price they name & give in return what provision they like, always arranging the prices so that there is nothing on the credit side."[37] Grenfell's views would have been well known and resented. Nevertheless, although Grenfell as an individual helped to set up a co-operative store in Red Bay, Labrador, in an effort to introduce cash by providing some goods himself, the truck system did not occupy the IGA agenda during its first fifty years, and this form of credit payment had little relevance to the organization's activities.

With some attention to this and related issues, the essays in this collection confirm not just the large numbers of Americans involved in Grenfell mission activities within Newfoundland and Labrador, but also the American nature of their activities – from sports to health care, Americans definitely had a tremendous impact on the everyday lives of people in the region. The ten contributions are arranged thematically and roughly chronologically in two groups. Part I, from James K. Hiller's discussion of Wilfred Grenfell and Newfoundland that sets the scene for the study of the Grenfell enterprise politically and historically, through the chapters by Jennifer J. Connor, Ronald L. Numbers, and Heidi Coombs-Thorne, explores its social, religious, and organizational shape. They emphasize the increasing role of American support from the beginning until 1940, with particular focus on the activities of Grenfell himself in recruiting help from American colleges and his personal connections to notable Americans. Importantly, as he drew so much on Americans for support, Grenfell increasingly adopted and employed American notions of philanthropy. His mission activities therefore reveal a shift in approach from Victorian-style charity, in which those from the middle class distribute free provisions and goods to the less fortunate, to the empowerment of the working poor to become self-sufficient, which occurred through active engagement of the middle class. As Coombs-Thorne indicates, these notions were pervasive in the American Progressive Era, when the largesse of extremely wealthy Americans such as Andrew Carnegie and John D. Rockefeller was keyed to benefiting society through public health measures and social and educational institutions, and when the systematization of voluntary organizations took place modelled on the business corporation. Rompkey noted as well that these large-scale trends and improvements were well under way when Grenfell visited the United States to spread the word in 1903.[38]

In Part II, John R. Matchim, Emma Lang and Katherine Side, Mark Graesser, Helen Woodrow, Rafico Ruiz, and J.T.H. Connor raise similar themes about the shift from charity to social reform in the Grenfell mission. Together they demonstrate the Grenfell enterprise in motion through sport, clothing, education, building, and health care, while highlighting the degree to which the support of Americans materially influenced the whole operation. Most importantly, they illustrate the Grenfell enterprise from within and in action, with studies of the people – both local and volunteer – associated with them, their beliefs and influences, and their routines. Sometimes examining the same activities – such as the contributions of the American architect of the Seamen's Institute and the new St Anthony hospital – from different perspectives, they reveal the degree to which Americans and their notions of progress and social uplift influenced recreation, survival, training, education, and treatment of people in the region for decades. John Matchim indicates how the mission formed a meeting place of international and local influences in sport, with attendant notions of muscular Christianity; Emma Lang and Katherine Side analyze the impact of clothing donations from the United States on a rural population, with attention to gendered clothing requirements of mission staff as well; Mark Graesser examines a unit, led by a Vassar College graduate, that loosely linked to the Grenfell mission to integrate health care and education in White Bay; Helen Woodrow extends the discussion of education specifically to explore the mission's work in sending young people from Newfoundland and Labrador to the United States for training in New York and, notably, in Kentucky – where comparison with the Appalachian region was made explicit; Rafico Ruiz focuses on the builders of the new hospital in St Anthony, in part through an interview with the daughter of its key builder, Ted McNeill; and J.T.H. Connor demonstrates how aid from the United States enabled development of a health-care system in northern Newfoundland that would later be absorbed by the government.

As this collection clearly conveys, Grenfell relied heavily on the United States for staff, funds, and materiel to complete his vision of a reformed society in Newfoundland and Labrador. His reliance on American support for the region was not the first, nor the last, however. As scholars have long demonstrated, the American influence on culture and life in Canada in general, and in Newfoundland in particular, is deep and pervasive. Canadians in the nineteenth century often saw themselves as having a continental identity.[39] And in publishing, libraries, and post-secondary schools, especially by the middle of the twentieth century, American foundations such as the Carnegie and Rockefeller had provided substantial financial support to Canadian institutions.[40] Moreover, the first collaborative research projects in Canada and their extensive book series were funded in large part by American agencies.[41] With respect to Newfoundland and Labrador, from the late nineteenth century, Americans from New England had strong economic ties through their active development of the region's resources: it was American firms that employed thousands of Newfoundlanders in mining and logging, often in seasonal rotations to accommodate fishing. As W.G. Reeves noted in his analysis of this resource development, Americans also arrived annually in Newfoundland communities to fish, distributing "significant amounts of money among a cash-poor population."[42] Americans travelled to the region as well for hunting and pleasure[43] and, later, during the Second World War, to establish military bases – both activities augmenting economic success in the colony before it joined Canada.[44] Americans retained strong connections to the region, marrying into local families or buying property for vacation or retirement. In addition to these trends, thousands of Newfoundlanders themselves have moved away or commuted for work elsewhere and thus have longstanding ties with the Maritime provinces and with cities along the northeastern American seaboard, which they dubbed "the Boston States"; the money they often sent back home had significant impact on local communities.[45] In Massachusetts in 1905, Newfoundlanders were in occupations of fishermen, oystermen, draymen, servants, and labourers; in the blue-collar trades such as carpenters, dressmakers and tailors, machinists, and painters; or in the lower middle class, as salespeople, clerks, bookkeepers, accountants, merchants and dealers, and nurses and midwives.[46] When American firms moved into Newfoundland to develop its natural resources, Newfoundlanders often returned for work in a "sizeable repatriation" that, Reeves suggests, "likely had a double-edged impact on the home society," for they brought new skills and financial savings that enabled them to establish small businesses, while they expected higher, more modern standards of living.[47] During the 1920s, Newfoundlanders were building skyscrapers in New York City.[48] Given the "common history" of Newfoundland and eastern American states,[49] by the time of Confederation with Canada in 1949, journalist Richard Gwyn later suggested, "Newfoundland's ties with the United States were far stronger and far more affectionate than those of Canada."[50] If it was debatable that Newfoundland in 1911 was "untainted by American ways," by the middle of the twentieth century this categorical statement by a colonial governor surely was a questionable claim. Indeed, by Grenfell's death in 1940, his distributed social enterprise in Newfoundland and Labrador capitalized on transnational movements of the early twentieth century and epitomized transnational ideals of a North American identity that would become more pronounced in global aid endeavours after the Second World War.

Part I

Shaping the Grenfell Mission

1

Wilfred Grenfell and Newfoundland

James K. Hiller

Dr Wilfred T. Grenfell arrived for the first time in St John's, Newfoundland, on 9 July 1892. He found the town stunned and in crisis, devastated by the fire that had gutted much of it the previous day. He had crossed the Atlantic on the *Albert*, a vessel owned by the Mission to Deep Sea Fishermen,[1] the British organization for which he then worked. So who was Grenfell? And why had he come to Newfoundland?

Wilfred Grenfell was twenty-seven years old in 1892, the son of an Anglican clergyman who had decided to give up his position as headmaster of a family-owned private school in Cheshire to become chaplain at the London Hospital in Whitechapel, in that city's East End.[2] Wilfred enrolled there as a medical student in the same year, 1883. He was an enthusiastic player of whatever sports were on offer – cricket, rugby, rowing – and was often absent from his classes. He was never an original, systematic, or profound thinker, but he qualified as a doctor (though failing the London MB exam). Through the influence of Frederick Treves,[3] a prominent surgeon at the London Hospital and a medical advisor to the Royal National Mission to Deep Sea Fishermen (RNMDSF), Grenfell went to work for the mission and became its superintendent at Great Yarmouth on the Norfolk coast, an important fishing port, looking after its activities on the North Sea.

By this time, Grenfell had experienced a religious conversion through attending a meeting held by the American evangelists D.L. Moody and I.D. Sankey and was convinced that his medical training should be dedicated to the public good. This was reinforced by attending another meeting some time later at which the speakers were the outstanding cricketer C.T. Studd (1860–1931) and his brother J.E. Studd, both of whom had been "born again." The former, one of the famous "Cambridge Seven," became a missionary in China, India, and later Africa. "They were natural athletes, and I felt I could listen to them … [I] went out feeling that I had crossed the Rubicon."[4] The result was that Grenfell became a prime exemplar of "muscular Christianity," the mid-Victorian movement lasting well into the twentieth century that stressed the importance of Christian manliness to Britain and its empire, a manliness that could be encouraged by games (especially team games).[5] The movement was embedded in the British public schools, almost all of them Protestant, and rapidly spread to North America and the English-speaking world.[6] It was a reaction against what was widely seen as the "effeminacy" of contemporary religious practice and closely allied with the Social Gospel crusade. Less attractively, muscular Christianity became associated with British and American imperialism, the eugenics movement, and a belief in Anglo-Saxon superiority (the term was used loosely). The influence of muscular Christianity in Newfoundland has not yet been explored, but similar tendencies no doubt existed.

The key figure who made the link between the RNMDSF (founded in 1881) and Newfoundland was Francis Hopwood.[7] A member of the mission council and a civil servant at the Board of Trade, in 1891 he met in London the premier of Newfoundland, Sir William Whiteway. The latter apparently mentioned the possibility of assistance from the RNMDSF in a general way, and Hopwood arranged to visit St John's later that year. He stayed at Government House and spoke with a number of local people, his main informant being Rev. Moses Harvey, an Ulster-born Presbyterian minister, then retired, who had become a prolific author and journalist.[8] Hopwood gathered information about the different Newfoundland fisheries and concluded that, given its capabilities, the RNMDSF could make the greatest contribution in the migratory Labrador fishery where, he was told, conditions were particularly appalling for those involved. This was, it seems, a suggestion made by the governor, Sir Terence O'Brien.[9] He so recommended to the mission council in a report that was widely circulated and publicized. The result was Grenfell's 1892 voyage.[10]

The *Albert* stayed in St John's for a few days to help fire victims and then set off northwards to follow the migratory fishers. Grenfell travelled along the Labrador coast as far north as the Moravian mission station at Hopedale and became convinced both that there was a real need and that the Labrador fishery should become part of the RNMDSF's work. The young John Richards from Bareneed (Conception Bay), later the Anglican priest at Flower's Cove from 1904 to 1945, encountered Grenfell at Indian Tickle, where he was fishing with his brothers:

> When it was announced that this strange doctor would hold a service on Sunday, and in the night display a magic lantern, something extremely rare in those days, the building was literally crammed. I can see him now standing there, and in the simplest language, telling the old, old story ... There was something unusually attractive ... in the voice, the fervour and the personality of this young English doctor ... I have never forgotten ... the text of the first address I heard him give: "Noah was a just man and perfect in his generations, and Noah walked with God."[11]

Clearly, Grenfell was immediately able to establish a close connection with the fishers at Labrador. He arrived back in St John's on 21 October, determined to make things happen.

THE REGION OF NEWFOUNDLAND AND LABRADOR[12]

Except on the island's south coast, where there was a small offshore bank fishery, Newfoundlanders for the most part fished inshore. For many years, at least since the 1820s, some fishermen from the east coast had extended their fishery to Labrador, sailing north in late spring or early summer, and returning in the fall. Some were "floaters," able to move around in their schooners if they so chose, who usually brought their catch, known as "shore-cured Labrador," back to Newfoundland for processing. "Stationers" were taken north as passengers, fished from a fixed location, and sold their catch on the coast; it was known as "soft-cured Labrador." As the inshore fishery on the island became more crowded, more people joined the annual Labrador migration, pushing further and further north, even though the season became progressively shorter. A St John's newspaper in 1885 estimated that between fifteen and twenty thousand people made the journey each year, men, women, and children.[13] This was the historic peak of the Labrador fishery, which declined during the years that followed.[14] The 1891 Newfoundland census tabulated 859 vessels participating in the Labrador fishery during the 1890 season, carrying 13,300 persons, of whom 2,900 were women and children.[15] Detailed lists in Grenfell's papers for 1894 and 1895 – the source is unknown – give another count.[16] On the basis of this evidence and an average of these two years, 955 vessels of about forty tons made the voyage to Labrador from Newfoundland at that time. Nearly 80 per cent were floaters. There were about 7,000 crew members, and passengers numbered 4,895 males and 2,132 females. This adds up to about 14,000 persons in all. Whatever the source and whatever the discrepancies, this was an enormous exodus. Grenfell's figures for 1895 show that 257 vessels came from Conception Bay, 449 from the northeast coast (Trinity, Bonavista, and Notre Dame Bays), and 78 from elsewhere on the island.[17]

The annual migration caused only a degree of concern on the island. A doctor was sent north on the mail steamer each season, the reports complaining of rushed consultations and inadequate facilities.[18] Legislators were concerned by overcrowding on Labrador vessels, especially the accommodation provided for women at sea and on shore. A specific act was passed in 1882,[19] and following a tremendous storm in October 1885, a select committee was asked "to consider the operation and effectiveness of the present Law." It reported that there had been inadequate enforcement, and the legislature agreed that there should be proper rules and stricter, more frequent inspections, to ensure that there were "suitable separate apartments" for women.[20] Whether there was any effective result is unlikely.

Labrador was (and is) a huge territory with a small population, which in this period hovered around four thousand – Inuit in the North, Innu in the interior, Southern Inuit and settlers of European descent in central and southern areas. The interior boundary was disputed between Newfoundland and Canada,[21] but both agreed that the "coast of Labrador," which had originally been placed under Newfoundland jurisdiction in 1763, extended from Blanc Sablon to Cape Chidley. There was little if any formal administration. For the most part, Labrador was under the control of the Hudson Bay Company and the Moravian mission in the North and central areas. There were no policemen and no political representatives. South of the Moravian settlements, the 1891 census listed only three clergymen and five teachers. For the whole coast, the census reported a population that was overwhelmingly Protestant.[22] *Mutatis mutandis*, the situation was similar to the relationship between the English West Country and Newfoundland centuries earlier. Labrador was a neglected territory, seen on the island only as a place to fish and its permanent inhabitants as of marginal importance.

Grenfell also became deeply involved with Newfoundland's Northern Peninsula, creating a headquarters at the little settlement of St Anthony in 1899, which had about three hundred inhabitants.[23] It was part of the single-member electoral district of St Barbe, an enormous coastline extending from La Scie on the Baie Verte peninsula north about to Trout River, just outside Bonne Bay in the west. Its total population was about eight thousand in that year, living in 161 places. Like Labrador, it was largely Protestant, with burgeoning numbers of Methodists and Salvationists. However, there was a substantial Roman Catholic minority, concentrated in the Baie Verte area and on the east side of the Northern Peninsula – a reminder that the coast from Cape St John in the east to Cape Ray in the southwest was part of the French Treaty Shore until 1904, and that the French had generally preferred Irish Roman Catholics as *gardiens* to look after their premises. The Grenfell mission, as it became, could not serve the whole district and concentrated on the area between Flower's Cove in the west, and White Bay in the east.

The island of Newfoundland had a population of about 198,000 in the early 1890s, of which 18 per cent lived in or near the town of St John's, the colony's economic and administrative hub and capital.[24] Most inhabitants lived along the coastline, for the most part in the east and southeast, and were largely dependent on the fisheries, though there was some mining and forest activity and great hopes for new industries in these and other sectors. Railway building had begun in 1881, the expectation being that a trans-island line would open up the interior to settlement and stimulate new industry. This did happen eventually to some extent, but when Grenfell first arrived the railway was unfinished and was steadily driving up the public debt. Indeed, the colonial economy as a whole was not doing well. The all-important price of fish in foreign markets was low as the result of severe competition, the Labrador and seal fisheries were in slow and erratic decline, and the government was finding it difficult to make ends meet. Apart from these overall economic difficulties, the colony had to deal with the 1892 St John's fire and the collapse of the two local private banks late in 1894. It was, to say the least, a difficult decade.

Constitutionally, Newfoundland ranked as a settler colony with responsible government, meaning internal self-government. The question of confederation with the Canada that had been created in 1867 was the central issue in the 1869 election. The confederates were overwhelmingly defeated, and Newfoundland seemed determined to continue as a separate political unit within the British Empire. The option of confederation lurked in the background – even though Canadian governments were ambivalent – and it remained a controversial topic. The British government controlled external affairs, which in Newfoundland's case were complicated because they involved international fisheries agreements. Eighteenth-century treaties had awarded France an ill-defined right to fish in season on the so-called French Shore, and the return of French fishermen after 1815 was one reason for the emergence of a Labrador fishery.[25] In addition, the United States possessed fishing rights under an 1818 treaty on part of the south coast, the west coast, and at Labrador. French rights were deeply resented, American rights less so, but an important issue in the 1890s was whether Newfoundland would be allowed to negotiate a reciprocity treaty with the United States separately from Canada. An attempt had been made in 1890 and quickly squashed at Ottawa's insistence, but many in St John's saw ready access to the American market as a key to the future, even though trade with the United States represented only about 17.5 per cent of the colony's total[26] – that, and the ending of French rights on "their" shore.

GRENFELL AND LOCAL AFFAIRS

Whether Grenfell was aware of these issues in 1892 in any more than a general way is improbable. But on his return to St John's, he began his education about local affairs under the tutelage of Governor Sir Terence O'Brien. A former Indian Army officer and police superintendent, O'Brien was impatient with the requirements of responsible government and generally critical (if not contemptuous) of the Newfoundland political elite. He thought that Newfoundland should not have been given responsible government, and that the existing system was riddled with corruption, conflict of interest, and inefficiency.[27] It was an attitude largely shared at the Colonial Office in London. So, at the start, Grenfell received a negative and condescending view of local politics and society that he absorbed without criticism. An upper-class Englishman, he shared instinctively the prevailing British snobbery concerning colonies and colonials, especially those with pretensions. On the other hand he apparently had no problem with the "ordinary people," whom he tended to romanticize. Grenfell also seems to have rapidly adopted the one-dimensional view that Newfoundland fishing people were exploited by rapacious local merchants, whose excesses had to be curbed. Against this, he relied on members of the St John's mercantile class for support. He had to tread a fine line.

There was some truth to O'Brien's strictures on local society, though they reflected a distinct lack of sympathy with how Newfoundland, a small, divided, and scattered society, had chosen to arrange its public affairs. To his credit he was a strong Grenfell backer, used his influence accordingly, and went to work to help set up a local organization to support Grenfell and the RNMDSF. An immediate difficulty, though, was the colony's entrenched religious denominationalism. Interdenominational rivalry and prejudice was commonplace everywhere in this period, and Newfoundland was no different. But the colony had settled on an unspoken but generally observed agreement that had evolved since the 1860s, that provided that each church should have a proportionate share of place and pay in the public service and the legislature, and that each major denomination should have its own schools. It was

a sensible arrangement in the circumstances, though it had costly dis-
advantages in several respects, and it certainly helped to prevent overt
sectarian strife.[28] The problems in this instance were that the RNMDSF
was officially non-denominational, though obviously Protestant and
evangelical; and that Grenfell himself was not only Protestant, but entirely ecumenical in spirit – William Gosling wrote that "all shades of
belief are alike to him."[29] Both he and the future mission did not fit
easily into the existing religious matrix.

The result was that the churches in the colony did not become
actively involved in any official way. Relatively few Roman Catholics
participated in the Labrador fishery, but more important to the bishop
(later archbishop) Michael F. Howley was religious and denominational
control. Native-born, he was a conservative nationalist (though a con-
federate) who was suspicious of "outside" interventions and fiercely
protective of his country's reputation. On the Protestant side, Dissenters
were generally supportive, as were many Anglicans of the low church
persuasion. However, the hierarchy was high church, and the Church
of England bishop, Llewelyn Jones, told Grenfell in 1895 that the
RNMDSF "should come out in its true colours as a dissenting institution" – and "I ... maintain that Dissent is a Sin." "Why should a
Churchman go out of his way to connect himself in religious work with
those who are bitter foes to the Body of Christ?"[30] Grenfell wrote that
"the Church of England is highly ritualistic and doesn't care about
Evangelical preaching" and was "our most bitter antagonist. Alas,
Alas."[31] The local committee was exclusively Protestant and included
a fair number of Dissenters.[32] In 1892 the committee promised and provided hospitals at Battle Harbour and Indian Harbour, and this was the
beginning of "the Grenfell mission," which steadily expanded in geography, scope, and ambition.[33]

Grenfell himself had found an opportunity to create his own adventurous and individual niche far removed from the RNMDSF brass in
England, on a little-known imperial frontier, where he could fully indulge
his love of boats and the sea. It would not be a mission to Indigenous
peoples in the classic sense. He was not converting people to Christianity,
and in any case, he never showed great interest in the Innu or Inuit peoples, whom he clearly viewed as racially inferior.[34] The former were tit-

Not FN mission

ular Roman Catholics, looked after by that church. The Inuit had been the responsibility of the Protestant Moravian Church since the late eighteenth century.[35] Grenfell's movement would be a mission to the descendants of British immigrants in need of assistance and uplift, Christians who lacked the wherewithal to live decent and healthy lives. It was frequently claimed that Grenfell worked among Anglo-Saxons, but this is not altogether accurate, since the mission also helped people of Celtic and mixed-race ancestry. In its day, though, the term *Anglo-Saxon* was potent, both in Britain and the United States, and was assumed to apply to the English-speaking world as a whole. There was a linked, pervasive background assumption that "Anglo-Saxons" were racially superior. This muddled concept, based on a false reading of history, helped the rapprochement between Britain and the United States at the turn of the century and no doubt helped Grenfell as well.[36]

Newfoundland and Labrador was an obscure corner of the settler empire where Christian social action could make a difference. It was exotic to outsiders in its own way, and importantly, a relatively accessible route to "the northern experience" – this was, after all, the age of Robert Peary, Frederick Cook, and other explorers. Labrador, a subarctic region, is the most southerly part of the Canadian north, and because of the Labrador Current, much of the island of Newfoundland, especially the northeast coast, experiences cool temperatures and harsh winters. There are icebergs, heavy snowfalls, and pack ice. This enabled Grenfell to promote and represent a northern image, and in this he was very successful. He never spent a winter in Labrador, though he was often resident at St Anthony. His promotional skills made the most of these advantages, and the notorious, fetid east London slums were left far behind. The focus now was on the privations experienced by the people of Labrador and northern Newfoundland and by those who participated in the migratory fishery. Both *the coast* and *Labrador*, words heavily used in mission speeches and literature, were left ill-defined, one suspects deliberately.

Besides the churches, Grenfell had to deal with the Newfoundland government. It was willing enough to support the RNMDSF in various ways, since it promised to provide services that the colony could not afford.[37] This was a period when the role of the state was assumed to be restricted, and in any case the colonial government had very limited resources. Grenfell also arrived at a time of severe financial difficulty. The situation improved after 1900, but the local government had to be sensitive to public opinion. The major churches were ambivalent, there was a general sensitivity to charitable condescension, and the mission was by no means universally popular. As a result the colonial government tended to be co-operative but cautious. It was sensitive to the potential impact of Grenfell's lecture circuit portrayals of Newfoundland, was not overtly enthusiastic, could not afford to be financially generous, and had (in the end) to be pressured into providing a basic grant. In general, Grenfell seems to have understood these limitations and usually did not malign the local political situation. He also avoided direct political involvement.[38] However, in private, and in the depictions of the fishery and outport life in his writings and lectures, there was a great deal of indirect and implicit criticism. It was not always appreciated.

Grenfell disliked denominationalism, but he equally disliked the mercantile system, if not more. A merchant would advance supplies to a dealer on the understanding that he would buy that dealer's catch at the end of the season. The price of the supplies, the grading (or "cull") of the cured fish, and the value of the voyage would be set by the merchant, who could also decide whether or not the dealer might be advanced winter supply.[39] Largely cashless, the system was deeply ingrained, had its advantages for both sides, and was prevalent throughout the colony. Grenfell rapidly became an opponent. He thought it was fundamentally unfair to ordinary fishermen and prevented them from making a decent living. Moreover, he and his staff saw many patients whose health would have been improved by a better diet, and he saw the credit system as a problem in this regard as well. His viewpoint was shared by many visitors to the colony but was less enthusiastically accepted within it. Grenfell could not do anything about the management of the migratory fishery, but he thought he could help the people who lived year-round in Labrador and northern Newfoundland by promoting co-operative stores.[40] He also helped fur trappers avoid the Moravian stores and the Hudson's Bay Company by selling their furs for them elsewhere. Grenfell was especially critical of Moravian trade practices, given that this was a religious organization, which (like the

RNMDSF) paid no import duties. Writing to the Reverend Paul Hettasch at Hopedale in 1900, he was quite explicit: "If you can't do better then in God's name close your trading."[41]

Grenfell's commercial initiatives proved to be a trespass that was not readily forgiven, even if the impact was local and, over time, relatively insignificant. It was one thing for the RNMDSF to alleviate pain and suffering, but quite another for it to question established mercantile practice and encourage commercial competition.[42] The colonial government did not want to intrude on current practice, and supply merchants great and small had always assumed that relationships with their dealers were in some sense private. There were many resentments involved, especially concerning the culling of fish, but the system was understood and entrenched. In 1896, W.A. Munn of Harbour Grace, a merchant long involved in the Labrador fishery, advised Grenfell to steer clear of any sort of commercial activity and to work with local traders.[43] He was referring to Red Bay, where the first co-operative store was nevertheless established that year, apparently an initial attempt to introduce cash dealing in a largely cashless economy. Grenfell himself advanced the initial capital.[44] Other such stores followed. In 1910 he complained in frustration, "At one time I'm a knave because I'm making money and at another a fool because I'm losing. It is the same with the [Roddickton lumber] mill, the same with the schooners, and with the distribution of old clothes. While religious men, so-called, criticise you for mixing material work with spiritual, business men condemn you for interfering when you ought to be holding a prayer meeting."[45]

Very soon after his first encounter with the Labrador coast, Grenfell had moved far beyond the original assumptions of the first voyage. In his new vision, the RNMDSF would do much more than provide medical assistance and shore facilities: it would be an agent of social change on both the Labrador coast and the island's Northern Peninsula. In time this encompassed an orphanage and schools as well as hospitals and nursing stations. There was an industrial program, farming was encouraged, and there was a remarkable (and unfortunate) experiment in reindeer herding. Grenfell was also the force behind the creation of the King George V Seamen's Institute in St John's, where seamen could find affordable and alcohol-free lodging.[46] Not surprisingly, Grenfell

met opposition from some mainline churches and from some merchants, and there was also resistance from local inhabitants.[47] J.T.
Richards wrote that he had seen Grenfell "very angry because a man,
whom he wanted to help, failed to respond and do his part in the doctor's plan. He could not see the validity of the man's reasons for not
responding."[48]

Overall, Grenfell and his colleagues and workers saw little need to
cooperate or work with Newfoundland and Labrador institutions. He
and his allies thought that they had found the solutions to the region's
social and economic problems and sought to implement them. Local allies were warmly welcomed, but the agenda was Grenfell designed and
imposed. This attitude was typical of the period. In effect, the mission
treated their "Anglo-Saxon" clients as though they were "lesser breeds"
– but within "the law."[49]

Tensions also developed internally, between the RNMDSF and Grenfell, and between the Labrador and Newfoundland areas of responsibility. The parent mission became increasingly impatient with the erratic
Grenfell and by 1914 was starting to lose its enthusiasm for the overseas
adventure. It was becoming very expensive, beyond anything that it
could realistically afford, given that it was itself expanding in the United
Kingdom. A second tension developed from the move to centralize mission activity at St Anthony. This made sense in many ways, but it seemed
to marginalize Labrador and its fishery, the original reason for the mission. Labrador found its champion in Dr Harry Paddon (1881–1939),
who had arrived from England in 1912 and soon established himself as
the senior physician in the region. Paddon was insistent that the mission
had to maintain hospitals in Labrador and fought hard for the North
West River and Indian Harbour stations. He also became deeply attached to Labrador as a place, thinking that it had immense economic
potential.[50] Indeed, the continued Grenfell presence in Labrador owes
a great deal to the Paddon family. For Grenfell himself, though, the
Labrador coast was increasingly a summer-time distraction.

Grenfell had to raise funds devoted specifically to the Newfoundland
and Labrador initiatives. As a result he not only looked to Britain, but
to Canada and then to the United States. In 1918, the total expenditure
of the International Grenfell Association was $70,083.68 (excluding

the George V Seamen's Institute) and would have been higher were it not for the extensive use of volunteers. Against this, the IGA had raised $63,355.50, of which about 59 per cent came from the United States, 25 per cent from Britain, 16 per cent from Canada, and 2 per cent from Newfoundland.[51] The link with the United States was therefore crucial and became firmly cultivated over the years. Grenfell's marriage to the capable and well-connected Anne MacClanahan of Chicago in 1909 was of central importance in this respect. The mission became in essence an American operation, with adjunct organizations in Britain, Canada, and Newfoundland. As Grenfell said in a confrontational meeting with the RNMDSF council in 1926, "England has not done nearly her fair share towards our work; America has been giving 7/8ths of all the work. I have to raise that money in America, or else close up the Labrador work."[52] In 1928 Harry Paddon spent some weeks at St Anthony as a patient. It is "an American colony," he wrote. "I spent 5 weeks there ... The medical officers have been American there for over 20 years. Just as the USA is nominally a Democracy but really an Oligarchy, so St A. boasts ½ a million of real estate in an area where there is no more than 4 months employment in the 12 for the great majority of the men & has rigid caste barriers. Further, after 37 years of work, not a single native holds any better position than an artisan's. At St Anthony, take away I.G.A. and the people must clear out or go on govt. relief."[53] He intended to do better at North West River.

Newfoundlanders had always been mobile, moving to and from the economic opportunities presented by New England and the Maritime provinces, sometimes permanently, sometimes for short periods. They went elsewhere on the mainland as well, but northeastern America, both the United States and Canada, was the most usual destination.[54] Hard economic times in Newfoundland in the later nineteenth century led to a substantial out-migration, especially from southeastern districts, and by 1905 there were over ten thousand Newfoundlanders living in Massachusetts alone, the largest concentrations being in Boston and Gloucester.[55] There were more Newfoundlanders living in Canada, however. Using census data, R.A. Mackay and S.A. Saunders put the Newfoundland-born population in the United States at 9,311 in 1910, and at 15,469 in 1911 in Canada.[56] Not surprisingly, there was sometimes talk of joining the

United States or developing a "special relationship," but the Newfoundland identity was strongly infused with loyalty to Britain, the monarchy, and the empire. The British connection was fundamental, and such talk was ephemeral, even among those with Irish roots.

Nevertheless, many Newfoundlanders hoped for and applauded American investment in the forest and mining industries from the late 1890s. There was, however, no heavy industry as the government of the day hoped and encouraged.[57] At the turn of the century there was as well strong support for an independent reciprocity treaty with the United States – seen as "a sort of El Dorado," says Mackay – which would give ready access to the American market for local products of all kinds. This initiative failed, mainly because of protectionist opinion in Congress, the opposition of American fishing interests, and continued hostility in Ottawa – all of which led to a short-lived confrontation between Newfoundland, the United States, and Britain after 1905, and an important arbitration in 1910.[58] In the years before the Great War the United States supplied about 30 per cent of the colony's imports but took only 10 per cent of its exports. The situation improved after the war with the development of the newsprint mill at Corner Brook; taken over by American interests, it sold much of the product in the United States, but the balance of trade remained adverse.[59]

Grenfell first visited Canada in 1893 and was warmly welcomed in Halifax, Montreal, and Ottawa. The Montreal link proved to be especially important. A branch of the Canadian Foreign Mission Society and members of a Congregational Church there had supported a mission on what is now known as the Quebec North Shore between 1858 and 1880. The initiator was an American clergyman, the Reverend C.C. Carpenter. He was now in New England and the children's columnist for the *Congregationalist*, published in Boston.[60] Grenfell also received the highly influential backing of Sir Donald Smith (soon to be Lord Strathcona), who had spent twenty-one years in Labrador working for the Hudson's Bay Company. He was now president of that company, the Bank of Montreal, and the Canadian Pacific Railway – in short, he was at the centre of Canadian business.[61] Smith opened doors that Grenfell could not have done. The first American tour took place in 1896, paid for by the Toronto Grenfell committee, and facilitated by

Carpenter.[62] Other tours followed, but as Ronald Rompkey points out, the cause does not seem to have really taken off until 1903.[63] There were both Canadian and American reasons.

In Ottawa, Grenfell met the ambitious William Lyon Mackenzie King, then deputy minister in the Department of Labour and widely seen as "a coming man." A Presbyterian social gospeller, King was impressed by Grenfell and used his connections to help the mission. Among them were friends from his University of Toronto days, a group that included the journalist Norman Duncan, now on the staff of the *New York Evening Post*. Duncan had already visited Newfoundland and met Grenfell in 1903.[64] The result was a series of articles and two books that idealized Grenfell and became immensely popular: *Dr Luke of the Labrador* (1904) and *Dr Grenfell's Parish: The Deep Sea Fishermen* (1905).

Another significant boost came from the Pomiuk story, which Grenfell carefully cultivated. Pomiuk was a child among a group of fifty-seven Labrador Inuit exhibited at Chicago in 1893 and then left to their own devices. Some returned, and Grenfell found a crippled Pomiuk at Nachvak in 1895 and brought him to Battle Harbour, where he died in 1897. The boy had already been noticed at the exhibition by Carpenter, known as "Mr Martin" in the Children's Corner of the *Congregationalist*,[65] and the story was given additional impetus by Rev. William Forbush's book for children, *Pomiuk, a Waif of Labrador: A Brave Boy's Life for Brave Boys* (1903). Forbush called Grenfell "a Christian Viking," guided by God to assist Pomiuk.[66] Grenfell always referred to "Prince Pomiuk," as the boy had been known at the exhibition, a saintly romanticization that increased his general appeal and reinforced the Northern image. Grenfell was a natural and highly successful publicist, though vitally assisted by others.

One further book needs to be mentioned in this context: Grenfell's own *Adrift on an Ice Pan* (Boston, 1909).[67] In late April 1908, he set off from St Anthony by dog team to visit a patient. Impetuously and imprudently, he tried crossing Hare Bay on an ice bridge, which broke up – it was spring, after all – and Grenfell found himself floating out to sea. He had to kill his dogs to survive and was lucky to be rescued, at some risk to those who came to his aid. The result of this bungled dog-team journey was first a sensational article and then a short book that proved to be a blockbuster – a huge publishing success that went through three editions by the end of 1909. Grenfell became a folk hero.[68]

The publicity and romance that now surrounded Grenfell and the mission attracted people to his lectures and made them readier than ever to donate money and goods to the mission. This was true in Britain and Canada, but his celebrity in the United States was exceptional, and that was where he found his most important backers. Grenfell liked the United States, and Americans liked him. They also had the deeper pockets. This was the period when "scientific philanthropy" was coming into fashion, meaning charitable foundations based on a corporate model – the IGA was an example. Generally, such philanthropists were not so much concerned with religious conversion as with top-down social engineering, education, health, and related fields.[69] Grenfell's activities had an obvious appeal – and glamour – that resonated with "young idealists" and many others.[70] This was not so much the case in Britain, and it is possible that Grenfell did not want to compete with the RNMDSF.

The early twentieth century was also a time when the British and American governments were settling differences. The Canadian and Newfoundland governments had their own problems with the United States and each other, but the underlying trend was towards rapprochement and the elimination of transatlantic disputes, often facilitated by British concessions. It was a period of mutual reconciliation, which eventually led to the "special relationship." Like Anglo-Saxonism, this was also very much to Grenfell's advantage.

The situation in Newfoundland was more problematic and came to a head in 1917. For some time there had been critical rumblings from the Roman Catholic Church, clergy of other denominations, and merchants involved in the Labrador fishery. As early as 1894 the Reverend Jabez Moore, an Anglican who had worked in Labrador, attacked Grenfell for his portrayal of Newfoundlanders and for speaking and writing "as if he alone put forth heroic effort to benefit Labradorians."[71] Bishop Howley had made critical public remarks in 1899, and in 1905 the *Trade Review* had attacked the mission's involvement with trade, sparking a controversy that prompted Howley to renew his assault in a series of letters to the *Daily News*.[72] The Reverend F.W. Colley, another Anglican minister who had been in Labrador, wrote in 1916, "It seems most unfair to Newfoundlanders that an impression should be abroad that Labrador was permitted to remain in heathen darkness, sin, and wickedness until it was discovered by one Dr Grenfell in '92."[73] Such complaints came together in a petition to the legislature, signed by a number of St John's and Conception Bay merchants.[74] The central allegation was that regular traders had to compete with a privileged charitable organization that, as a result of "misrepresentations that this dependency of Newfoundland is largely composed of paupers," gained the support of United States charities in money and in kind. This constituted "a menace to all other mercantile concerns on that coast who have to pay duty and freight." IGA trade concessions should be abolished, and its connection with the co-operative stores, allegedly financed by American philanthropists, should be examined. In a separate submission, W.B. Grieve – an original supporter of the Battle Harbour hospital – claimed that the mission had "largely developed ... into a merchantile [sic] concern."[75]

The dominant theme of the petition was, obviously, that the IGA was improperly competing with established traders. Though the local economy did reasonably well during the Great War, merchants remained very concerned about competition, and the activities of the mission were seen as potentially damaging. Much more serious, in fact, was the equally resented competition coming from stores operated by William Coaker's Fishermen's Protective Union (FPU), which not long after its foundation in 1908 became an important force in the colony's economic and political life. Coaker and Grenfell, on the surface, had much in common. They both wanted to improve the lives of outport fishing families and had ambitious agendas. Yet Coaker was not thought to be "an upholder."[76] The essential difference was that Coaker, a Newfoundlander who had lived for many years on the northeast coast, chose to work within the system and to try to reform it, seeking to ensure that the fishermen who supported the FPU got a fair deal. For this he was vilified by the mercantile establishment and their political allies, and the churches – especially (then) Archbishop Howley – strongly disliked his ideas concerning education and allied matters.[77] In contrast, Grenfell was independently funded, was allied with much of the Protestant upper class, and applied ideas that largely came from elsewhere. He could do as he saw fit. His critics seem to have thought that in his independence lay his vulnerability, their indignation apparently increased by the establishment of a co-operative store at Cape Charles in 1914.[78]

The attack was also fuelled by affronted nationalism at a time when Newfoundland was strongly backing the war effort and making considerable sacrifices to do so, both financial and human – the Newfoundland Regiment suffered severe losses. Grenfell went to France for three months early in 1916, but with a Harvard Surgical Unit that was supporting the Royal Army Medical Corps. He held the temporary rank of major. So far as is known, he did not contact the Newfoundland Regiment, even though fifty-five Labradorians enlisted, and sixty-three from the Northern Peninsula.[79] A well-publicized visit would have been a wise move in the circumstances.

The petitioners clearly thought that Grenfell had slandered the colony both in his writings and on the fund-raising lecture circuit. This was nothing new, and clearly some had problems with the mission on cultural as well as economic grounds, and the passage of time did not make these feelings disappear. The immediate cause of indignation this time were sensational reports of a lecture Grenfell had given in May 1916 to the Canadian Club at the Montreal Ritz Carlton. In a statement issued in June, Grenfell aggressively defended himself. Young reporters were to blame, he did give credit to other workers, he was not a cheap seeker after heroics by giving the coast an "evil reputation" ("my friends" cruise there in their yachts), and the money came from outside the colony, which – an unpleasant taunt – did nothing to support outport hospitals.[80]

In response to the petition, the Newfoundland government established a commission of enquiry, which was carried out by R.T. Squarey, the magistrate at Channel. Grenfell treated the whole business with condescension and clearly thought the enquiry was a waste of time. Giving evidence at St Anthony he firmly denied making misrepresentations and asserted that the co-operatives were essential. He had assisted some of them to get started, but this was a personal matter and nothing to do with the mission.[81] The report was remarkably positive and uncritical, and dismissed the petitioners' claims. Squarey reported that there was no connection between the IGA and the co-operatives, and that while "the religious aspect" of the mission caused much "suspicion and misunderstanding," he had received no complaints. As for the Montreal incident, he blamed the reporter (as did Grenfell) and, more generally, "the over-enthusiasm of the students" who worked as volunteers in the summer. His single recommendation was that imported clothing should be liable for duty, which the government would rebate. This was "a burning sore and a source of constant friction and bitterness" that had to be dealt with.[82]

Not surprisingly, Grenfell and the mission staff were delighted by the report and rightly saw it as a complete exoneration. The report had "silenced the lying mouths of saloon men, cheating traders, and lower class political hangers on."[83] Whitewash it may well have been though, since Squarey (an Englishman) seems to have been charmed by the welcoming atmosphere of the mission, overawed by Grenfell himself, and impressed by the relative absence of serious, factual opposition. The legal counsel in attendance were equally cautious. There were certainly legitimate questions to be pursued about Grenfell's connection to the co-operatives, and about his portrayals of life in outport Newfoundland and Labrador, but these were not directly confronted. Nor did Squarey address a central question: How should a largely independent agency relate to the legitimate government of the colony?[84]

Grenfell and his allies would have thought such a question tiresome and irrelevant. The important point was that the mission had been vindicated, accusations against it dismissed, and its position strengthened as it faced a troubled postwar world. The relatively prosperous times, which had existed in Newfoundland since about 1900, were over. The colony was saddled with a large public debt that had been inflated by the war, and related financial responsibilities continued. In 1914, the debt had been about $30.5 million; in 1918–19 it was $42 million and continued to climb steadily, reaching $100 million by the early 1930s.[85] The gross export value of fish declined from $15.7 million in 1915–19 to $13.3 million in 1920–24, $11.6 million in 1925–29, and $7.0 million in 1930–34.[86] This reflected not only a general trade depression, but more particularly severe difficulties in the fish markets, especially in Italy. The Labrador fishery continued to contract.[87] Out-migration persisted, at least until the Great Depression,[88] the Newfoundland Railway was in severe financial trouble – it had to be taken over by the government – and it seemed that the only positive development was the establishment of a newsprint mill at Corner Brook in the mid-1920s. It did not help that the political scene was unstable. The wartime National Government had collapsed in 1919, and public life became fragmented, the factional chieftains competing for power, circling each other, looking for place and power. There were many who despaired for the future.[89]

To a considerable extent the mission was insulated from this dismal situation by its financial and administrative independence. But the people of northern Newfoundland and Labrador were not so fortunate and faced genuinely hard times. Grenfell, it seems, had learned little from the crisis of 1917, and in 1921 he began to issue reports of famine and destitution, which were energetically disseminated and exaggerated by the wire services. The reaction was immediate. The time had come, said the prime minister, Richard Squires – who was trying to float bonds on the American market – when "the people of Newfoundland ought to rise up and drive the blackmailers of the Grenfell class out of the country." There was "a dirty trail left by a man named Grenfell, who, to get money for the various institutions ... is continually portraying Newfoundland as being a country of the direst poverty and the basest ignorance."[90] Grenfell also seems to have become involved with the New York philanthropist William Willard Howard in a scheme to purchase and sell fish. More than that, Grenfell began to promote confederation with Canada as a possible solution to the colony's problems, and that placed the governor (Sir Charles Harris) in a very difficult position – he resigned as chair of the local Grenfell association, and invitations to Grenfell to stay at Government House ended.[91] The criticisms did not cease. In 1922, the *Evening Telegram* complained, "The people of this country are heartily sick of being held up as fit subjects for cast off garments, as starving, as suffering from all sorts of incurable diseases, as ignorant, as inept, by men who drift into this island and remain but for a short period."[92]

Political chaos was not confined to Newfoundland in the 1920s, nor were the shabby aspects of public life about which Grenfell and others

Mission integrated into
fed Gov't
Public healy

incessantly complained and grumbled. There were plenty of examples elsewhere. But he was starting to become distanced from Newfoundland and from the mission that he had founded. He did not winter at St Anthony after 1918–19 and spent more and more time on the lecture circuit and at his home in the United States. He suffered from angina after 1929, his wife died in 1938, and like many others in this period, he came to favour strong and decisive government, even at the expense of democracy. So far as Newfoundland was concerned, Grenfell supported the suspension of responsible government – which had been a failure in his view – and the imposition of the appointed Commission of Government in 1934. There was even talk of him becoming governor.[93] He had never had an easy relationship with successive elected Newfoundland governments and was very critical of them for not giving his mission the support he thought it deserved.

Grenfell was, in any case, a figurehead by this time, and "his" mission came under increasing government control thereafter. It retained much of its original character until the 1950s, however, though it is now fully integrated into the provincial health-care structure – and "Newfoundland and Labrador" is now a Canadian province. The "Grenfell" name remains. The nagging and persistent question is how much actual difference Grenfell and the mission, in its various forms, really made.

GRENFELL'S LEGACY IN NEWFOUNDLAND AND LABRADOR

The few relevant studies of the mission's impact that have been done concentrate on the Labrador side of the Straits. Otto Junek studied the village of Blanc Sablon in the 1930s and concluded that lasting benefit from Grenfell work occurred only "wherever the missions are located," and that "the educational and clinical work accomplished … is meagre, sporadic and ephemeral in its influence on the lives of the folk."[94] This may be a harsh judgement based on a single example, but it is telling. John Kennedy has written more recently that while local people appreciated the mission, "their accommodation … was also tinged with resentment."[95]

The mission was an outside institution, a colony within a colony. Staffed almost entirely by people from the United States, Canada, and Britain, assisted by a flood of eager volunteers in the summers, it never genuinely sought to work alongside and with the people of "the coast," their churches, their institutions, and their government. It was a paternalistic, top-down affair, essentially colonial, dictating solutions to local problems derived from models developed elsewhere. Kennedy speaks of the cultural distance between local inhabitants and the Grenfell staff. Older people, he says, recall "the inflexible, patronizing manner of many mission personnel. Mission land was fenced ... Grenfell staff did not hesitate to tell families where to move."[96] Grenfell – who died in 1940 – received a mixed reaction within the colony, and his workers were not always greeted with enthusiasm. In essence, he and his supporters tried to impose an alien model on a traditional and conservative society, and it is arguable that their success was limited. The fundamental, structural problems that beset "the coast," economic and social, are as intractable now as then. Grenfell and his supporters recognized that the problems of "the North" had to be confronted in many ways; they undertook many positive initiatives, transformed many individual lives, and founded a lasting health-care system; but in hindsight, they were perhaps working against a stubborn reality. Current analyses provide gloomy prognoses for what was once Grenfell's sphere of operations, especially the Northern Peninsula.[97] The population is declining and ageing, the fisheries are far less productive, the provincial economy is not doing well, and the harvesting of seals and fur-bearing animals has come under intense international criticism. The future is not bright.

"It was a paternalistic, top down affair, essentially colonial, dictating solutions to local problems derived elsewhere"

2

"We Are Anglo-Saxons": Grenfell, Race, and Mission Movements

Jennifer J. Connor

That Wilfred Grenfell masterfully crafted his northern enterprise from transnational trends is understood among scholars familiar with his work. He drew upon various "movements" at the end of the nineteenth century and early twentieth century: a mission movement, including the settlement house movement; other social reform movements, including the Social Gospel; a student volunteer movement; and even incipient aid activities of later non-government agencies. Yet although the origins and evolution of his eponymous mission have been situated within these large social movements – most notably by Grenfell's biographer, Ronald Rompkey[1] – the degree to which the movements shaped the social and organizational architecture of the mission itself has not been explored. Indeed, the Grenfell mission has been overlooked in histories of all kinds of missions, whether overseas or at home. Such historical oversight exists in part because, as historian Andrew Porter has observed, religious missions themselves were not examined but "pushed to the margin" in a historiographical interest in mission history that favoured them as a way to appreciate instead the non-European societies in which missions were based. Their history thus needed to be larger than one missionary society to study the development of these local societies; at the same time, the histories of individual missions continued to be written by insiders in the vein usually associated with this kind of literature (hagiographic, teleological, etc.) – the kind of literature, in fact, that has been associated with the Grenfell mission. In general, as Porter

Yeo

observes elsewhere, a Canadian historiography on religion, missions, and empire is developing but is "rarely considered ... in tandem with the patterns produced in other mission fields." Even with a more nuanced approach to the study of religion and the British Empire, Porter's own brief mention of Canada and its Protestant missions excludes Newfoundland, which he shows only as part of the Anglican diocese of Newfoundland and Bermuda from 1839 in order to identify the Moravian (Protestant) mission stations to the Inuit along the northern Labrador coast from the eighteenth century.[2]

Grenfell's mission, however, clearly emerged during a massive Anglo-American mission movement in the second half of the nineteenth century, a period that Porter describes as "a great age of religious expansion": by 1900, about ten thousand Christian missionaries from Great Britain alone were supported overseas by voluntary Protestant missionary societies.[3] The mission movement has been widely recognized and studied, with historians now generally dismissing earlier views that missionaries actively participated in, if not represented, the aims of imperialism. Rather, although British missionaries did believe that the empire promoted British culture and Christian civilization and thus often, as Phillip Buckner explains, "defined their mission in imperial terms," they were, in Porter's terms, "profoundly egalitarian." Furthermore, Porter continues, missionary societies were determined to "avoid involvement with trade, government, and politics. The missions began by explicitly distancing themselves from expanding colonial rule, wary of its chauvinism, secular authority, and often flawed commercial ambitions."[4] At the same time, missions established connections that cut across national boundaries, placing them "outside the limits of any nationally based empire building."[5] Additionally, the complex history of the mission movement indicates that an anti-imperial spirit at the end of the century influenced missionaries' interest in inter-denominational cooperation.[6] In this historical context, with the Grenfell mission operating across several national boundaries – Great Britain, Newfoundland, Canada, and the United States – combined with the evolving international mission movement at the end of the nineteenth century, it would therefore be difficult to maintain that the missionary impulse of its founder in Newfoundland and Labrador had direct association with imperialism, regardless of his British origins. Indeed, Grenfell himself suggested – somewhat hyperbolically – that the coast of Labrador is international, "in that the British, Canadian, Newfoundland, and American fishermen have equal fishing rights there"; moreover, he declared, it was difficult to estimate the importance of the fishery not just to the British Empire, but to the entire world.[7] As well, a survey of missionaries in 1899 revealed that 338 American missionary physicians served in 348 hospitals, almost 800 dispensaries, and forty-five medical schools around the world, a reminder that imperialistic impulses in any event did not necessarily represent the British Empire.[8]

Nevertheless, Grenfell's mission differs from other missions in many ways. This chapter explores those differences while uncovering ways that Grenfell the man – who had international celebrity status and charisma – recruited vast numbers of volunteers to work in Newfoundland and Labrador. Many were young people from elite American universities and colleges, who undertook manual labour that they would never perform at home. It demonstrates the degree to which Grenfell created a unique amalgam of mission activities to serve the unique needs of an occupational group that he and his followers emphasized was Anglo-Saxon, like them, in a land of ice and snow.

Fundamentally, his was not a church-based mission, nor was it a university-based mission. Rather, it blended many of the late-nineteenth century approaches to missions as they repositioned themselves.[9] Unlike church-based missions overseas, the Grenfell mission focused on a single geographic area along hundreds of miles of Atlantic coastline. In keeping with later trends in "applied Christianity," it was a non-denominational, though essentially Protestant, mission; it was also based on medical aid.[10] In other words, it was not a religious mission with medical missionaries attached: it was a medical mission with social activists attached. The demand specifically for dedicated medical missions arose from the 1870s, when medical missionary societies were established in Great Britain, and soon after in the United States, and the numbers of medical missionaries quickly grew. By Grenfell's time in the 1890s, there were 680 medically qualified Protestant missionaries worldwide. After setting up makeshift quarters for dispensing medical care in their regions, these missionaries worked toward constructing purpose-built hospitals, activity that involved them in planning, fundraising, and eventually staffing and running the institutions. Grenfell's mission clearly reflected this trend toward building new structures for medical care, along with many other purpose-built institutions; as one supporter noted, it was "the first bit of institutional Christianity" the area had seen.[11] An important difference perhaps involved the greater extent of local voluntarism and less government involvement in the development of such institutions: unlike more populated and long-settled regions, such as Hong Kong, where land was provided by the government for hospitals, Newfoundland had limited political or legal (including municipal) infrastructure with which Grenfell had to contend. He indicated that he had been "given an excellent site" to construct the first hospital building in St Anthony; since all the land was owned by the Newfoundland government, presumably this gift was easily acquired from the government in St John's, followed by a government grant for the hospital.[12] Moreover, there were no competing medical activities outside of St John's: Grenfell could "import" medical staff to any part of the colony at will.

Medical missions by and large, however, typically were developed in tropical countries where they aided – and often religiously converted – non-white, non-Christian, Indigenous peoples. Grenfell's mission, on the other hand, catered to Christians of a particular occupation and class. In spite of the fact that Grenfell was associated for decades with the Royal National Mission to Deep Sea Fishermen for this specific aim, from the time of his arrival in Labrador he wrote extensively not just about members of this occupational group, but also about Indigenous peoples. His books such as *Down to the Sea: Yarns from the Labrador* contained tales and especially images of Inuit – sometimes with captions "The Native Eskimo – still almost prehistoric in their customs" – that perhaps attempted to key into readers' expectations about bringing a medical mission to an exotic locale. Certainly some of his tales substantially promoted his personal image and acclaim as a Samaritan to exploited and injured Inuit children such as Pomiuk.[13] After the IGA formed in 1914 (if not before), it appears Grenfell had to overcome this international impression of his now self-named association by ensuring that a more powerful message of affiliation with his Anglo-Saxon supporters would keep the funds and upper-class personnel flowing into his mission.

Again and again, Grenfell and his supporters took care to emphasize that their work was among English-speaking white Anglo-Saxon Protestants: "It was among these white fishermen that I came out to work primarily," Grenfell recalled, "the floating population which every summer, some twenty thousand strong, visits the coasts of Labrador. It was later that we included the resident settlers of the Labrador and North Newfoundland coasts."[14] In 1893 his report to the Mission to Deep Sea Fishermen in London had made his findings clear: "At L'Anse au Loup we found people who had themselves come out direct from Devonshire and Somerset, from Chard, Dartmouth, Torquay, &c., and some at one place from Bude in Cornwall"; these people, an Anglican clergyman attested, were already "far from a condition of religious unenlightenment."[15] For British readers, Grenfell projected a romanticized view of fishermen and their Anglo-Saxon race as being admirable: as masters of the sea, they represented the refinement of human nature in their innate ingenuity, perseverance, daring, and virility.[16]

To businessmen in Toronto in 1920, Grenfell suggested that, if given a chance, the people prove "their inherent possession of that peculiar ability that has made the Anglo-Saxon predominant in modern history"; at the same time, he distinguished the people of Labrador, whose long isolation required educational intervention, from people of Newfoundland, who "are in the same class exactly as are those who reside in the Maritime Provinces."[17] To potential donors in 1925 – in particular to Shriners, who had recently begun to build hospitals for children in the United States and opened the first in 1924 – Grenfell emphatically declared, "We are Anglo-Saxons." More than this, "We live in North America. Many of the patients of the States and Canada are far less American and Canadian than we."[18] Grenfell's evident appeal to the common lineage of the people he helped with those who aided them and who read his New York–based magazine occurred at a time when immigration was a major concern for both the United States and Canada. North America had experienced large immigration from countries in eastern Europe, but after the First World War immigrants from

Europe were discouraged; indeed, in Canada, according to Donald Avery, "The purpose of the Dominion government now was to re-establish the Anglo-Saxon character of the country."[19] Clearly, Grenfell felt the need to differentiate this population seeking medical care in North American hospitals from the ancestrally related population he wished his readers to support. His intent, while implying racism today, was in keeping with openly discussed concerns among white, Anglo-Saxon colleagues of his day – especially those associated with elite institutions and medical practices.

By 1933, Grenfell's refrain was also in keeping with British parliamentary debate about the political future of Newfoundland, which as a result of economic crisis had just given up self-rule and was overseen by a British Commission of Government. As Declan Cullen has recently shown, any decision about returning political independence to Newfoundland rested implicitly, according to Scottish politician James Maxton, on an attitude towards British protectorates as peopled by "lower breeds without the law," rather than on a right to democracy based on British origin. Maxton argued forcefully in the House of Commons, "These are not coloured people. Perhaps I ought to explain that the natives of Newfoundland are not black men, or yellow, or some inferior breed. These are men of English, Scottish, Irish, and even Welsh descent. And though perhaps some of them have deteriorated, like others, by absence from their own soil, none the less they are people of exactly the same type as those of us who sit in this House."[20]

Regardless, many mission volunteers still expressed surprise at their encounters with residents in the region, in comments that often echoed Grenfell's description of the people's Elizabethan form of English. In 1920, when she first joined as a summer volunteer teacher from Vassar College in New York state, Elisabeth Greenleaf noted the English origins of the people in Newfoundland – especially from the West Country – and the form of their speech: "All British Newfoundlanders, except those who have been sent away to school in Canada or the United States, use an old form of the English language, which sounds strange but yet not unfamiliar to an American. They still use commonly expressions obsolete elsewhere which I recognized with a queer shock of pleasure as phrases explained in footnotes to Shakespeare."[21]

The "quaintness" and "charm" of the dialect led another volunteer teacher from Dartmouth College, Fred P. Carleton, to publish a glossary in an annual report of the activities of the Columbia University College of Physicians and Surgeons station in Spotted Islands, Labrador. "To make things clear at the start," he told readers in 1922, "the language spoken on the coast is English. The isolation of the country and the conditions of life and livelihood have produced a dialect wholly unlike that of any other English people. Many of the people are of Dorset and Devonshire stock and the presence of a number of the terms is explained by this fact."[22] Carleton's glossary then listed terms under headings by topic according to work, domestic life, and medicine.[23] In 1928 Donald McI. Johnson, a physician from England who served in Harrington Harbour, reflected on the strong resemblance of the people to those he later came to know well in the "southern English countryside": entering the harbour, he remembered, "it was no longer French-Canadian, or even English-Canadian, that we now listened to, but voices with an unquestionable English South Country accent ... it was as if we had travelled right round the world and ended up where we had started."[24]

Explanations about the British heritage of these peoples increasingly distinguished them from other peoples, sometimes to offset misconceptions that may have been promulgated decades earlier by Grenfell himself. Indeed, Bess Armstrong, who hawked Labrador handicrafts around summer resorts in New England in 1930, observed, "Everywhere people were enthusiastic and interested, but everywhere we found great ignorance about the North. Many believe, as I myself believed long ago, that the inhabitants of northern Newfoundland and Labrador are all Eskimos. We had great difficulty in convincing some of our inquirers that they are of English extraction." Furthermore, she provided an unusual anecdote: "Of all the remarks of our customers one so overwhelmed me that I shall never forget it. Many people naturally thought that Sir Wilfred had brought us down from Labrador to sell the goods. I must explain that I am sun-tanned in summer. One day an old lady came up and gazed at us and then said to me, 'My dear, your friend looks English, but by your coloring I can tell that you are pure Eskimo.'"[25]

More than "English extraction," it was Anglo-Saxonism that supporters highlighted was shared with these people. In 1924, when an

American volunteer found it difficult to hear the quietly spoken names of children, she explained, "Fortunately for us, they were good, old Anglo-Saxon names for which our ears were well attuned"; in 1932, a report of the British and Irish Grenfell association described the work along the Labrador coastline that was "mostly populated by Anglo-Saxons"; and in 1937, a speech at Vassar College by Eleanor Cushman, secretary of the Grenfell Association of America, took pains again to clarify this point: "Contrary to popular belief, 'we really don't work with the Esquimaux; we work with the Anglo-Saxon fishermen.'"[26] At the time, "Anglo-Saxon" for all these mission workers alluded to British heritage, despite the ethnic origins that we would now recognize; however, even the distinctions – including correctly identifying French settlers – were described in 1916 by Marian Cutter, a librarian volunteer: "These people are descendants of Welsh, Scotch, French and English who settled along the coast of this desolate country, attracted by the fishing opportunities."[27]

In this regard, the Grenfell mission built on a tradition of maritime missions for sailors, at sea and in port. Grenfell joined the Mission to Deep Sea Fishermen for those on the North Sea, which had formed in 1881 as an organization akin also to the friendly society that particular groups of workers in Great Britain founded in order to provide poor relief and benefits for their aged colleagues and for their families in the event of their deaths.[28] The friendly society in addition acted as a means in which workers "without political power sought to protect themselves" from exploitation, as historian P.H.J.H. Gosden explained.[29] During Grenfell's time with the Mission to Deep Sea Fishermen, it changed name to add *National*, then soon after the *Royal* designation, to become the Royal National Mission to Deep Sea Fishermen in 1896; now named the Fishermen's Mission, it has continued to offer financial, pastoral, and emergency response support to fishermen and their families to the present, though its full history remains to be written.[30]

Freedom from exploitation was similarly one of Wilfred Grenfell's early aims as representing the Mission to Deep Sea Fishermen to aid those who fished between Newfoundland and Labrador to become self-sufficient, for he believed they were kept in poverty by merchants who set credit amounts for the fishers' harvest in this cash-poor society in exchange for supplies. This "truck" system was an ancient form of payment that Grenfell knew well from England: in his view, this nasty form of paternalism was tantamount to peonage and slavery.[31] He therefore determined to encourage the establishment of co-operative stores by local residents, based on a successful model used in England – a rallying move that engendered such hostility for Grenfell from merchants that he later described the co-operative stores as having "lent more thrills to a 'missionary life' than has the Arctic [*sic*] Ocean."[32] (By 1917, as discussed in the introduction, chapter 1, and especially in chapter 6 with respect to clothing donations to the mission, an independent investigation into the IGA activities found no direct link to the co-operative stores to support the merchants' claims of commercial competition.)

Under Grenfell, the mission in Newfoundland and Labrador also adapted the activities of urban missions – especially those associated by his time with the settlement house movement. The settlement movement focused on the community and was widely modelled in North America and Europe on Toynbee Hall in London and Hull House in Chicago. The concept involved houses in underprivileged neighbourhoods of large cities, lived in and staffed by middle-class volunteers from church congregations as neighbourhood centres and schools in which religious preaching and charity were replaced by community involvement. Communities served by the settlement house differed for Great Britain and the United States: the British settlement house focused on urban communities divided by social class; the American settlement focused on ethnicity and race of immigrants in urban neighbourhoods.[33] As Rompkey has indicated, Grenfell not only was influenced by this movement but became close friends with William Lyon Mackenzie King, then deputy minister of the new Canadian Department of Labour (and later prime minister of Canada), who had worked at Hull House "and understood the possibilities for social change in an urban setting."[34] By building solid structures in impoverished communities of Anglo-Saxon people in Newfoundland and Labrador – not just hospitals, but schools and orphanages – complete with separate community centre for recreation in St Anthony, Grenfell clearly applied the idea of the British urban settlement house to a rural context. His volunteers lived in these structures, after they were built, for the periods that they worked with and for the local residents of the community.

In addition, for other aspects of his mission Grenfell tapped into social reform concepts such as industrial (or "cottage") activity, including those associated with American settlement houses, that had emerged especially in the United States. The notion of "profitable philanthropy" espoused by Helen R. Albee of New Hampshire encouraged the handcrafting of furniture, woven items, and most especially, rugs by people living in rural areas. This kind of activity was integrated in Hull House, for immigrant women in Chicago to create and sell their handiwork, and run by Jessie Luther, an artist and teacher from Providence, Rhode Island, who adhered to the Arts and Crafts style that rejected the industrialism of Victorian society. Luther then briefly established workshops in Marblehead, Massachusetts, where she met Wilfred Grenfell on one of his fundraising tours in 1905. Grenfell immediately invited Luther to Newfoundland to teach crafts. After taking responsibility for the occupational therapy program at Butler Hospital in Providence, Luther began to travel to St Anthony to undertake this volunteer work. She eventually founded six weaving centres in Newfoundland and Labrador, and marketed their goods in shops in Boston, New York, and Philadelphia.[35]

Grenfell's ideas and the approach to his mission were thus grounded in a complex amalgam of several strong historical and contemporary trends related to friendly societies, religious missions, overseas and urban missions, settlement houses, and social reform activities such as home industries. They, with Grenfell himself as exemplar, also drew heavily on "muscular Christianity" notions espoused by Victorian Anglo-American schools and the British Empire that emphasized manly activities and social responsibility; in contemporary literature, these notions simultaneously keyed into late nineteenth-century anti-modern sensibilities that inspired "true adventure tales" of the romance and lure of the pristine, reinvigorating northern climate.[36] Additionally, Grenfell's world view reflected the Social Gospel movement: along with other Christians who averred that their primary goal was the reform of society, from within, Grenfell's work to aid self-improvement was less for individuals than it was for communities.[37] As a contemporary explained, "His program was to make Christianity practical to the whole life of the people, so he organized his faith in beneficent institutions that touched and still touch the life of our people, industrially, socially, intellectually and religiously."[38]

Significantly, the Grenfell mission also capitalized on an "exploding enthusiasm" at the time among "young, middle-class volunteers, many of them university students" for whom reform activities were viewed as character-building.[39] Indeed, the formalized Student Volunteer Movement rapidly expanded from home missions to overseas missions as the numbers of volunteers swelled in North America and Great Britain. As Porter indicates, the significance of this movement was enormous: "More than anything else in the 1890s it was the chief source of fresh ideas and enthusiasm for the traditional overseas societies. It generated recruits, funds and inspiration sufficient to survive even the great hiatus and missionary reconstruction imposed by the war of 1914–18. It represented the latest of the many successive injections of revivalism into Protestant missions since the early eighteenth century and its leaders either took advantage of existing institutions or created new organisations to channel its energy and commitment towards constructive missionary ends."[40]

Among the many to be deeply influenced by this movement and imbued with its global evangelizing aim at the time was Wilfred Grenfell. When he was still a medical student in London, Grenfell attended a religious meeting led by Dwight L. Moody, the famous American evangelist who held meetings at elite universities in the United States and Great Britain. The immediate impact of this event on the young Grenfell was life-changing. As he recalled decades later, Moody imparted a "spiritual impetus which was still influencing my reactions to life"; what Moody did for Grenfell was to show "a vital call in the world for things that I could do.... He started me working for all I was worth, and made religion real fun – a new field brimming with opportunities. With me the pendulum swung very far."[41] Grenfell would later receive an honorary doctorate from Moody's son, then president of Middlebury College in Vermont. Other contacts between the two men are not mentioned by Grenfell or his biographers; however, the fact that Moody was in-

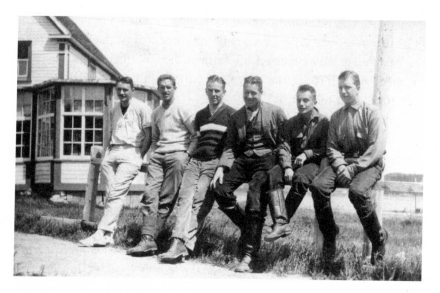

Figure 2.1 Student volunteers, 1915; Harold D. Finley, Yale; William Adams Jr, Yale; Charles MacPherson Holt, Williams; Philip Garey, Newark Academy; Waldo L. Tucker, Yale; William A. Rockefeller, Yale. Mary Schwall Photographs, MU-ASC, 1.01.108

strumental in establishing the Student Volunteer Movement in the United States at a meeting in Massachusetts in 1886[42] suggests that Moody's influence on Grenfell extended far beyond this initial impetus. Soon after beginning his work in Labrador in 1892, Grenfell attended a hugely successful foreign mission conference in Toronto that provided him with a widely publicized platform to spread the word. The conference was front-page news, with summaries of Grenfell's presentation joining others in newspapers and religious periodicals[43] – including that of Arthur T. Pierson from Boston, a "leading missionary promoter of the day," who addressed the foundational meeting of the Student Volunteer Movement.[44] This remarkable achievement and aspect of Grenfell's life and mission organization has not been recognized but is beyond the scope of discussion here. Suffice it to say that whether through his continued exposure to developments in the evangelical missionary field, or through contacts with other Americans involved in the mission and student volunteer movements, Grenfell quickly applied Moody's ideas to the practical aspects of operating a mission on volunteer help, particularly one that was overseas for both British and American university students, and of undertaking regular lecture tours for support.

Grenfell's lecture tours regularly targeted American Ivy League institutions, where his speeches not only raised funds but also recruited young men and women for voluntary work of all kinds in Newfoundland and Labrador for decades through the early part of the twentieth century (figure 2.1). Consequently, according to Cushman, almost all of the IGA work was done by volunteers: "Harvard, Yale, and Princeton are actually represented in that particular ditch," she told her Vassar audience about an image depicting road construction.[45]

Vassar itself had already taken on a significant role in supporting the mission through volunteer teachers (chapter 7 in this volume) who then gathered traditional (that is, folklore) information from Newfoundlanders, encouraged by the college president, funded in part by college trustees, and led by Elisabeth Greenleaf, that eventually would help to keep longstanding oral traditions alive through scholarship. As Neil V. Rosenberg and Anna Kearney Guigné noted, in addition to her own collecting of folk songs in northern Newfoundland, Greenleaf drew on a wide network of contacts as additional sources for songs, many of whom were mission volunteers from Vassar;[46] the result was the publication by Harvard University Press of the most significant collection of folk songs from Newfoundland. For its part, by 1932 Harvard had apparently sent over 150 students, raised funds, and purchased at least one ship.[47] For its student readership, an article in the *Harvard Crimson* in 1919 perhaps best described the "modern missionary," in the guise of Grenfell:

> The prevalent picture of a modern missionary in the mind of the average educated man is the idea of a long-haired individual, with a Bible, standing under a palm tree trying to "convert the heathen." Many people have a strong antagonism to the work of missions, and believe that people in foreign countries are happier without than with the missionary.
>
> The fact that this opinion exists is due to the ignorance of the advances made by the missionary movement during the last few decades. No longer is a true missionary a man whose purpose is

to force his religion upon someone else. The modern missionary makes life easier where it is hardest. It may be that he is a physician in a country like India, which has fewer doctors than the city of New York.... Or he may be an economist, educator or business man who works to make living conditions better in countries where people have difficulty in finding the wherewithal to live. The spirit of modern missions is one of service and reconstruction, not of dogmatism.

"The true missionary of today," this writer concluded, "is well represented by Wilfred Grenfell."[48]

Grenfell acknowledged the contemporary connotation of *mission* and *missionary*, though for him it was a "sorry comment" that the tops of his lecture posters in 1928 had been cut off because organizers maintained "the average man is not interested in the popular idea of missions." He subsequently praised a local resident for becoming a missionary in India, in terms that stressed the unrecognized value of this work: "My readers may be saying," he wrote in the IGA magazine, "'I loathe missions. Missions are obsolete.' Maybe they are right. But anyone whose face betrays a beautiful nature cannot be doing harm really, whether her intellectual attitude to religion is ours or is not."[49] However, it was this "modern" view of the missionary as social service worker that suffused his supporters' publications; as early as 1910, for example, a volunteer physician from Philadelphia, Emma E. Musson, directly equated the missionary with the college student: "The missionary generally numbers about fifteen or twenty and hails from Harvard, Princeton, Williams and many other colleges. He can be first assistant to the doctor, he can dig a ditch, help build a house, take charge of the lumber mill, go off to capture caribou to swell the reindeer herd, look after the sheep or garden, and be delegated to unpack boxes sent from all over the land. When he spends a day delving into a box filled with the debris of some one's garret his language is not that of the seasoned missionary"[50] (figure 2.2).

Student newspapers reveal the mechanisms of recruitment, fundraising, and organization for Grenfell's mission on campus. While the *Harvard Crimson* published dozens of items over about three decades, the

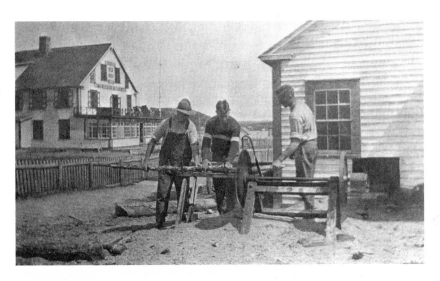

Figure 2.2 Student volunteers sawing wood, St Anthony, ca 1915. PAD,
IGA Photograph Collection, VA 106-26.2

Yale Daily News carried well over three hundred routine items about
Grenfell from about 1904 until the 1950s (extending to a couple in
1960 and 1971).[51] Annual calls for volunteers appeared in the papers,
accompanied by promotional information about the mission, Grenfell,
Labrador, its peoples, and the value of a working summer vacation in
the North, all of which illuminate the themes of this discussion. Student
volunteers displayed pride in working collegially alongside students
from other Ivy League schools, whose own mission activities they sometimes reported, and to call themselves WOPs (Grenfell's term that sup-
posedly meant workers "With-Out-Pay").[52] The IGA staff selection
committee itself published an article in the *Harvard Crimson* in 1921
that highlighted the camaraderie among these students:[53]

> The trip down [north] is a get-to-gether party and by the time St
> Anthony is reached, the Princeton, Yale and Harvard men have
> forgotten their college rivalry, all have become one unit and as-
> sumed the name of "Wops." Their work is mostly out-door labor.
> A new road to be built, vessels to be unloaded, launches and boats
> to be taken to other ports, patients to be carried from the boats to

the hospital – such is the work of the "Wops."... It was at this station [St Anthony] that last summer the "Wops" under Professor Gillespie of Princeton, excavated for the foundation for the new Orphanage. This coming summer the Orphanage is to be built – and who is going to lend a hand? The Wops.

Articles explained the work of the wops for prospective volunteers (figure 2.3). In 1925, observed the *Harvard Crimson*, "Harvard men are known as 'waps' in Labrador":[54]

At least such is the official title of four Harvard students who have been with Dr Grenfell's mission in Labrador for the past summer. According to G.D. Krumbhaar '26, the foreman of the "waps," their job is anything from scrubbing floors in the hospitals to preaching sermons in the churches.... From the one hospital on the ship, the mission has grown to have four hospitals on land, and in addition to this a number of churches, schools, and libraries. It is in order to run these establishments that the mission each year calls for volunteers who pay their own expenses to come to Labrador and work as "waps."

Similarly, Gibbs W. Sherrill, who had worked three summers with the mission, reported in the *Yale Daily News* that

from the very first the "Wop" (as the volunteer worker is invariably called) has always been an integral part of the staff. At a first glance it is hard to understand of what real service the average college boy or girl could be to such an organization, but when we realize that a hobby such as sailing a boat or tinkering with motors can be made into a very definite step in saving a life or giving back sight to a blind man we begin to see why, as the work enlarges, not only the number but also the proportion of jobs for the Wops increases.[55]

For Yale readers, Grenfell himself had expanded on these notions, with an added comment about the particular advantages of American volunteers: "One of the best characteristics to my mind of Yale men, and

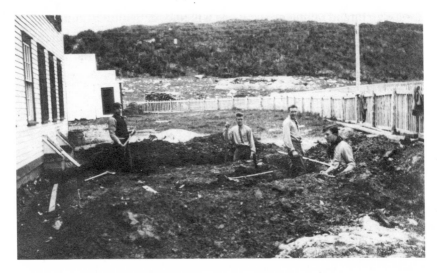

Figure 2.3 Student volunteers, 1912, digging hospital foundation, St Anthony: William Logan Fox, Harvard; S. Frederick Cushman, Amherst; William Moore Carson Jr, Harvard; Mr Raley, Oxford. PAD, IGA Photograph Collection, VA 107-43.1

of all university men for that matter, is their keenness to do things, and their catholicity in tackling any job that turns up.... The rotten distinction of a job being menial and unfit for a gentleman has never been an American bugbear."[56]

Many articles also attest to Grenfell's stature and power to attract students to such laborious work in an isolated northern locale. In 1922, when Phillips Brooks House, a social service organization at Harvard, took on the task of recruitment for the Grenfell mission, the student paper outlined the proposed work:

Volunteers will leave in the latter half of June, and remain in Labrador until early in September. This year they will be assigned to St Anthony, Newfoundland, and Battle Harbor, Indian Harbor, and Harrington on the Labrador coast. They will engage in boat trips to secure supplies and transport urgent medical cases, and do such work as digging foundations, unloading vessels, or painting and machine shop jobs. Volunteers who are in the Medical School, or who intend taking up medicine will find many opportunities for helpful service.... Men are wanted who are willing to work hard, and who have the necessary physique to accomplish the needed labor most efficiently.[57]

It also encouraged students to volunteer in order to meet the man behind the mission itself: "One of the chief attractions of the work is the personal contact with Dr Grenfell, who visits all the mission stations during the summer. It is his inspiring personality that has been the mainspring of the work of the Labrador missions, and it is due to him that such keen interest has been shown by college men in this from [*sic*] of summer service. It is with the view of rekindling this interest that Phillips Brooks House is making special effort to secure a large enrollment of students from the University for the coming season."

Clearly, college students did all kinds of work in Newfoundland and Labrador, and they were posted wherever they were needed. Detailed information about student volunteer activities on site is found in the annual reports of one station in Spotted Islands, Labrador, that was established and routinely run by students. This station was started in 1912 by a Cornell medical student who wished to find a place "where he might spend an enjoyable yet useful summer in the open" to do "real servicable [*sic*] work." Furthermore, he was directed to Spotted Islands where "fisher folk" were in need of medical attention and someone who could "start their youngsters on the way to more healthful manhood."[58] After two summers, during which he erected a building out of lumber and supplies he brought himself, he turned the work over to the P&S Club (of Columbia University College of Physicians and Surgeons). For medical students, this club supported co-curricular activities, including community service.[59] Each winter subsequently, a medical student was chosen to accompany his predecessor to Spotted Islands, where they maintained a dispensary and answered medical calls on the *P&S*, a twenty-eight-foot motor boat, over a hundred-mile coast containing 1,200 people. Over the next dozen years, a dozen medical students travelled to the station, along with teachers, and the station expanded to include a school, dental clinic, and clothing store (to distribute donated clothing in exchange for work or crafts). The activities were financed each year by faculty and students of the College of Physicians and Surgeons. Published annual reports appealed for funds while describing all the station's activities, including statistics of medical care to patients, articles by volunteers, photographs, etc. As a result of their well-known activity, other units were established along the Labrador coast by Yale, Harvard, and Johns Hopkins.

Of note are the appeals to persuade university students to join the cause, especially after 1914 when the International Grenfell Association was formed. Supporters and mission staff alike drew particular attention to race, place, and therapeutic work for vacation. Routine visiting lectures at Yale by Grenfell, with accompanying slide images, along with those by mission staff such as Harry Paddon, indicate a rapid decline from early emphasis on the "Eskimo" inhabitants of Labrador to a focus on the Anglo-Saxon population instead. Their intent was to draw well-to-do young Americans to the aid of their poor distant relatives. Articles in the *Yale Daily News* – no doubt with material provided by the IGA – repeatedly told readers in the 1920s and 1930s that the mission catered to white men, "largely of English extraction," descendants of "Englishmen" or of "the British fishermen" or of "the fishermen from Devon and Dorset," or of "the old stock" "who began to settle there in the seventeenth century," or who came over to Labrador "during the last four centuries" or came out "in the employ of sailing companies of a century ago": the "true" Labradorian is "a mixture of white and dark, British servants, sailors, carpenters, coopers, tinsmiths and shipwrights." "These people," in short, summarized Grenfell in one interview, "are descendants of Scotch and Devonshire settlers, and they are a fine race." Furthermore, observed two other writers, although once "originally Esquimaux, this race forms but a minor portion of the inhabitants" because the "Indians and Whites have intermarried, and sometimes strains of Eskimo blood can be detected." By alluding to the growing attention paid to eugenics and race in this era,[60] the latter writer continued, "Whether this combination of peoples is eugenically sound or not, it produced a happy race of men." In short, as another remarked, "The natives are Anglo-Saxon. Their customs and habits, however, are often very different and more simple then [*sic*] American conventions."[61]

These descriptions were also stressed in reports of presentations and in editorials. Dr Harry Paddon, medical officer in charge of the Indian Harbour hospital, often wrote and spoke glowingly of both Labrador and the people. "Convinced that Labrador's hardy and self-reliant trappers, her splendid mariners, and her capable workmen are worth preserving," he told the *Yale Daily News* in 1920, "Dr Grenfell appeals to citizens of the bigger Anglo-Saxon communities to ensure to their kinsmen, speakers of their tongue, pocket editions of Canadian and US institutions.... American parents to-day are exulting in the shaping, under happy conditions, of their own children's splendid destinies. Would they wish to see the humble cup dashed from the lips of Labrador's little ones?"[62] Paddon expanded on notions of race a few years later, noting, "While the population includes relics of two oborignal [*sic*] and several more of mixed blood, while the white civilization looks down on these people with a supercilious eye," he could attest to the "courage, endurance, enterprise, and self-sacrifice [that was] unsurpassed and usurpassable in our own civilization."[63] Over a dozen years later, an article that praised Paddon and his significant contributions to the mission as "head of Yale-in-Labrador" described the people as "mostly of Anglo-Saxon stock, with a little Indian or Eskimo blood intermingled, the men of the region are of a genuine frontier type and as interesting a race as any in the world."[64] Grenfell declared in a similar vein that fundraising for the IGA was carried out by "the four countries that have contributed to the International Grenfell Association: namely, Canada, Newfoundland, the United States, and England." Therefore, "the Directors are justified in the conviction that these Anglo-Saxon nations that have made possible the work in the past, will not fail to meet this opportunity for helping, both now and in the future, the more needy people in the north of Britain's aldest [*sic*] colony, and dependency, Labrador."[65]

The appeal to a common Anglo-Saxon ancestry could not have been made clearer to student readers. Nevertheless, an editorial in 1925 vigorously defended the IGA, and Grenfell's approach, against critics who might impute imperialistic aims: "Because of its association with institutions whose chief aim is to convert more people to Christianity, the word, 'mission' has acquired especially among undergraduates an opprobrious sense." However, if the "Grenfell Mission" were more commonly known by its more accurate name, "The International Grenfell Association," people would be quicker to realize that it is primarily a medical rather than a religious mission. Indeed, people who know Dr Grenfell personally, realize that his claim for divine favor lies not in converting more heathens to the true gospel, but rather in adhering closely to the unwritten doctrines of the Church of the Good Samaritan which combines all practical religions.

But as a "missionary" Dr Grenfell has been further criticized for bringing the "white peril" to natives and especially esquimaux who would be better off without the contaminating influences of civilization.

In fact, this writer maintained, unlike the Moravians, who since the late eighteenth century tried to prevent the mixing of "Esquimaux" blood with white, Grenfell's activities were "comparatively recent" and dealt "little with esquimaux but almost entirely with white population of fishermen, 'planters,' and 'livyeres.' The ancestors of the latter class were the original sailors and traders who first visited the coast, settled, and gradually diluted esquimaux blood."[66] Prospective volunteers, this editorial implied, should not be deterred from associating themselves with this inherently secular organization.

Paddon's reference to a "frontier type" to describe the Labrador people conveys another of the significant appeals used to attract student volunteers from American cities. Labrador, students were told in the 1920s, "offers itself as an ideal place to spend a summer vacation," and the "desire to join Dr Grenfell's mission for a vacation has become increasingly great in the last few years."[67] Moreover, the latter article from *Yale Daily News* continued,

Men have not only recognized the natural advantages that Labrador offers for enjoyment, but they have taken an absorbing interest in the work....

But the work is varied enough with diversions to keep it far from being drudgery. The invigorating climate is always cooled by an ocean breeze and the temperature seldom rises about seventy degrees

Fahrenheit. On some afternoons the "wops" may drop their work and jump into a heavy dory which is rowed a mile or so beyond the entrance of the fiord where cod may be caught. Or in the noon of some unusually warm day there is the lake on the hill for bathing. There are always enough congenial people among the "wops" and nurses of St Anthony to organize occasional dances in the evenings and picnics in the day time. On Sunday evenings Dr Grenfell is in the habit of inviting the workers up to his house.

Attesting to their social class, along with the concept of a working vacation, the students generally paid their own travelling expenses (as they did from Columbia as well). In 1920, the cost of the trip was quoted as being reasonable at $160 to $320; in 1928, the total expenses for three months were estimated as $300 to $400.[68]

The recreational emphasis in its call for volunteers by the Yale Grenfell Association (formed in 1920)[69] was criticized in an editorial in the student paper that contrasted the typical European wanderlust that undergraduates exercised in "fords in Scotland, waves on the Lido and gala nights in Paris" with "useful labor in a world-recognized philanthropic organization that takes only red-blooded men": "After nine months of sublime inactivity of the undergraduate, a summer of cutting pines, navigating boats, and hoisting freight will to many be a conscience-easing remedy.... Is there not a certain satisfactory feeling which one experiences on returning from Battle Harbor or St Anthony in the Fall that is missing in the vacationist just back from Europe, Newport, or Madison?"[70] The value of such a working vacation was reinforced in an item reprinted in the *Harvard Crimson* from the *New York Evening Post* in which a businessman extolled the experience of "open air work" in the young college graduate he had just hired: it put him "in good physical condition and in touch with all sorts and conditions of men. He used only twenty-six of the forty-eight free weeks at his disposal, but I don't care what he did with the others," this businessman remarked, "Those twenty-six weeks were what I call a 'vacation cum laude.' They gave him an unusual equipment for success and I only wish I could find more young men who possessed it."[71] Grenfell himself had said as much many years earlier: of his volunteers, "we review their records in terms of what they did. It forms a very interesting guage [*sic*] by which to estimate values, which have so often been judged by other standards."[72]

An editorial in the *Yale Daily News* then elevated the appeal from the American physical and social success story to one addressing the American psyche: Labrador was, for these students in 1925, a novel terrestrial frontier: "The American frontier is historical legend to us now. But in Labrador has sprung up a new one. Here there is an outpost with rigor of life, opportunities for service, and a more extraordinary and untroubled beauty of natural scenery than former generations knew in 'the States.' Here is an almost inconceivable land of torrential rivers and great falls, of uncut timber, and unmolested peace. Here, where mountains rise sheer thousands of feet from the surf, is what is virtually a new country."[73]

Wilfred Grenfell would speak to the students about this "frontier community." Interestingly, some of this appeal to the – what some might consider a quintessentially American characteristic – "desire for producing, rather than always consuming,"[74] was keyed to the economic and commercial promise of the settlement in North West River at a time of boundary dispute between Quebec and Labrador. In 1925, Yale established a school there when it was perceived that education would benefit the local population after the dispute was settled, for it had been proposed that a railway would be built from Quebec to North West River, turning this settlement not just into the capital city but also a gateway to the Atlantic.[75] Thereafter, "Yale-in-Labrador" (as it became known) was a going student concern, with funds regularly allotted for decades from the University Budget that supported various charities and Yale projects overseas (including "Yale-in-China").[76] From the beginning of the "intimate connection" that Yale had with "bleak Labrador,"[77] however, was the *Yale* boat, which frequently appeared in the student paper as needing funds for either repair or replacement.

As these student publications from Yale, Harvard, and Columbia reveal, Wilfred Grenfell, and his organization's activities among people of Newfoundland and Labrador, reaped substantial benefits from the volunteer labour of students. More than this, they emphasized for contemporary, by then ambivalent readers how much his original mission was not a religious one, but a medical one that offered means to support local residents who – apart from their lower education and economic status – outwardly resembled the volunteers in language, religion, colour, and customs. Grenfell's idiosyncratically designed mission keyed into several reform movements of the time, blending, adapting, borrowing, and employing approaches that accorded with his view of non-denominational Christian social reform to extend the work of his complex enterprise far beyond medical and surgical care. Moreover, just as the Student Volunteer Movement was a significant component of the mission movement that also led, in Clifton Phillips's terms, to "transatlantic cross-fertilization,"[78] so too did Grenfell's mission capitalize on student volunteers to forge international connections, within continental North America and the Western Hemisphere. It did so by appealing to American traits of useful activity, productivity, economic and even potential commercial improvement, all for a "race" of people who landed on a shore around the same time as the students' own ancestors. But for circumstances of geography, in this view, these people might have fared as well as those who landed on the shores of new colonies that became the prosperous United States.

In these ways, Grenfell successfully tapped into an American ethos to operate his enterprise for decades. Not only did predominantly American volunteers provide tangible support for residents, but in turn they also received intangible benefits of satisfaction in honing their own leadership, team, manual, and other skills, while participating in a kind of co-curricular program of character building. At an early period, Grenfell's mission for Newfoundland and Labrador therefore perhaps anticipated global secular trends in aid and development that would become more pronounced in the latter part of the twentieth century with the establishment of non-government organizations and other agencies for student volunteer work overseas. Indeed, in 1914, as an astute student editorial had indicated, the Grenfell mission affirmed its distinction when it adopted its name as an international association rather than a mission.

3

The Gospel of Right Living: Wilfred Grenfell's Association with John Harvey Kellogg of Battle Creek

Ronald L. Numbers

The flamboyant John Harvey Kellogg – inventor of flaked cereals and peanut butter, promoter of frequent bowel movements, best-selling author of sexual and dietary manuals, and prolific sanitarium builder – was the leading health reformer and one of the most famous physicians in late nineteenth- and early twentieth-century America. During the last quarter of the nineteenth century he turned an obscure water cure in Battle Creek, Michigan, into the world-famous Battle Creek Sanitarium and in 1895 opened a medical school, the American Medical Missionary College, with campuses in Battle Creek and Chicago.[1] Among his many associates was the like-minded medical missionary Wilfred Grenfell of Newfoundland.

Over the years both men turned increasingly from evangelical religion to eugenics and the Social Gospel. Kellogg had grown up in the Seventh-day Adventist Church, a small religious group headquartered in Battle Creek best known for believing in the imminent return of Jesus Christ, observing the Sabbath on Saturdays, and accepting of the visions and "testimonies" of the prophet Ellen G. White as revelations from God. Mrs White and her husband, James, had virtually adopted twelve-year-old John Kellogg, who set about learning the printing business in the denomination's publishing house. In the fall of 1872 the Whites sent young Kellogg, along with two of their own sons, to study hydropathic healing at Russell T. Trall's degree mill in New Jersey. Later, again with the Whites' support, Kellogg went on to study for two additional years at reputable regular medical institutions: the College of Medicine and Surgery of the University of Michigan and the Bellevue Hospital Medical School in New York City. In the spring of 1875 Kellogg returned to Battle Creek and joined the staff of the Western Health Reform Institute, the Adventists' struggling water cure. The following year, at age twenty-four, he took over the superintendency of the institute, quickly expanding it into a popular Medical and Surgical Sanitarium. As his profile and power in the denomination grew, he clashed increasingly with Mrs White's son, William, and his ministerial associates over access to the prophet. By the early twentieth century Kellogg was sharing his discovery that Mrs White had plagiarized some of her allegedly inspired writings – as well as his growing conviction that she was not what she claimed to be. In 1907, amid exaggerated charges of having embraced pantheism, Kellogg was dis-fellowshipped (that is, excommunicated) from the Adventist Church.[2]

Grenfell's spiritual journey had begun differently, but he ended up in a place similar to Kellogg's. Although raised in the Church of England as the son of an Anglican minister and educator, Grenfell converted to American-style evangelical Christianity while in medical school in London. Returning to his lodgings after making an evening house call, Grenfell slipped into a tent meeting being held by the visiting American evangelist Dwight L. Moody and his singing sidekick Ira Sankey. Profoundly influenced by their message, he responded to the "altar call" inviting the convicted publicly to show their intention to devote their lives to following Jesus Christ. He vowed to become a medical missionary and soon thereafter joined the Mission to Deep Sea Fishermen, a charitable society that "saw itself primarily as an evangelical organization in search of souls, and only secondarily as a philanthropic agency." In a locale where Methodists battled Anglicans for influence, and other denominations held sway – notably the Moravians – Grenfell's mission remained officially un-denominational. While raising funds in the United States, Grenfell fell under the influence of the liberal Congregational minister Lyman Abbott, editor of the influential *Outlook*, which promoted the union of social reform and Christianity. According to Grenfell's biographer, Ronald Rompkey, about 1903, with Abbott's endorsement, "the myth of the heroic, adventurous Labrador doctor was launched."[3]

In 1910 Grenfell wrote a booklet titled *What Life Means to Me* in which he confessed to having no theology. "What is beyond life's spectrum is a mystery to me." He now lived for the present. Not surprisingly, such candour did not sit well with some of the folks back at the mission. Despite Grenfell's break with orthodox Christianity and his once warm feeling for Methodism, he remained a nominal Anglican. As he wrote to his mother about 1918, he and his wife, Anne (Anna), were experiencing "a lessening value for the emotional doctrines of Methodism &c. than we had. I never quite understood your own love for the old Church [of England] prayers & service. But I'm getting it now – this easy, cheap, emotional religion does *not* produce trustworthy men.... So we rejoice in our dear little Church of England here."[4]

Kellogg seems to have first met Wilfred T. Grenfell in February 1906, when the now-famous Labrador doctor visited Kellogg's Battle Creek Sanitarium on a fundraising tour in the United States, the first of a number of visits to Battle Creek. In reporting on Grenfell's two lectures, which raised $760 for the Labrador mission, Kellogg's *Medical Missionary* described the visiting celebrity as

> a man of quiet and unassuming nature and disposition. As a public speaker he is, perhaps, not fluent and verbose, but his simple direct style combined with his evident sincerity, produces a strong effect upon his hearers who listen with great interest to the plain recital of experiences. There is an absence of sanctimoniousness, sense of humor, a disposition to look upon his chosen work as a very pleasant calling.... He has gained the admiration of the whole world in his heroic self-denial for the good of a suffering and obscure people.[5]

In promoting Grenfell's return visit in February 1907, the Battle Creek magazine hyped the story of his life as reading "like the wildest romance, exposed as he is to constant danger and hardship and brought into contact with suffering in all its worst forms."[6]

On the occasion of this visit Grenfell confessed to having previously harboured suspicions about his self-promoting host and his Battle Creek operation. Kellogg lived his professional life precariously on the cusp between scientific medicine and quackery. Before his visits Grenfell had been inclined to associate the Battle Creek Sanitarium with Sunny Jim, a popular cartoon character used to promote Force cereal, a variety of wheat flakes, "but since I have come here, I have learned that 'Sunny Jim' was a pirate [used to promote a knock-off of Kellogg's own flaked cereal] and has nothing whatever to do with the Battle Creek Sanitarium. I am glad to know of that, and I am glad to see the broad, liberal, un-denominational Christian spirit in which the work of this institution is being carried on.... I believe thoroughly in the ideals and principles for which Dr Kellogg and this institution stand."[7]

Later that year Kellogg announced that Grenfell would be joining the editorial team of his long-running magazine *Good Health*, along with such luminaries as the Yale economist Irving Fisher; the "Great Masticator" Horace Fletcher; Harvey W. Wiley, the father of the recently passed Food and Drugs Act; and the muckraking journalist Upton Sinclair, author of *The Jungle*, which exposed the dreadful conditions in the meat-packing industry.[8] The Good Health Publishing Company also began distributing Grenfell's spiritual autobiography and guide, *A Man of Faith*.[9]

When Grenfell returned to Battle Creek in 1909 for what had turned into an annual fundraising event, *Medical Missionary* proclaimed that "it can truly be said that there is possibly no living man who would meet a heartier welcome than he received." Kellogg and the students at his American Medical Missionary College enthusiastically welcomed "their fellow missionary who had come from the Icy North, if not actually 'From Greenland's Icy Mountains,'" the title of a popular evangelical hymn. The editors promised soon to publish "an account of the terribly thrilling experience" he had passed through, nearly "losing his life" – speculating that "perhaps it was only by some such suffering and possible martyrdom that the Christian church could be awakened to its duty." Indeed, a short time later the magazine carried Grenfell's heroic tale about going sixty miles with a dogsled to care for a dying boy. On the way he found himself trapped on an ice pan and near death from the cold. To survive, he killed several of his dogs and skinned them to make a coat. For sharing this and other experiences with the people of Battle Creek, Grenfell collected $600. In return, Grenfell agreed to serve on the advisory board of the American Medical Missionary Board, which Kellogg had established with a gift of 5,000 shares of Toasted Corn Flake Company stock to support the American Medical Missionary College and other charitable activities.[10]

Over the years, in his numerous publications, Kellogg energetically promoted the "heroic missionary work" of his new friend. The *Medical Missionary* closely tracked Grenfell's career: his engagement and marriage to Anna C. MacClanahan, his new home in St John's for visiting fishermen, and accommodations for "fishermen's daughters who come to the city to seek employment" (often in the saloons), and, of course, his repeated visits and lectures in Battle Creek. In one piece, reprinted from the *Outlook*, the magazine portrayed Grenfell as a man for all seasons: "surgeon, master-mariner, magistrate, agent of the Lloyds in running down rascals who wreck their vessels for the insurance, manager of a string of co-operative stores, general opponent of all fraud and oppression," to say nothing of his frequently repairing "his little iron steamer." Grenfell's "muscular Christianity" – to which the five-foot, four-inch Kellogg also aspired – enabled "him to knock down and drag out the human beast that comes into Labrador to add the illicit whisky-bottle to the other sources of the suffering which the inhabitants have to endure."[11]

Grenfell returned the favour, puffing Kellogg in his own writings. In a major endorsement of Kellogg's work in the journal *Modern Hospital* he declared that "a long experience of Battle Creek has forced me to class it as one of the vital forces now working for righteousness in the world." He revealingly recalled his first meeting with Kellogg:

Some years ago, while in Chicago, I received an invitation to visit and inspect the methods of the best-known simple food protest in America, known to the public as the Battle Creek Sanitarium. With an inbred hatred of cant and quackery, and thinking that the institution might be merely a means of advertising patent food and a new sect called Seventh-Day Adventism, I at first respectfully declined. Later, however, I decided to go, feeling that there must be some germ of good in a system which had produced such wonderful physical improvement in some of my personal acquaintances.

Grenfell continued to address Kellogg's controversial reputation:

> Every prophet or protestor makes enemies.... The assertion that a
> surgeon has no right to invent breakfast foods is almost a cardinal
> canon of medical lore. But the fact that Battle Creek food products
> have come as a benefactor to many digestions, and that Dr Kellogg,
> so far as I know, has not any personal financial interest in the sale
> of any patents, has not yet altogether modified the offense inventing
> them.... [T]he declaration by Battle Creek that it dispenses almost
> entirely with all drugs is regarded with no little suspicion.... It is
> an improved and successful "Brooks [*sic*] Farm" experiment.

Kellogg, a distinguished surgeon, had, according to Grenfell, surrounded himself with equally accomplished colleagues: James T. Case,
a "world famous" roentgenologist (radiologist); Martin A. Morensen,
"one of the ablest of diagnosticians" in the field of cardiovascular diseases; William H. Riley, a neurologist, who reported "the first case of
Friedreich's ataxia." In short, Grenfell concluded, "The profession has
no fear, and the public need have none, of the scientific ability of the
staff." The Battle Creek Sanitarium promptly reprinted this article as a
fifteen-page pamphlet titled *The Soul of Battle Creek*.[12]

Writing in ADSF, Grenfell credited Kellogg with having been "again
and again ... a good angel to our work." Although Grenfell stopped
short of following Kellogg into thoroughgoing vegetarianism, arguing
that living in Labrador without eating fish "would spell starvation," he
never used alcohol and "eschewed tobacco and hot condiments, and
meat to as large an extent as possible." He repeatedly praised Kellogg's
meatless food products for "how easy they are to assimilate, how easily
prepared, how large a value in nourishment small quantities carry, and
how relatively inexpensive they are. All these attributes of foods are
particularly valuable to our work in Labrador – portability, easy cooking
and high nutritive value with small bulk."[13] On one occasion, according
to the visiting director of the Battle Creek Sanitarium's nutrition laboratory, various Kellogg enterprises contributed to Grenfell's mission
twenty-one cases (500 pounds) of Kellogg's All-Bran cereal, eight bags
(200 pounds) of sterilized bran, four cases (20 pounds) of Savita yeast

extract, two weighing machines, and one carbon arc light. On another, the Battle Creek Sanitarium sent "large supplies of cereals, tinned milk and other foods to be used for the people up and down the coast, as well as a variety of vegetable seeds for their gardens."[14]

Grenfell's reluctance to condemn the eating of fish also reflected the values of the community, where fish were the lifeblood of the economy. In 1910 Kellogg's *Good Health* reported that the travel writer Felix J. Koch, who had recently investigated the codfish industry in Newfoundland, "seems to have made the discovery that Newfoundland is a great incubating center from which tubercle germs are scattered all over the earth." Indeed, Koch had estimated that 90 per cent of all cod fishermen and processors suffered from "incurable" consumption. Local officials, fearing that if word got out it would threaten the island's economy, urged immediate action to rectify the embarrassing situation.[15] Despite their commitment to healthful living, both men laboured long hours on little sleep. On the occasion of his first meeting with Kellogg, apparently on the train from Chicago to Battle Creek, Grenfell recalled being introduced to "a short, wiry, keen-looking man ... Dr Kellogg, superintendent of the sanitarium. Though well over 50, he had not a wrinkle in his skin.... When I turned in to sleep he was dictating to a secretary, and when I turned out again in the morning he was still dictating, presumably to another secretary. 'Don't you ever sleep?' I ventured to ask. 'Oh, yes, when I need it,' was the cheerful reply." One admirer described Grenfell himself as "one of the people who don't seem to need more than three or four hours of sleep and worked both himself and his associates at full pressure."[16]

In the late 1920s Grenfell's health began to decline. On one occasion he collapsed in Labrador while working and, according to Rompkey, became "a patient in his own hospital ship."[17] In the late 1930s, Anne Grenfell wrote to Kellogg, who from time to time advised the Grenfells on matters of health, that her husband was suffering from "arterial spasms," memory lapses, hallucinations, and melancholia. Grenfell spent the winter of 1936–37 trying to recuperate on the South Carolina coast, accompanied by his wife and a trained male nurse who was an Adventist from the Takoma Park Sanitarium. Anne Grenfell praised this nurse, for "by temperament and training this young fellow is an ideal companion for Sir Wilfred, as he is a strong idealist, a very hard worker, and keenly interested in scientific subjects – all of which appeal strongly to my husband. Among other things he is a trained physio-therapist, and gives Sir Wilfred such excellent treatments."[18]

When Kellogg learned of his friend's condition and proximity to Florida, he invited him to come to his Miami Battle Creek Sanitarium, which he had opened in 1931 and where he himself wintered. Offering to treat Grenfell as an "honored guest," Kellogg wrote, "Nothing would afford me so much pleasure as to have an opportunity to render some service to those who had been of so great service to so many." On this occasion Grenfell declined, but, according to Rompkey, during the winter of 1938–39 he spent "a spell at Dr Kellogg's sanatorium [*sic*] in Miami, and he felt reinvigorated by the vegetarian diet and regular massages."[19]

In 1940 Grenfell celebrated his seventy-fifth birthday as a guest-patient at Kellogg's Miami institution. The sanitarium made the most of the occasion, organizing a series of "Labrador days" in Florida. As reported in ADSF,

> Daily sales and lectures were held at churches, clubs, resort hotels, county fairs.... At Homestead, the Grenfell truck was driven on to the County Agricultural Fair Grounds.... The presence of Sir Wil-fred and the enthusiasm aroused made many new friends for the Mission.... Sir Wilfred's seventh-fifth birthday was a real event. A friend in Coconut Grove sponsored a successful sale to celebrate that day. The Miami Battle Creek Sanitarium, where he was a guest, helped by having a sale – a Sunday afternoon meeting and a very beautiful cake was presented to the tune of Happy Birthday, on February 28th.... Sales of Labrador industries were arranged and held on the Florida west coast and at several vacation spots on the coast of Georgia and South Carolina.[20]

Just months later Grenfell died from a heart attack. Kellogg, though thirteen years his elder, lived another three years. Thus the world lost two of its most enterprising apostles of the "gospel of right living."

4

To Prevent "the Otherwise Inevitable Catastrophe": American Philanthropy and the Creation of the International Grenfell Association, 1905–1914

Heidi Coombs-Thorne

In 1912, the continued success and longevity of the Grenfell mission in northern Newfoundland and Labrador was not a foregone conclusion. The organization had expanded at a remarkable rate since 1892, under the frenzied leadership of its founder, the charismatic Dr Wilfred Grenfell. It consisted of four hospitals, a nursing station, a hospital ship, an orphanage, an industrial department, a series of co-operative stores, and the new $150,000 King George V Seamen's Institute in St John's. Each summer, the mission attracted an array of doctors, nurses, teachers, college students, and other volunteers, drawn to "the Coast" because of Grenfell and his increasing appeal throughout North America. However, as Ronald Rompkey argues in *Grenfell of Labrador*, Grenfell's growing network of support in Canada and the United States made him increasingly independent of his parent organization, of which he was superintendent, the Royal National Mission to Deep Sea Fishermen. By 1912, Grenfell raised the vast majority of funding for the Labrador Branch of the RNMDSF in North America, especially through the Grenfell Association of America in New York. However, the GAA had no administrative authority over the mission, despite being the most significant contributing financial interest in the Labrador Branch. On the other hand, notwithstanding their position of authority, the executive of the RNMDSF had difficulty keeping Grenfell under control; they worried about Grenfell's careless bookkeeping practices and felt that the Labrador branch was drifting away from the evangelical approach that was central to their mandate. Both sides were moving towards restructuring the Labrador Branch in relation to the RNMDSF, especially in light of its North American focus, when an international scandal broke around the immensely promoted Seamen's Institute and its superintendent, Charles F. Karnopp[1] (figure 4.1).

In August 1912, Karnopp was charged and convicted with misappropriation of mission funds related to his management of the Seamen's Institute in St John's. His arrest was based on the results of an audit conducted by Cecil Ashdown of Price, Waterhouse of New York (board member of the GAA), which found that Karnopp had "pocketed many of the subscriptions" for the institute without keeping any record.[2] This was not the first occurrence of questionable accounting practices with the mission. At the time, the financial operations of the Labrador Branch in general were vague and disorganized, there was often no clear source of revenue besides widespread generic fundraising, and bookkeeping practices were disorganized and ambiguous. In fact, confusion over accounts led to a crisis in 1909–10, prompting Grenfell to bring in an American accountant and issue an audit of the co-operative stores. Ashdown's audit in 1911 was a follow-up to the smaller 1910 audit and was conducted at the suggestion of Chicago banker William R. Stirling, guardian of Grenfell's wife, Anne MacClanahan, who became Grenfell's trusted friend and confidant. In 1911, when the RNMDSF suspected financial mismanagement of the Labrador Branch and "hinted at the misapplication of funds," Stirling suggested an audit to satisfy the RNMDSF (who were worried about being financially liable for Grenfell's impulsive and expensive activities) and the GAA (who wanted more administrative control over the Labrador Branch).[3] The audit was also an important step towards the potential transfer of authority for the Labrador Branch from the RNMDSF to a new North American organization. On the basis of the audit, and after Grenfell consulted with the mission's legal counsel,[4] Karnopp was arrested, tried, and convicted, and served a six-month prison sentence in St John's.[5]

This chapter examines the events surrounding the arrest and conviction of Karnopp and the growing influence of American philanthropy on Grenfell and his activities, leading to the incorporation of the International Grenfell Association in 1914. These events must be understood

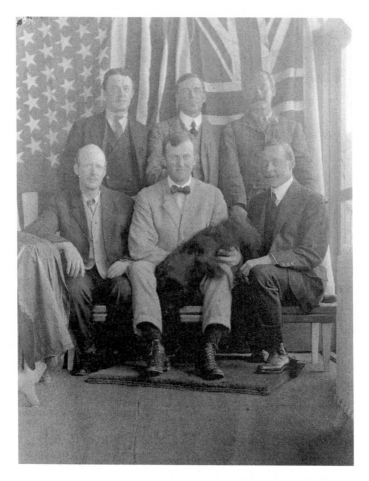

Figure 4.1 Charles F. Karnopp, *front centre*, flanked by Dr Grieve and Dr Walter Seymour Armstrong, with Dr John Mason Little, Francis Wood, Dr Wilfred Grenfell, *second row*, ca 1909. Location unknown, but possibly the Grenfell Association of America. The flags of both the United Kingdom and the United States provide a backdrop. PAD, IGA Photograph Collection, VA 118-192

within the framework of the new mass philanthropy movement in the United States during the Progressive Era. At the beginning of the twentieth century, American industrialists like Andrew Carnegie and John D. Rockefeller Sr turned towards a concept of "scientific giving" and began investing large sums of money into new foundations and endowments designed to foster social progress.[6] They administered these activities based on the principles of the Efficiency Movement and with the same business acumen that led to their success in industry. This brand of philanthropy differed greatly from the traditional "distributive" charity of the nineteenth century, with its "more modest goals" and its charity givers who "did not expect much in return for their generosity."[7] By contrast, the new philanthropy was "a capitalist venture in social betterment, not an act of kindness as understood in Christianity."[8] During the Progressive Era, the small-scale, local charitable organization was being superseded by the large, ambitious, and efficient philanthropic organization. Yet the one form of giving did not preclude the other and indeed, as Ruth Crocker argues, there was "no neat break in the history of American philanthropy between the old-fashioned gifting by individuals and the beginning of the foundations."[9] However, the philanthropic organizations were increasingly attractive for the large scale of their financial giving.

It was within this context that the Grenfell mission found itself the centre of an international scandal and at an administrative crossroads in 1912, in both a practical and theoretical sense. Grenfell's Victorian-era medical mission fit the traditional charity model, with Grenfell holding the entire operation together, and the vast majority of financial support flowing through networks of individual giving. However, with its expanding services and increasing costs, the mission needed greater revenue and, encouraged by board members of the GAA, many of whom were well connected to American society, Grenfell began reaching out to the new philanthropy. In 1907, Grenfell's friend in Boston, Reginald Daly, approached Olivia Sage for support, but was declined.[10] That same year, Grenfell himself began petitioning Rockefeller to support a seamen's institute in St John's. In his analysis of this appeal, Rompkey found that "although the Rockefeller Foundation admired Grenfell personally it shied away from an organization that depended for its existence on the personal appeal of one man. The Labrador mission, it noted, lacked the supervision and management of a missionary society whose history tended to create a feeling of confidence."[11] In March 1911 Grenfell finally met with Rockefeller,[12] who was happy to have met Grenfell and "to learn informally more of [the] splendid work of which [he had] known generally for many years."[13] But he was not prepared to support the cause, despite further petitions from their mutual friend and future Canadian prime minister, William Lyon Mackenzie King.[14] Grenfell had more success with Carnegie, who donated money for loan libraries in Labrador as well as $500 towards the library in the Seamen's Institute.[15] Carnegie and his foundations have been described as having "bridged" or "[straddled] the worlds of traditional and scientific philanthropy," which could account for his willingness to donate to Grenfell where Rockefeller would not.[16] So, in its early appeals to American philanthropy, the Grenfell mission had limited success, but members of the GAA continued to push in that direction.

Although Grenfell and aspects of the Grenfell mission have been the topics of numerous academic studies, the early administrative history of the mission leading to its incorporation as the IGA has not been examined in depth. Rompkey has provided the most academic detail on this history in *Grenfell of Labrador*, albeit from the perspective of events within Grenfell's life rather than an analysis of structural change. In his chapter titled "Running a Railroad Accident," Rompkey framed the Karnopp incident as one of several stressful administrative and financial issues Grenfell faced in that period. Grenfell's own expansive writings were vague on the details of the Seamen's Institute and the administrative crisis of 1912. In his autobiography, *Forty Years for Labrador* (1932), he discussed his reasons for building the institute and the support he received from the Newfoundland governor and the merchants of St John's. He hinted at some resistance, such that "reports were circulated by ill-wishers that the whole thing was a piece of personal vanity" and that despite his success with the institute, "the hostility of enemies was not over."[17] But otherwise he focused the institute section of his autobiography on King George V's laying of the cornerstone via transatlantic cable. He effectively avoided the entire period from mid-1912 to the end of 1913. In his revised autobiography, *A Labrador Doctor*, Grenfell acknowledged Karnopp's prosecution in a short, but telling, paragraph: "On arrival [at St John's] we found that trouble had arisen concerning the funds of the Institute and a prosecution was to follow. It was the worst time of my life. Things were readjusted; the money was refunded, punishment meted out – but such damage is not made right by reconstruction. It left permanent scars and made the end of an otherwise splendid year anxious and sorrowful."[18]

With the exception of Rompkey's contribution and Grenfell's not-unbiased biographies, the early history of the Grenfell mission remains shrouded in the literature, eclipsed by the dominance of Grenfell the man and the myth. This chapter will broaden our understanding of this pivotal moment in the mission's history and the mission's pre-1914 administrative deficiencies that led to the establishment of the systematized and long-lasting IGA.

BACKGROUND: "A GENERAL UNREGULATED SYSTEM OF BEGGING"[19]

The Mission to Deep Sea Fishermen sent Grenfell to spend the summer preaching and providing medical care to the people involved with the Labrador fishery in 1892, and Grenfell returned to continue the work the following year. In 1894, he then began petitioning for financial assistance to expand the mission's activities and received limited support from the Newfoundland government and the local merchant community.[20] He also appealed directly to the MDSF and its supporters through that organization's magazine, *Toilers of the Deep*, recounting riveting tales of poverty and hardship on the Labrador coast. However, the MDSF was not prepared to take on the full expense of Grenfell's Labrador activities, so Grenfell began raising money for the venture himself. For this, he looked increasingly to Canada and the United States. Through the winter of 1894, he toured Canada from Nova Scotia to Ontario, raising money, building support, and establishing local branches of the MDSF, and his lecture tours became crucial to the continued growth of his work. By 1903, he had established sixteen offices of the MDSF in Canada and two in the United States, each of which participated in ad hoc fundraising specifically for the "Labrador Medical Mission."[21] The Canadian branches were especially active in the first decade of the twentieth century and led the way in fundraising, organizing Grenfell's tours, and shipping donations to the Labrador coast. In addition, in 1903, Julia Greenshields of Toronto established and edited the mission's quarterly magazine, *Among the Deep Sea Fishers*, which became the official voice of the Grenfell mission.[22]

In the meantime, Grenfell was determined to increase his exposure in the United States, and in February 1905 he arrived in New York to begin an extensive lecture tour. He had visited the United States on previous occasions and in 1903 had spent almost two months lecturing in Boston, Chicago, and New York.[23] For that tour, he had met with some success, especially in building his American base. His lecture at Holy Trinity Church on 19 April triggered widespread publicity – the event itself was covered by the *Sun* (New York), and lengthy articles about Grenfell subsequently appeared in other newspapers and magazines.[24] Rompkey noted that in the *New York Times* interview, "Grenfell demonstrated how well he understood his American audience, for he carefully distanced himself from the traditional missionary."[25] He had begun to emphasize Christian actions, deeds, and "heaven on earth," as opposed to eternal salvation. However, it was the 1905 tour and his connection to Lyman Abbott (editor-in-chief of the *Outlook*) and Norman Duncan (author of *Dr Grenfell's Parish*, 1905) that marked the tipping point for Grenfell's American ambitions.[26] He spoke at numerous churches and private clubs throughout New York and Boston; he met with ministers, medical students, and nurses; he spoke at Young Men's Christian Association (YMCA) gatherings; and he gave the Trask Foundation lecture at Princeton University, through the invitation of Henry van Dyke. But the greatest achievement of the 1905 tour was the establishment of an association in New York in aid of Labrador (the Grenfell Association of America), with van Dyke as chairman, Eugene Delano as treasurer, and "about ten members, numbering among them some of the best known names in New York,"[27] carrying with them, according to Rompkey, "the unmistakable stamp of Fifth Avenue liberalism."[28] By 1912, Grenfell had undertaken additional lecture tours throughout the United States, established ten American offices (in addition to the GAA in New York), and activated widespread interest in the mission – and by doing so, he had tapped into a significant network of American millionaires and philanthropists.

The administrative transition from a small charity to a large systematized organization that would appeal to twentieth-century philanthropists was not easy or straightforward, and was especially complicated by Grenfell's careless accounting practices, lack of business acumen, and his non-medical activities. Until the mid-twentieth century, the fishing economy of Newfoundland and Labrador was structured on a truck method in which residents sold fish and purchased supplies through merchants who decided both the value of the fish and the cost of the supplies, a method that tended to hold people perennially in debt. In order to combat this system of payment, which Grenfell viewed as a significant contributing factor to the widespread poverty in the region, he initiated a series of co-operative stores – the first in Red Bay in 1896 – and a lumber mill in Roddickton. Grenfell supplied goods to the stores, and the local families entered into a bond to purchase the goods and maintain the co-operatives; they were then able to sell their fish to whomever they chose after they had paid for their salt.[29] Any profits were divided among shareholders or used towards improving the stores. Along with Red Bay, Grenfell started co-operatives in Braha, Englee, West St Modeste, Flower's Cove, and Forteau, and provided loans/supplies to individuals at Nain, Turnavik, Boulter's Rock, and Long Tickle. He appointed W.H. Peters as agent and manager of the accounts.[30] However, the co-operatives and the mill met with criticism, since they involved the mission in trade and made Grenfell vulnerable to charges of personal profiting, even though he provided personal loans to the stores to get them started and subsequently bore financial losses from the ventures.[31] They also competed with the merchant establishments, which jeopardized Grenfell's support from the merchant elite of St John's. Furthermore, as early as 1897, there was confusion surrounding mission accounts, including the Red Bay co-operative. That spring/summer, Grenfell hired a college student, Edgar Jones, to preach along the coast and to straighten out the accounts for the Red Bay store. In April, Jones was already confused by the accounts, and he sought clarification from Grenfell:

> I understand from the accounts that the Expenditures & Receipts of last year were abt equal, plus the amt of goods on hand etc. This I understand to be apart from the working capital of $800.00. Yet toward the close of your letter you use these words: "I know there is $234.75 left in Bank now, there may be more, I don't know, I am sending another $350.00 and the $320.00 in stores make the

capital." Does this refer to the working capital? This amt in total amts $854.75. These figures don't correspond with the capital placed in by your friends $800.00 plus 95.70 + 75.00 which you referred to as shares & profits, to be added to the working capital. Now if this capital remains in the bank all the time as the basis on which we work, what do you mean by the sending of $350.00 to the bank as is stated in quotation above. Where do this money come from? Is it your own? etc. I daresay you will see what I am drifting at. If you would kindly explain in a few statements abt this capital etc I am sure I will understand alright.[32]

Grenfell's response was vague, and in subsequent correspondence Jones was still uncertain of the particular arrangements.[33] Grenfell was not a bookkeeper, and his financial management of the various activities on the Coast were "muddled" from the start.

FINANCIAL CRISIS 1910: "THE TROUBLES THAT HAVE ARISEN IN THE MISSION"[34]

With the rapid expansion of activities on the coast and the increase of American interest in the work after the turn of the century, Grenfell's lack of financial sense became even more obvious and problematic. William Adams Delano, treasurer of the GAA and architect who designed the Seamen's Institute, and other members of the GAA were particularly worried about Grenfell's haphazard business methods.[35] Grenfell had his staff on the coast and elsewhere involved in ordering supplies and transferring checks and donations to himself and Peters;[36] and he himself did not always keep track of orders for supplies, nor did he regularly keep vouchers or receipts.[37] The finances of the stores and the lumber mill caused particular problems in 1909–10 and prompted subtle American interventions. Apparently, the co-operatives were carrying significant debt, and Peters mixed up several accounts. After consulting with the GAA about the finances, Grenfell agreed to have an American accountant, W.H. Webster, conduct an investigation and help Grenfell straighten out his practices. Grenfell referred to Webster as "a hot headed IRS man and difficult to control,"[38] and indeed in some ways he aggravated the situation. He directed blame exclusively towards Peters, and subsequently Grenfell began to blame and distrust Peters, especially concerning the stores and the mill for which Grenfell was personally liable.[39] However, even Webster could not fix the situation, and in June 1910, Grenfell was warned that, because of outstanding debts, "creditors were about to take an injunction on the Strathcona"[40] (the mission's hospital ship donated by Donald Smith, Lord Strathcona). Grenfell vaguely referenced the financial problems in a letter to Jennie Gray in New York, office secretary for the GAA, that June: "Peters has muddled us up awfully. An inquiry is going to be held this week. I do hope it is nothing worse than muddled. I am dreadfully afraid it is."[41] Then, in August, he and/or Peters missed or overlooked a payment of $300 to the Marconi Wireless Telegraph Company that Grenfell thought they had paid "ages ago."[42] Grenfell informed the company that he did not receive funds or pay bills for the mission, and that it was all done through a finance committee.[43] However, in a letter to Francis Wood (secretary of the RNMDF), Grenfell admitted that "there was never a finance comm^ee except on paper. It *never met.*"[44]

Meanwhile, perhaps influenced by Webster or members of the GAA, Grenfell began to see that the organization needed financial restructuring, and he wrote to the RNMDSF in June:

> As I found the methods of doing business for the Mission here utterly inadequate I asked Mr Wood to come out here to arbitrate on that matter and arrange some new one. I find Mr Peters, who disburses all the money has an arrangement by which he signs the checks himself. There really is no finance committee whatever. It has never once met and it has been Mr Peter's [*sic*] custom to get blank checks signed by one of the nominal members and fill them in as he needs. While I don't impute any dishonesty to Mr Peters yet the impossibility of getting what we order and paying for only that we receive and the mix up that Mr Peters made with many other accounts he was managing led me at the advice of the New

York accountant, who has been down with me for twelve months to ask Mr Wood to come out here and arbitrate and suggest new methods.[45]

As a result of Webster's inquiry and the discovery of Peters's apparent autonomy, Grenfell wrote to his major suppliers in the city, telling them he was not responsible for orders coming to them from anyone associated with the mission, the stores, or the mill unless the order was counter-signed by him personally.[46] He also wrote Greenshields in Toronto, telling her not to pay any money to anyone without a signature from him and not to send any more money to Peters, because they were making new business arrangements for the mission.[47] However, contrary to improving the financial situation with the mission, Webster's involvement caused more anxiety for Grenfell because he found it impossible to determine which of his advisors was advising him best.[48] In the end, John Munn, a merchant in St John's, and Stirling in Chicago steered Grenfell towards a solution. Grenfell had the co-operative stores audited to determine their indebtedness,[49] and he took steps to reduce his outstanding debts; as Munn suggested, "All the Creditors here who are owed money for the past eighteen months to two years, will soon begin to look about for a means to get their indebtedness considerably reduced, and I think it is necessary that every effort was made now for the Co-Operatives to reduce their Liquidations."[50] Within a week, Grenfell had transferred $5,000 to Munn to dispense to creditors, had given him a schooner to sell and put the proceeds towards his debt, and had paid him the bank balance from the Roddickton mill.[51] Meanwhile, Grenfell began to trust Stirling's judgment and advice in particular, and when the crisis with the co-operatives had passed, he admitted, "I've had a bitter lesson over Cooperatives & I'll be more guarded in my references but I do believe they can succeed, & are the only real solution – *but* they want possibly more overseeing than I can give – that is why I first got Peters, & later Webster. Of course the real secrets are larger capitals & cash dealings – & no debts."[52] Grenfell credited Stirling with helping to ease the "endless day & night mental strain of Webster," and he had Webster sent back to the United States in the winter of 1910–11.[53] By the end of 1911, Grenfell had most of his debts on the co-operatives repaid and was feeling optimistic about the work and the atmosphere of the mission, which was greatly improved since Webster's dismissal.[54]

However, straightening out the business practices of the mission required more than paying off debts and providing Grenfell's signature on appropriate documents – the accounting practices of the entire Labrador Branch required restructuring. The financial crisis of 1909–10 exposed Grenfell's inability to manage his ongoing operations, which was worrisome to his American supporters, and also increased discussions of a new North American organization to oversee the work. Even Grenfell's physician in charge at St Anthony, John Little, privately expressed concern that Grenfell was financially "irresponsible" and, with reference to the 1910 situation, he stated, "'The poor man has a frightful muddle to straighten out. It is of his own making I am sorry to say.'"[55] Little reflected the new American philanthropy and felt the organization should be restructured with "modern business methods," and the New York committee agreed.[56] In 1909, Willis Lougee, secretary of the GAA, admitted in the *ADSF* that the mission had been considering for a long time the need for more systematic and comprehensive bookkeeping practices.[57] And in August 1910, he reiterated these thoughts privately to Grenfell: "I am very much disturbed over the situation at Labrador … Personally, I can see no other way out of it than the Grenfell Association of America take over the work at Labrador, or rather the management of it."[58] In 1910, the RNMDSF sent Wood to New York to explore the possibility of transferring administrative authority to the GAA, and Jennie Gray informed Grenfell that the English committee would be glad for New York to take over the work.[59] Grenfell increasingly expressed misgivings and frustrations about being bound to the RNMDSF in London and told Stirling in December 1911 that he wanted a committee like the one in New York, which took a practical approach to "heaven on earth," rather than the staid approach of the RNMDSF and their focus on future salvation.[60] These discussions were important, because without new arrangements, and leaving Grenfell responsible for finances, the Labrador Branch would likely continue to experience intermittent problems and "muddled" accounts, which would jeopardize the entire operation.

THE SEAMEN'S INSTITUTE: "A CENTER FOR EVERY SORT OF HELPFUL AND UPLIFTING AGENCY".[61]

In the midst of this financial turmoil, Grenfell initiated his most ambitious undertaking with the mission: the construction of a large seamen's institute in St John's. The King George V Seamen's Institute was built on the east end of Water Street and officially opened on 15 July 1912 (figure 4.2).[62]

It was modelled on the Rowton Houses of London, a chain of hostels that offered clean accommodations to working-class men who otherwise lived in squalor.[63] The institute's primary purpose was to provide "wholesome" temporary accommodations for the estimated 85,000 outport fishermen, sealers, naval reservists, and international fishermen who visited St John's throughout the year. Grenfell felt these men needed an alternative to the local boarding houses, which left men susceptible to the temptations of nearby liquor saloons.[64] According to the mission, in the early twentieth century, "there [was] not a place in St John's

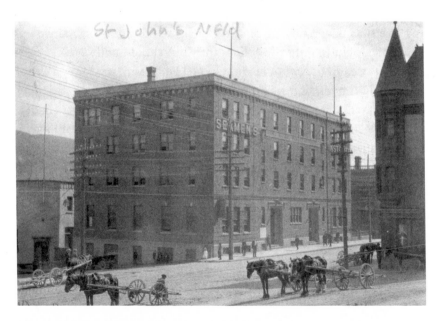

Figure 4.2 King George V Seamen's Institute, St John's.
WGP, Photograph Album

where one of these men can spend an hour of innocent recreation or sit
down with a friend and be decent. The harbor [was] encircled by fifty-
seven saloons where warmth and companionship [was] extended to all
strangers."[65] In keeping with the widespread social reform and temperance sentiments of the day, the institute provided a variety of alcohol-
free activities to help mitigate against the "perils" of the city, where
men's lives could be ruined by alcohol and its associated entertainments.
The institute also provided moving pictures, musical concerts, and educational lectures. In this way, it was intended to provide more than
clean and affordable accommodations – it was an enterprise in social
uplift, with the building as a "radiating center of helpfulness, an object
lesson in cleanliness, and a power for righteousness."[66]

The institute was designed, free of charge, by renowned New York
architects William Adams Delano (member of the GAA) and Chester
Holmes Aldrich. (Delano was the architect for the later St Anthony and
Twillingate hospitals, as discussed by Rafico Ruiz and J.T.H. Connor
in chapters 9 and 10 of this volume.) Delano and Aldrich were well connected to the elite of America's east coast, being members of prominent
New England families. They designed townhouses and country estates
for wealthy clients, such as the Rockefellers and the Astors, as well as
gentlemen's clubs, public buildings, private schools, and several buildings on the campuses of Yale and Cornell Universities.[67] Many Delano
and Aldrich buildings have become landmarks and notable historic sites
in the United States. The Seamen's Institute in St John's was a characteristic Delano and Aldrich building – minimalist neoclassical in style
and constructed with their trademark feature, brick with limestone
trim. It provided accommodations for men and women, with a "Girls'
Department" on the top floor.[68] The building had a variety of amenities,
some of which were not common in St John's at that time, including a
bowling alley, a gymnasium, an auditorium, an elevator, and a swimming
pool. The pool served the dual purpose of encouraging bathing and offering swimming lessons to the many fishermen in Newfoundland who
spent their lives on the sea but could not swim. The institute contained
a restaurant and temperance bar, an officer's room with chess boards
and a globe, a games room with billiard tables, and a Lend A Hand Society (Boston) reading room with a library donated by Andrew Carnegie

(figures 4.3, 4.4).[69] Beds were rented out at twenty cents per night.[70] The institute was also partially inspired by the YMCA, which at this point in its history was moving away from the theology of personal salvation towards a muscular Christianity version emphasizing character and service, or the practical application of ethical deeds and a form of "social evangelism."[71] Karnopp had been secretary of the International YMCA in New York when he was recruited in 1908 to assume charge of the new Seamen's Institute in St John's.[72]

From the outset, the institute was high profile for the Grenfell mission. There was tremendous enthusiasm about the new venture, especially from Karnopp, who reportedly stated that "if [the institute] was built sufficiently generously to offer a reasonable hope of being successful, he and his wife would be willing to devote at least the next few years of their lives to the carrying out of the work."[73] The mercantile and professional elite of St John's were involved with the building and formed the local Advisory Committee, which held its inaugural meeting at Government House in October 1908.[74] There was significant local and international support for the new venture, and the building was highly promoted on both sides of the Atlantic, especially through Grenfell's fundraising tours and associated media coverage. In fact, with the assistance of Newfoundland's prime minister, Sir Edward Morris, the mission arranged for King George V himself to "lay" the cornerstone for the building on the same day as his coronation. On 22 June 1911, at a predetermined time, the King pushed a button at Buckingham Palace that sent a telegraph signal to the site on Water Street that triggered a switch to lower the cornerstone into place.[75] Furthermore, Karnopp arranged for a number of dignitaries to speak or send messages to the formal opening in July 1912, including King George V; Prince Arthur, Duke of Connaught; and American President William Howard Taft.[76] The King and Queen Mary also provided signed portraits, which were displayed in Grenfell Hall at the institute.[77]

However, the institute was also a costly venture. Grenfell began raising money for the building during his lecture tours as early as 1905 and published several appeals in the ADSF. With Karnopp involved, in 1908–09 Grenfell launched a more aggressive fundraising campaign across Canada and the United States to support construction of the

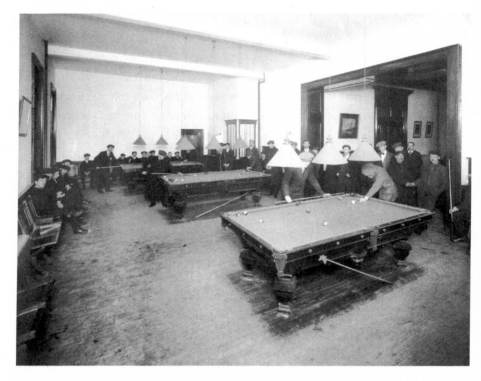

Figure 4.3 Billiards Room, King George V Seamen's Institute.
PAD, IGA Photograph Collection, VA 118-234

building. Karnopp himself toured Newfoundland, promoting the institute and selling subscriptions for the Seamen's Institute Building Fund.[78] In Toronto, Greenshields promoted the institute through her own impressive network of friends and acquaintances and became the Canadian media contact for information on the mission and the institute. The *ADSF*, to which her name was intimately attached, frequently reported on fundraising efforts and the progress of the construction (figure 4.5).[79] Greenshields was also directly involved with the finances of the institute and maintained an "Institute Account" at the Bank of Montreal.[80]

However, as with the mission's structure at the time, the finances of the institute were also vague, as Grenfell wrote to Lougee: "The matter of the institute has hitherto been left in Karnopp's hands and he drew money for institute purposes himself. I simply cant [*sic*] add to my labors the detailed care of a building five hundred miles away. I always

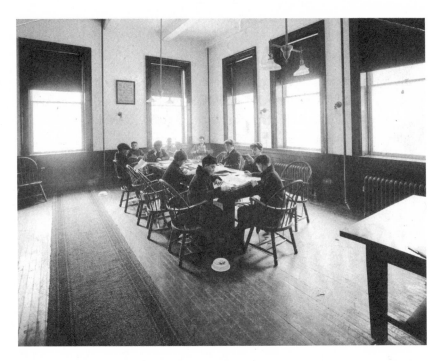

Figure 4.4 Reading Room, King George V Seamen's Institute.
PAD, IGA Photograph Collection, VA 118-233

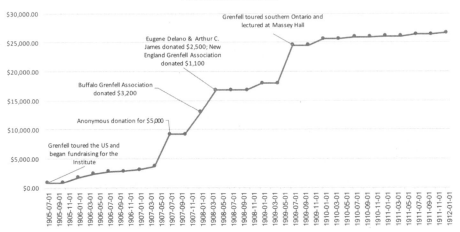

Figure 4.5 Fundraising for the King George V Seamen's Institute.
Derived from *ADSF*, 1905–12

wanted to make the Institute Karnopps [*sic*] life problem. It is a big problem and one well worth while a man's giving his whole energy to. Will you let him know in future how he is to get the money he needs."[81] It appears that from the outset, the institute suffered from the same ambiguity in its finances, sources of revenue, and accounting practices as the Labrador Branch in general. And bookkeeping for the institute was ad hoc and as unstructured as Grenfell's other operations.

MISMANAGEMENT OF FUNDS: "WE HAVE HAD TROUBLE AT THE INSTITUTE"[82]

In the summer of 1911, Ashdown spent several months in Newfoundland and Labrador conducting an audit of the Labrador Branch.[83] The main purpose of this audit was to examine the workings of the hospitals and stations on the coast with a view to updating the mission's business practices and as a step towards implementing a new international organization. As Ashdown explained to media outlets in New York, "I was sent north because it was realized that the work which was started in London twenty years ago had grown by the process of evolution from a one man mission to a large proposition. It had got to be such a big thing that it was found necessary to put it on a business basis with a central headquarters."[84] The mission had outgrown its traditional charity structure and, in order to effectively manage the work, especially in light of significant American interest in the venture, it had to transition into a modern, systematic, philanthropic organization. The audit was also a response to complaints surrounding the mission finances, especially from customs officials with the Newfoundland government who charged that certain items were brought into the country for philanthropic purposes, such that customs duties were waived, but those items were diverted to private use and sold or given away.[85] Ashdown uncovered the misappropriation during his audit. He returned to St John's in the summer of 1912 and confronted Karnopp about the customs charges and missing stubs in his receipt book, whereupon Karnopp panicked and destroyed the book. Ashdown summoned Grenfell to return to St John's as soon as possible.

Grenfell had been in St Anthony with William McDonald, professor at Brown University, who was conducting his own study of the Grenfell mission. McDonald was also a special correspondent with the *Times* (London). When they arrived in St John's, they met with Karnopp and the local committee, and Karnopp apparently admitted to the misappropriation. The matter was reported to the minister of justice, and Karnopp was arrested.[86] Grenfell, Ashdown, Miss Barnes (the mission's stenographer), McDonald, and Abram Sheard (secretary of the institute) all testified at the hearing. According to the *New York Herald*, "Grenfell was loath to prosecute [Karnopp], but the businessmen who are back of the association felt that public confidence could only be restored by cleaning house and punishing the man who had been guilty of a breach of trust."[87] Grenfell was in a difficult position. He had just weathered the financial crisis with the co-operatives in 1910, during which time he faced significant criticism from the GAA for his careless business practices. The fundamental purpose of the audit was to prepare the mission for transfer of authority from the RNMDSF to a new organization based on sound principles and systematic management. On the other hand, Grenfell was at least partially responsible for Karnopp's unfortunate situation. Karnopp arrived in St John's in the fall of 1908 as a young man highly recommended by the International YMCA in New York and was unwittingly drawn into Grenfell's financial chaos. As he proceeded to raise money and focus his efforts on the institute, he also witnessed first-hand the problems with the co-operative stores, the "muddle" with the accounts involving Peters, the attempt to remedy the situation through Webster, the audit of the stores, and finally the closing of some stores and the dismissal of Webster. And it was a statement of Karnopp's reflecting on the crisis of 1909–10 that captured the crux of the overall financial problems with the mission: in September 1910, he told Grenfell that, with reference to the mix-up of the accounts, "Word has certainly made a mess of it!"[88]

Up to this point, the mission had been functioning in a traditional and honourable manner, relying on individuals giving their word, rather than on rigorous bookkeeping practices. Karnopp himself fell into this pattern. He arrived in St John's with the understanding, or verbal agreement, that the mission would cover his accommodations, but it did not.

And when his wife took ill, he spent money sending her back and forth to the United States for treatment, increasing his own debts and forcing himself to find alternative sources of financial support. He charged some of his expenses to the institute account, with the intention of paying the money back. Karnopp was a devoted Christian committed to the ideals of the Grenfell mission and a man who thought extremely highly of Grenfell, such that he admitted to Grenfell, "You are my hero and always will be. God bless you. Your life has meant so very much to me."[89] He assumed that others would trust him when he gave his word.[90] Karnopp was, by all accounts, "the soul of honor,"[91] and the charges against him were widely met with disbelief; for example, upon hearing of the scandal, van Dyke told Grenfell, "He was the last man from whom I should have expected anything like this, and even now I cannot understand or fully realize it."[92] Some of Karnopp's defenders felt the accountants were too eager to find guilt where there was error.[93] At Karnopp's hearing, Grenfell stated that "the prosecution did not wish to press the matter very hard, and also spoke very favourably of the prisoner's character during the time he had known him."[94] And the judge expressed his regret at having to pronounce a sentence because, according to some sources, he was not convinced that there was wrong intent.[95] When the sentence was pronounced of six-months in prison, "the American Consul and Dr Grenfell both expressed their sorrow for Karnopp's fall and shook hands with him, whereupon he broke down. He was then removed to the lock-up."[96]

News of Karnopp's arrest and conviction made international headlines, and a public relations crisis ensued.[97] Ashdown's confidential report from the audit was leaked to the media on 2 September 1912, and the *New York Herald* printed an inflammatory story on "misuse of funds," "employe [sic] in jail," and "food stations on barren coast abandoned."[98] Another article in the *New York Herald* listed the members of the GAA by name and highlighted their affiliation with the mission, stating that "some of the most generous benefactors of the work are prominent in business and social circles."[99] In an attempt at damage control, Ashdown met with the media and outlined a plan for reorganizing the mission along modern business practices. He admitted to irregularities with the mission but assured readers that it involved only one person handling petty cash and minor subscriptions and that the work of the mission overall was not affected. Lougee also spoke to the media and informed the public that "a lack of coordination has been the only drawback to the great philanthropy established by Dr Grenfell along the barren coasts of Labrador and Northern New-foundland, and the mismanagement at the Seamen's Institute was made possible only because of the divided responsibilities."[100] Ash-down took the opportunity to emphasize the new organization that was in development, such that the entire Grenfell system would be "reorganized along international lines, with a view to bringing about greater economy and efficiency of management."[101] The organization would have a central office in St John's to control contributing and distributing interests and would have representation from all four countries involved in the enterprise.[102]

However, the arrest and conviction of Karnopp caused a temporary divide within the mission itself, both between and within the various offices. The Toronto office was particularly outraged at the treatment of Karnopp. In January 1913, Sheard informed Stirling in Chicago, who had become an important confidant to Grenfell and guided him through the Karnopp scandal, "The attitude of Mr [R.S.] Cassels has been a cold one, if not unfriendly, on account of the Karnopp prosecu-tion, and I fear with some affect upon Miss Greenshields. I used to send along carbons, etc. etc., to Miss Greenshields as I do to all, she in turn handed them to Mr Cassels, and he more than once wrote me there was no Association there."[103] Sheard hoped that a visit from Ashdown would result in "wrong conclusions being removed," since Toronto had been one of the most active centres of Grenfell activity in Canada.[104] But that January, Greenshields gave up her involvement with the Grenfell mission entirely, and Cassels took over all her correspondence.[105] Supporters of Karnopp in Toronto, St John's, and elsewhere argued that he was un-justly blamed for widespread mismanagement, perhaps best summarized by Wilson Naylor, professor of biblical literature at Lawrence College, Wisconsin: "Here is a given mission whose financial system was never put upon a budget basis, a young man comes in and at the time of sys-tematizing the mission he is made the scape goat of the lack of system which he inherited from the mission."[106] Meanwhile, in St John's, many prominent individuals associated with the mission staunchly supported and defended Karnopp after his conviction, and some of the most well-respected citizens of St John's remained loyal to Karnopp for their entire lives.[107] Karnopp's wife, Martha, developed a lifelong friendship with Phoebe Florence Miller of Topsail, and they corresponded until 1957. To Miller, in 1949, Martha reflected back on her years in Newfoundland: "The tragedy of our early years seems like an unreal dream. It has never laid its hand on our lives or touched our children. It is god's [sic] reward for the generous act of shouldering all the blame for a condition that was a shared responsibility."[108]

In August 1912, Charles Karnopp became at once compliant in, and a victim of, the careless accounting practices of the Grenfell mission in Newfoundland and Labrador. He joined the mission at a time when American interests in the venture had intensified, and the business practices of the traditional charity were inadequate to meet the demands of twentieth-century American philanthropy. When news of Karnopp's misappropriation, arrest, and conviction made international headlines, the accounting practices of the entire mission were called into question. The incident, and associated reports of mismanagement, exemplified the deficiencies of Grenfell's outdated nineteenth-century charity model and caused alarm within the American philanthropic community. Since Grenfell relied increasingly on the generosity of wealthy North Americans, the mission's financial success depended on a carefully crafted public image that was tarnished by the financial scandal. Viewed in this light, Karnopp's misappropriation of funds threatened to discredit the entire Grenfell mission and destroy the public favour that Grenfell had been building for twenty years. In the final estimation, Karnopp's prosecution, and the Grenfell mission's transition into the formalized IGA, appears to have been the result of Progressive Era influences within Grenfell's powerful American network of support. The GAA representatives in New York used the Karnopp scandal as an opportunity to promote the planned reorganization of the mission.

The IGA incorporated in St John's on 10 January 1914 as a "controlling association" to administer the mission's overall activities and to prepare consolidated statements of the accounts of the five auxiliary organizations – the RNMDSF in London,[109] the GAA in New York, the

New England Grenfell Association in Boston, the (Grenfell) Labrador Medical Mission in Ottawa, and the Grenfell Association of Newfoundland in St John's.[110] The Board of Directors included two representatives from each of these organizations.[111] This Board, as Rompkey pointed out, represented a wide range of business and financial interests, individuals who were used to "upholding sound financial principles."[112] The IGA created formal processes and a system of accounts, forms, and methods of record-keeping that had not previously existed in the mission. They established a new Medical Board consisting of all physicians stationed on the coast, who were expected to meet annually, keep minutes, and submit yearly reports of their medical activities. They introduced a uniform system of record-keeping at all mission hospitals and stations. (As J.T.H. Connor indicates in chapter 10 of this volume, clinical records in the main hospital in St Anthony had used printed forms of the Massachusetts General Hospital; these forms were afterward printed with the IGA name.) And they introduced a cost-recovery system, charging patients one dollar per day for treatment, with operations extra.[113]

Wilfred Grenfell became superintendent, responsible for overseeing the IGA activities on the coast. However, his financial involvement was curtailed. Reflecting on his own financial ineptitude and the role of his American advisors in guiding him through the crisis, Grenfell admitted to Stirling, "My business attributes, a long and somewhat sorry connection have made plain to you; and you have, with Ashdown and Sheard, possibly saved the otherwise inevitable catastrophe, when force of circumstances forces [sic] large business concerns and responsibilities on an unbusinesslike [sic] man."[114] The IGA created a discretionary fund for Grenfell, to allow him some of his previous flexibility in receiving donations from personal friends. Otherwise, finances were handled through Sheard, as secretary and business manager, and through a Finance Committee, with accounts audited annually and financial statements published in the ADSF. In light of the financial mismanagement highlighted by Karnopp's arrest and conviction, this new organization ensured accountability to the public and to its benefactors and "took on a distinctly American style."[115]

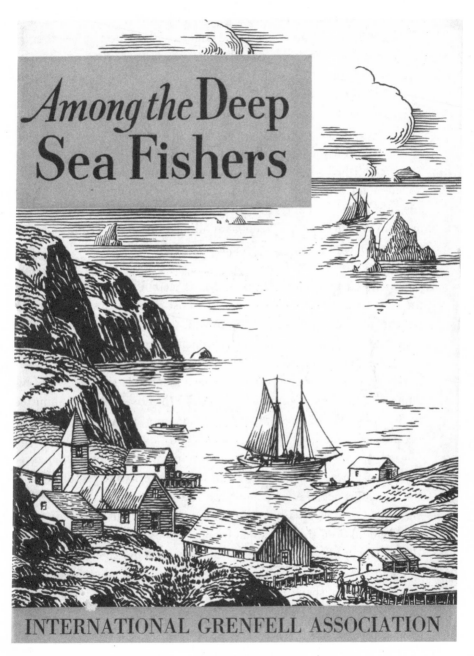

Cover of *Among the Deep Sea Fishers*. LeRoy Appleton, designer.

Part II

The Grenfell Enterprise in Motion

5

Sport in a Northern Borderland: A History of Athletics and Play in the Grenfell Mission, 1900–1949

John R. Matchim

This chapter examines the place of sport and physical activity in the communities of coastal Labrador and Newfoundland's Northern Peninsula that were serviced by the doctors, nurses, and facilities of the Grenfell mission. A visitor to the town of St Anthony, former headquarters of the mission, might consider the modern community almost inhospitably remote. One hundred years ago, however, St Anthony was not only a busy port of call for coastal steamers and fishing vessels sailing north to Labrador for the summer fishery, but home to an international community of medical professionals from Britain, Canada, and the United States. Only recently have scholars begun to move beyond the dominant personality of founder Sir Wilfred Grenfell to examine the remarkably diverse profile of the mission's staff and operations. Sport history offers a unique way to evaluate the cosmopolitan character of the Grenfell mission, for the mission brought together not only the medical expertise of an international cohort, but their national games and attitudes towards physical activity as well.

As the Grenfell mission grew, sport became an important part of life on the Northern Peninsula, and in the decades following Confederation with Canada in 1949, hockey, softball, and other games flourished. With massive levels of out-migration since the closure of the cod fishery in 1992, however, sport on the Northern Peninsula has withered. As journalist Terry Roberts wrote in 2016, "The cadet movement has all but disappeared. And minor hockey? A shadow of what it used to be in places like St Anthony. The ball field in Englee has never been so quiet. And Cook's Harbour feels hollow, cheerless."[1] To be sure, the fierce Straits–St Anthony hockey rivalry can still draw a crowd, but such events are only a shadow of the Northern Peninsula's former sporting landscape.

Sport and physical activity was an important part of the origins and ethos of the Grenfell mission. For members of the Victorian elite in Britain and North America (the class that was vital to the establishment of the Grenfell mission), sport was central to conceptions of social status, masculinity, and a proper education. In the context of rapid urban expansion and rural depopulation in the Global West, and accompanying concerns of emasculation and "race suicide," the prospect of working (and playing) on the frontiers of empire, such as that of the Grenfell mission, was appealing to generations of medical professionals.

However, sport was also an important part of governance and imperialism, a "form of social capital" that elites attempted to deploy within the areas they ruled.[2] Sport encouraged a sense of civic community and "inculcated notions of fair play and social peace,"[3] but in a time of imperial expansion sport also provided a means of engaging and assimilating subject peoples and reinforcing patriarchy.[4] While aspects of this strategy were evident where the Grenfell mission maintained a presence, it is misleading to argue that sport in Newfoundland, the Northern Peninsula, and Labrador was nothing more than an affirmation of an "elitist, masculinist account of power and social relations."[5] Sport here could be defined from below as well as above, and informal sports and games were played by people of all ages, played often, and often played without the direct intervention of the Grenfell mission. No matter how busy people were with the business of fishing and surviving, it seems, there was always time for play.

Defining sport in an area that was largely rural, scattered, and without codified sports can be difficult, but the near-total absence of organized sport within the territory of the Grenfell mission does not indicate a lack of sport or interest in sports. To limit our definition of sport to leagues, codified rules, and dedicated infrastructure is to dismiss older and predominantly rural forms of sport and physical activity. In communities that depended on the land and the sea for survival, demonstrations of bravery and physical prowess were highly prized. Dog-team races, snow-shoe races, rifle competitions, and even sack races provided a chance for participants to show off these skills in front of the community. The more formal and theoretical attitudes towards sport brought by Grenfell and his medical staff thus existed alongside much older and distinctly rural forms of sport. In addition, informal and impromptu versions of team sports such as rugby, soccer, and baseball were played by people of all ages in outport[6] communities, and not just children.

These were the games of the rural poor, but there was also sport for the urban rich. Encouraged by the Newfoundland government and the Grenfell mission, the rivers, bogs, and mountains of northern New-foundland and Labrador attracted the attention of "sportsmen" from the United States and Europe. These affluent anglers and hunters bought licences, used the railway and steamer services, lodged in hotels, and hired local boats, crews, and guides to win trophies beyond the pale of civilization. However, their arrival in ever increasing numbers forced Indigenous and settler subsistence hunters off the land and di-minished caribou populations that were an important source of food and material.

The variety of games and sports that can be found on the Northern Peninsula and Labrador during this period reflects a region best de-scribed as a "borderland." This does not mean that the region was peripheral in any way, but rather a "contact zone" or meeting place be-tween many peoples, nations, and other organizations and forms of au-thority. Borderlands history – first articulated in the early twentieth century by American historian Herbert Bolton – emerged specifically to better understand European (and American) expansion across North America. Where Bolton's mentor, Frederick Jackson Turner, believed that American democracy was forged in a vast, dualist confrontation between European "civilization" and native "savagery" on the western frontier, Bolton argued for a more nuanced approach involving many contact zones and many empires and peoples, "all of them important for the American nation."[7] The borderlands theory has lost none of its strength in the following century and continues to be applied by scholars to regions around the world, including the west coast of Newfoundland[8] and sport in the mining villages of Wales and Cape Breton.[9] The history of the Grenfell mission, with its Indigenous and settler communities, international (and especially American) medical staff, and imperial connections to the United Kingdom and Canada, is ideally suited to borderlands history and the study of sport on the Northern Peninsula and Labrador. As one Labrador magazine noted, the "games and other amusements of these people ... have been influenced by explorers, traders, missionaries, teachers, International Grenfell Association people and others."[10]

This chapter is organized into four increasingly specific levels of analysis. At the most general level, it examines sport and physical activity in the context of industrialization and the growing popularity of muscular Christianity in Britain and North America. The second level looks at organized sport in Britain and North America before moving onto the British colony of Newfoundland and the dominion's Northern Peninsula and Labrador coast. A fourth section briefly examines the history of sport fishing and hunting and its impact on local subsistence communities. While sport here was never an explicit part of the "colonial project" as it was elsewhere in the British Empire, we will see that the promotion of games and competition, and the celebration of athletic accomplishment, was nevertheless a feature of the Grenfell mission's operations and identity. The variety of games played in St Anthony and other communities attests to both the cosmopolitan nature of the mission (and the borderlands position of the colony of Newfoundland more broadly) and the importance of sport to the mission's staff.

SPORT AT THE TURN OF THE CENTURY: WHAT WAS IT AND WHO PLAYED IT?

Today we are perhaps more likely to interact with sport as observers than participants. Allegiances to team and nation, rather than positions played or styles practised, define our sport identities. Organized sport is a major entertainment business, and many of its most powerful brands – Montreal Canadiens, New York Yankees, Manchester United, Barclays Premier League, Superbowl, Wembley, Olympics – are universal. The real money in modern sport is reaped not at the gate but in merchandise, sponsorship, and broadcasting rights, and even spin-off industries such as real estate and construction. This hyper-commercialized world of sports first became recognizable after the Second World War, but it had its roots in the mid-nineteenth century.

The military, industrial, and scientific upheavals of the nineteenth century completely transformed the idea and practice of sport. Unsurprisingly, it has been impossible for historians to agree on what factors were most important in the formation of modern sport, and indeed what "sport" is now supposed to be. Some "distinguish sport from recreation, and focus their attention on formal, organized activities involving sports clubs and associations," while others take "a rather more inclusive view, arguing that any game, contest, or competitive leisure pursuit that involves physical activity ought to be designated a sport."[11]

Considering the rural nature of the Grenfell mission, the popularity of games of skill such as dog-team races and rifle shooting, the rich variety of children's games, the presence of visiting "sportsmen," and the amateur competitions organized by members of the mission staff, I will take the more inclusive view: *games, play,* and *exercise* are interchangeable with *sport* in this chapter. It is important to note, however, that while I would like to expand this chapter's scope beyond members of the local "elite" – the medical personnel and administrators of the Grenfell mission – and examine the sporting practices of European and Indigenous communities serviced by the mission, surviving accounts of sport and play in the rural north are largely those of mission employees and visitors. Nevertheless, in photographs, medical records, oral history projects, and community memoirs we can gain tantalizing glimpses into the sporting lives of settler and Indigenous communities, however incomplete those records may be.

THE GAME OF OUR LIVES: MUSCULAR CHRISTIANITY AND IMPERIAL EXPANSION

George Perkins Marsh, one of America's earliest conservationists, spent the mid-nineteenth century campaigning for the preservation of his country's eastern rivers, which were threatened by the effluent of urban industry. Marsh's concerns, however, were not driven by a desire to pre-serve the natural world, but to maintain an important training ground for America's future leaders. For Marsh, British imperialism owed its success to the training its officers acquired through hunting and fishing, and he feared that Americans were becoming "a more effeminate, and less bold and spirited" people.[12]

Despite Marsh's praise, however, many elites in the United Kingdom were not so certain about the health of the British race and its empire, but they would have agreed with Marsh's conviction that exercise and fresh air were fundamentally important to the preservation of both. Concerns about the relative decline of the British Empire coincided with a resurgence in church attendance, advances in the science and profes-sional standing of medicine, and the emergence of organized sport at both an elite and proletarian level. It was in this context that "muscular Christianity" emerged, and its leading proponents – England's Charles Kingsley, Canada's Ralph Connor, and American President Theodore Roosevelt – wished to "get religion out of the pale of the chapel into the fresh air of heaven."[13] For these men worship was more than kneel-ing in subservience to the Lord; their version of Christianity "symbolized God in *action*."[14]

Modern medicine, with its consensus belief that "physical health was linked with mental, moral and spiritual improvement,"[15] was par-ticularly important to the nineteenth-century ascent of both sport and muscular Christianity. As early as 1880 "mainstream medical and car-diological thought saw vigorous, manly exercise as entirely appropriate for vigorous, manly men."[16] This consensus, naturally, was wholly agreeable to proponents of muscular Christianity, and it is little wonder that so many of their number embraced sport and medicine as equal partners in religious propagation.

Industrialization and renewed imperial expansion in the United States and Canada (Central America and the Pacific in the case of the former, the western prairies in the latter) made North America equally welcom-ing of muscular Christianity. Roosevelt became a powerful advocate of federal intervention in sports programs across the country,[17] seeing ath-letics and missionary work "as symbiotic with a nation poised to con-quer."[18] For those frustrated with city life and affluent enough to escape it, missionary opportunities beckoned on the freshly seized frontiers of Hawaii and the Philippines, and (for a few) the forgotten British outpost of Newfoundland and Labrador. There was one blight on this new era of imperial expansion, however, for while Roosevelt's vision of an Anglo-Saxon empire was a male one, a disproportionate number of missionaries were women (60 per cent in 1893).[19] This was troubling for men like Roosevelt and Grenfell, the latter writing that "cutting out a Kingdom for Jesus" was a "tough job … a man's job."[20]

SPORT AND GAMES IN BRITAIN AND NORTH AMERICA

For muscular Christians, sport was a decidedly amateur pursuit. As the purpose of sport was to inculcate teamwork, loyalty, and determination, it was considered selfish and unbecoming of an athlete to play professionally, that is, for money. Whatever money happened to be accrued in the pursuit of sport was customarily donated to a charitable cause. But sport was not the preserve of European and North American elites, of men who could afford to play games for free. For athletes from proletarian backgrounds sport (and especially Association football and baseball) offered a rare means of escape from a life in heavy industry, but it could be pursued only if the game provided a wage. Fortunately for working-class athletes there was a huge appetite for Association football (hereafter soccer) and baseball in industrial Britain and America. Changes in technology and improvements in literacy also facilitated the popularization of organized sport. Electric lighting brought nighttime matches, urban railways and new construction techniques resulted in larger stadiums, and the combination of newspapers and mass literacy created an appetite for continuous media coverage.

This was a time of strong institutional affiliations, and in the United Kingdom allegiance to a soccer club was a mark of working-class identity. Sport, together with the nonconformist church, the trade union, and the Labour Party, constituted the pillars of (male) working-class life. For many a labour militant, one historian wrote, "Jesus Christ, Keir Hardie and Huddersfield United went together."[21] The growing importance of sport, and especially soccer, to working-class life is illustrated by a growing investment in sport medicine. Healthy players ensured a healthy gate, and by 1900 one Manchester institution was known as the "footballer's hospital" for the high number of injured players it cared for.[22] For the footballers admitted there, almost all of whom were from (skilled) working-class backgrounds, the hospital offered the best medical care they were likely to experience, and certainly better than that available to their peers in the terraces.[23]

In North America, baseball and ice hockey were similarly popular among working-class fans, although these sports also attracted a large middle-class following and sometimes enjoyed the patronage of elites (for example, Lord Stanley of Preston's donation of the Stanley Cup). Baseball became a truly national game in the United States during the Civil War, the humble Union soldier being its agent of dissemination. Like the United States, Canada developed its own sporting culture separate from the United Kingdom and the other white dominions. Canadian universities emulated the Ivy League in their adoption of American football as a respectable varsity game, but climate was the most distinguishing factor in the development of Canadian sport, and ice hockey was both practical and accessible to all classes and regions of the country, rural and urban.[24] To an even greater extent than Australia, South Africa, and New Zealand, sport in Canada became a way of forming an "independent – white – identity apart from Britain."[25]

In Britain, Canada, and the United States, women were also becoming increasingly involved in sport. While historian of sport Colin Howell argued that "the veneration of the 'manly' athlete left little ideological space for women to demand an equal place in competitive sport,"[26] there were notable exceptions. In early twentieth-century Britain, for example, women's soccer clubs enjoyed rising popularity, regularly attracting crowds of several thousand.[27] Sport also became an important part of the suffrage movement. Many suffragists "recognized that women's right to play was essential and inextricable from citizenship,"[28] and Susan B. Anthony rejected claims of physical inferiority by pointing out that women were not given a chance to prove themselves in athletics: "We cannot say what the woman might be physically, if the girl were allowed all the freedom of the boy, in romping, swimming, climbing, playing ball."[29]

SPORT AND GAMES IN NEWFOUNDLAND
AND THE GRENFELL MISSION

Despite being a thinly populated territory with only a handful of minor towns and an almost total absence of modern industry, Newfoundland was home to one of the first organized soccer leagues in the world.[30] Formed in 1896, ten years after a league was organized in England and two years before another one appeared in Italy, the St John's–based Newfoundland Football Association (NFA) routinely drew three to four thousand spectators from a city of thirty thousand people.[31] While the game's emergence was facilitated by visiting British warships whose crews issued challenges in the city's newspapers,[32] it was engineers and stone masons from Scotland and England who organized the first permanent teams and competitions. Though initially popular, soccer in St John's briefly declined before being revived by the denominational colleges at the turn of the century.[33] True to the spirit of amateur athleticism, the NFA hosted an annual Chaplin Charity Cup for the benefit of the city's three major orphanages.[34]

Impressive as it was, soccer was not the only game in town. Ice hockey, according to an entry in *The Book of Newfoundland*, was introduced "by Canadians who were employed here with the various banks and the Reid Newfoundland [railway] Company."[35] The first recorded game (although certainly not the "first" game) was played on Quidi Vidi Lake in St John's in February 1896 – the same year that the NFA was formed – with Dr Wilfred Grenfell playing alongside a number of other members of the colonial establishment. Two years later, in 1898, the Newfoundland Hockey Association (NHA) was formed in St John's, and the Reid family of Montreal supplied land on the site of their company's old railway terminus at Fort William (destroyed by fire) for the construction of a purpose-built arena in 1899.[36] In 1904 the young league was crowned with a beautifully crafted trophy donated by the governor of Newfoundland, Sir Cavendish Boyle. Although intended for use in an international competition between Newfoundland and Canada, the "strikingly magnificent"[37] Boyle Cup soon became a strictly local honour, and, after the Herder Cup, the most famous trophy in Newfoundland sport history.

Baseball was also popular in St John's from the earliest years of the twentieth century. While scratch games were played on the city's Parade Grounds (near the present Royal Newfoundland Constabulary headquarters) as early as 1901, it was not until 1913 that a dedicated league was organized. In February of that year the American manager of the Imperial Tobacco Company, J.O. Hawvermale, established the St John's Baseball League,[38] and teams with colourful names such as Cubs, Red Lions, Wanderers, and Shamrocks attracted loyal followings. The game was popular enough to survive the manpower drain of the First World War and was refined (like soccer before it) by visiting warships, this time American, whose crews "did much through a series of games arranged with city nines to popularize baseball locally."[39] As new single-industry towns grew alongside the colony's trans-insular railway baseball expanded outside of St John's, and for many years the Grand Falls–St John's inter-town baseball tournament captured the imagination of both cities.

Sport, as it was played in St John's and company towns along the railway, reflects the strong historical influence of Britain, Canada, and the United States on Newfoundland's cultural and economic development. With few exceptions, however, such as soccer on the Burin Peninsula and baseball in Grand Falls, organized sport hardly existed outside of St John's, even in communities very near to the city such as Bell Island, Conception Bay. One visitor's observations of that mining town are worth quoting in full, as they summarize the convictions of muscular Christians about sport and exercise, as well as their consternation upon finding an absence of it: "Sports and pastimes are unfortunately not in evidence at all [on Bell Island], despite the fact that there are some splendid sites, which with little trouble and expense, could be converted into admirable recreation grounds. Football, cricket, and other such sports should be at once organized, as they not only develop the muscle in its purely natural shape, but conduce to the cultured development of the intellectual faculties."[40] However, the absence of any kind of organized sport recognizable to this author does not indicate that sport and games were not played. While the largely rural demographics of Newfoundland and Labrador delayed the development of organized sport, they also preserved an eclectic array of traditional European and Indigenous games as well as informal versions of hockey, baseball, soccer, and rugby that barely adhered to any set of rules.

In Canada and the United States rural sport was giving way "to the more organized sports of the emerging cities and towns,"[41] but in Newfoundland and Labrador – where St John's was the only town with a population above 15,000 – "earlier sporting traditions tied to rural or village life" remained popular.[42] Some sports, such as marksmanship competition and dog-sled races, were played in rural communities across Canada. Other games, however, were unique to Newfoundland and shaped by its particular climate and geography. These games were especially evident on the island's Northern Peninsula and mainland Labrador, but they were by no means untouched by distant influences.

When we think of sport in connection with the Grenfell mission today – if we think of anything at all – it is perhaps an image of Grenfell, either adrift on an ice pan wearing only his public school rugby kit[43] or leaping over the side of his vessel in pursuit of a wayward cricket ball (figure 5.1). For those familiar with Grenfell's British colleague Dr Arthur Wakefield, the even more absurd image of the "Cambridge man" and "noted athlete" leaping from icebergs or diving in swimming pools "where he has to break the ice" may come to mind.[44] While these may be self-promoting tales, they reflect the important connection between sport and imperialism. While there were no soldiers, merchants, or railway engineers – the traditional agents of imperial sport – on the Northern Peninsula or Labrador, there was an abundance of medical professionals from Britain and the United States, and these men made their own attempts to impart (if not impose) athletic values.

Grenfell's presence at the "first" hockey game played in Newfoundland is not incidental. Educated at Marlborough, where "all athletics were compulsory," "Wilf" was the quintessential public school boy and muscular Christian.[45] Grenfell read "old boys" accounts in the Marlborough student newspaper that "endorsed the arduous but satisfying life to be encountered overseas," developing "a connection between the stamina and physical courage developed on English playing fields and the qualities required for pioneering success in Canada, soldiering in Burma, and baptizing in Melanesia."[46]

For Grenfell and Wakefield, demonstrations of athleticism and bravery reaffirmed their worthiness for work and life on the frontier, but for these men and others like them the entire ethos of serving on the margins of empire was itself part of a single, grand game. This attitude is illustrated in the 1931 book *Men of the Last Frontier* by the British trapper Archibald Belaney, who wrote that while his way of life was passing, "on the outskirts of the Empire this gallant little band of men still carries on the game that is almost played."[47] Given the physical and symbolic value of sport , it is natural that Grenfell, Wakefield, John Grieve, and other mission heads would want to share their enthusiasm for games with the local population.

Around 1910 Wakefield established an apparently short-lived Arctic Swimming Club "for the benefit of the fishermen, hardy in every other respect, but frequently drowned because of a natural antipathy to water."[48] In the winter Grieve "organized the same men into football teams, and they play soccer on the ice"[49] (winter was the only time a level playing surface was available, "flat" land being reserved for agriculture), while another mission employee, Agnes E. Hamilton, brought together "two stalwart teams" from Groswater Bay and Sandwich Bay in a "Labrador Public School football cup," a best out of three competition played on ice and refereed by Dr Paddon and his wooden whistle.[50]

Dr Wakefield also established a local branch of the Legion of Frontiersmen, a paramilitary organization found throughout the British Empire and self-styled as its most rugged arm. Founded in 1905 by Roger Pocock, the legion had as its president Lord Lonsdale, "the highly popular 'sporting Earl'"[51] – boxer, jockey, racehorse owner, chairman of Arsenal Football Club. As the choice of Lonsdale suggests, the legion prized physical fitness, even if formal training was irregular. Pocock fancied that his Legionnaires, because of their hardy frontier upbringing, would be misfits in the regular British Army but superb recruits for independent work such as scouting.[52] Newfoundland boasted two units, one in St John's and the other in the "isolated community" of St Anthony.[53] Wakefield's levy, organized in 1911, included telegraphists, farmers, teachers, and fishermen, and "sham fights" and demonstrations of "assault at arms" were organized for Empire Days.[54] Wakefield wrote

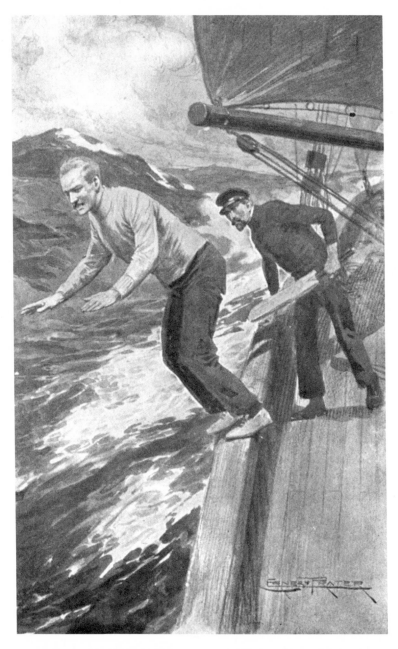

Figure 5.1 Grenfell pursues his cricket ball. Ernest Prater, "Frontispiece," in Basil Mathews, *Wilfred Grenfell: The Master Mariner: A Life of Adventure on the Land and Sea* (New York: George H. Doran, 1924)

in *ADSF* that "apart from its primary [military] object, and its secondary teaching of loyalty and imperialism," the legion is also "helping us to know and understand each other ... I have been deeply impressed by the earnest desire expressed by both Protestants and Roman Catholics that this movement may be the bond of union."[55]

No doubt Wakefield recognized (or thought he recognized) military potential in the marksmanship of his rural recruits, skills that were put on display during the mission's "most serious program of cultural intervention," annual Winter Sports Day.[56] Instituted by Grenfell "as a day when the people from all parts of this coast gather together – the men in particular – to demonstrate their ability in competitive athletics,"[57] Sports Day was the mission's most successful and enduring athletic effort. Held in mid-March, Sports Day featured games of skill that were often associated with work and survival in the country and on the ocean, and the competitions would have been recognizable to rural peoples across much of North America. Marksmanship competitions ("Naturally, these men are very good marksmen"),[58] dog-sled racing and snowshoe runs are obvious examples, but even such games as the two-mile race and the three-legged race showcased essential skills like endurance and balance (important in a trap skiff on a rough day) (figure 5.2).

Shooting was the first event and was, "as in other years, very popular."[59] On at least one occasion it was decided that two competitions should be held instead of one, a contest for rifles and another for the "old-fashioned muzzle loader, with its barrel about six-feet long, [which] has for some time held sway in this part of the world."[60] "The grand event,"[61] however, was the dog-sled race, sometimes featuring up to seventy-five teams, "the very barking and howling" of which "was enough to make one feel that a bedlam was let loose."[62] The "good and bad qualities of various dog drivers and their teams were discussed by the mission and harbour folks for many days prior to the event," one visitor noted, and "after the drivers were given instructions as to the conditions and length of the race – three times round the harbour – the signal 'go' was given" (figure 5.3).

In 1921 there was also the "very novel event" of a "ladies' dog race," introduced at the request "of several ladies of the staff."[63] Unfortunately,

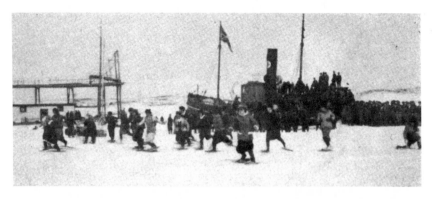

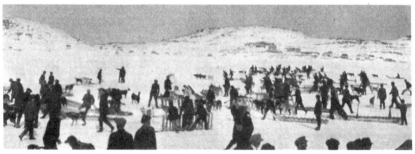

Figure 5.2 *Top* Ladies' Racquet Race, St Anthony, 1925. Note the hospital ship *Strathcona II* and the prominent Union Jack. Ilsley Zecher, "Annual Sports on the Ice in St Anthony," *ADSF* 23 (October 1925): 121

Figure 5.3 *Bottom* Lining up for the dog race, St Anthony, 1925. Ilsley Zecher, "Annual Sports on the Ice in St. Anthony," *ADSF* 23 (October 1925): 122

the race was not taken as seriously as the men's event, with "many a good laugh" being had by the onlookers.[64]

Sports Day was also hosted by mission stations such as the one at Harrington Harbour, Quebec. In 1927 a Harrington staff member wrote that there were "several dog-team entries" and "about 35 men took part in running, racquette, broad and high jump, sack and obstacle races," and even a greased pole competition (the pole, of course, being a schooner's mast).[65] "Besides bringing to Harrington considerable trade," the staff member wrote, "Sports' Day has taught the people something besides work and has given them an incentive such as bigger places in the outside world provide with annual tournaments and exhibitions."[66]

The benefits of trade and wholesome, worldly incentives represented the view from the top, but for most participants Sports Day meant other things: a rare reprieve from the hardships of winter and its seasonal work; an opportunity to meet friends and family from other communities; a chance to take on mission staff as equals on the harbour ice. Indeed, sport acted as a leveller between local resident-patients and medical professionals, providing an opportunity for locals to pit their native talents against mission staffers who were willing to participate, and perhaps have a laugh at their expense (which surely happened after Dr Hayden ran "head first" into a bush during a ski race).[67] As the excitement and discussions generated by the dog races suggests, Sports Day may have also furnished staff and locals with a topic of conversation that was accessible to everyone.

Sports Day, however, was not the only opportunity for sport and games, and the absence of other organized sports does not mean that team sports were not played. Baseball, soccer, and ice hockey (or variations of it) were played in many communities and throughout the year. Baseball was played (and perhaps introduced) by mission staff recruited from the medical schools of the northeastern United States, and ballgames were sometimes organized in St Anthony for special occasions such as Independence Day[68] (how many places hosted both Independence Day and Empire Day celebrations?). Grenfell was introduced to the game while touring the United States in 1905, writing in ADSF that while "it might seem frivolous in a Mission Magazine to be interested in these sorts of things ... One cannot but realize that they form a very large part of the life of the young men of America, and possibly their characters are altered as much by the games of the nation as any other individual influence."[69] Much later, in 1927, Grenfell would receive a donation and signed baseball from Cy Williams and the Philadelphia Phillies (which Grenfell mistakenly called the Nationals, the city's short-lived soccer team).[70]

While donations of baseballs, bats, and gloves were sometimes received from New England,[71] the game as it was played in the fishing villages probably bore little resemblance to that enjoyed by the mission's American staff. A visitor to Labrador's Spotted Islands, for example, observed that in a place lacking enough flat space "for even the infield of a baseball diamond," a stripped down version involving little more than batting and catching was popular.[72] Rather than baseball, our visitor may have observed a game of rounders, an English variation that was popular throughout Labrador and in Inuit communities in particular (see below).

Like rounders, soccer and rugby were particularly popular, perhaps because they lent themselves well to improvisation and frozen harbour surfaces. In the late nineteenth and early twentieth centuries, both soccer and rugby were referred to as "football," and in written records it is almost impossible to discern which sport is being played unless specified as "soccer" or "rugby."[73] However, both belong to the same family of games, and both could be played almost anywhere, in many kinds of conditions, and with only a single piece of equipment. In 1901 Grenfell received six soccer balls from Mostyn House School and distributed them along the Labrador coast, while he also attempted to instruct students in "the orthodox rules of Association football."[74] However, balls could be easily constructed out of locally available materials, and in spite of Grenfell's efforts one resident of Happy Valley, Labrador, recalled that "there was no such thing as rules or regulations, it was just a matter of who got the most goals."[75] Indeed, the same visitor to the Spotted Islands quoted above observed a game that used a soccer ball but was certainly not soccer: "The game is not especially complicated. Each player endeavours to kick a soccer ball higher than his opponents and tries to prevent its touching the ground."[76]

The popularity of soccer and rugby – or variations of it – is reflected in surviving Grenfell mission medical records, with a number of patients admitted after sustaining injuries while playing "football." These patients range in age from five to forty-eight, but most were in their late teens or early twenties. Indeed, while it might be assumed that in a labour-intensive economy adults could spare little time for sport, men (if not women) were known to participate whenever possible: "The men used to have their games of football too," one resident recalled, "when there was enough of them around, when they wasn't all gone in the woods."[77] The records also show that the game was played throughout the mission's "catch-basin," from southern Labrador to White Bay at the lower end of the Northern Peninsula.[78]

Soccer was also popular among the crews of large steamers that worked the seal fishery off northern Newfoundland each spring. While the communities of the Northern Peninsula and Labrador were more dependent on a smaller subsistence seal fishery, the steamers often visited St Anthony while their operations depleted local access to the resource (a concern Grenfell was aware of and wrote about).[79] Often trapped in thick ice and unable to work, crews organized soccer matches using bags of hard "duff" (a pudding made of flour and molasses) for soccer balls and following rules they had learned in their own communities.[80] Complete with boundaries and goalposts, these sealers played a game that was surprisingly formal, although teams were constantly changed as a way to mitigate unnecessary competition and conflict, a major concern in the confined space of a steamer.[81]

Strangely, although hockey was fast becoming the most popular sport in Canada and was already being played in St John's, it did not seem to take root in northern Newfoundland and Labrador until after Confederation with Canada. Skating was an undoubtedly popular pastime, with residents using discarded komatik runners and bucksaw blades to construct their own skates, and sometimes receiving instruction from Grenfell staff members.[82] However, although a mission employee noted in 1913 that "for a while in the autumn there was good skating and ice hockey was in vogue,"[83] there is not enough evidence to suggest that hockey was widely played until the 1960s.[84] While it is worth noting that the Canadian military organized an inter-service league in Goose Bay during the Second World War,[85] and that American servicemen donated sticks and skates to the mission shortly after it,[86] the influence of military hockey at this time seems limited.

Unpredictable winter conditions perhaps hindered the spread of hockey; a river, pond, or harbour surface that was ideal for hockey in the fall could be buried under a foot or two of snow by February. However, the likeliest explanation for hockey's limited presence was its cost: then, as now, hockey required a set of specialized equipment that was not cheap or readily available. Accounts of life in other Newfoundland outports certainly support this view, with one former resident of Rock Harbour, Placentia Bay, recalling that the "prosperity brought on by two world wars combined with successful fishing seasons allowed several members of the community to buy skates. The number of teenagers who could afford skates during and after W.W. II reflects the change to a cash economy."[87]

The popularization of hockey in the outports was furthered by the widespread introduction of radios in the 1940s, allowing Newfoundlanders to tune into National Hockey League games – and Foster Hewitt broadcasts from Maple Leaf Gardens in particular – for the first time. On the west coast of Newfoundland and its Northern Peninsula, the exceptional clarity of radio broadcasts from the eastern seaboard of the United States popularized Boston Bruins hockey, and a strong Bruins following remains there today. The larger number of teachers that followed Confederation also facilitated hockey's spread, with many teachers bringing their own hockey experiences and skills to new communities, including those of the Northern Peninsula. Nevertheless, for much of the period under consideration here, hockey appears to have been a relatively insignificant pursuit.

Hockey, baseball, soccer, and rugby were not the only team games played, however, with one old European pursuit called "piddly" being exceptionally popular. Although it has faded from popular memory, piddly was once played by people of all ages and with teams varying in size from ten to twenty.[88] Described as "a cross between cricket and hurly," piddly required no specialized equipment and was played using only two upright stones (or pieces of ice) and two sticks, one of about thirty centimetres called a "cat" and another of sixty centimetres called a "snig."[89] The stones are placed about a foot apart with the cat placed across them, and then flicked outward with the snig, while opponents try to catch it. Like soccer, piddly was also popular among sealing crews trapped in the ice and was played in parts of Newfoundland and Labrador as late as the 1960s.[90]

Other vernacular games included "staving" and "copying." The former was similar to skiing, with barrel staves being used instead of wooden skis. "In an unbelievably short time," one physician wrote, "the boys acquire the art of maintaining their balance while whirling down steep slopes and hills."[91] Copying was another winter game played by children (and especially boys) all along the Northern coasts of Newfoundland and Labrador when Arctic ice hugged the shoreline. The pursuit simply involved leaping from one ice pan to another without falling in between, and the dexterity (and daring) required for both copying and staving made them useful pastimes for children expected to learn small boat seamanship and seal hunting.

Sport and play in the Indigenous communities of Labrador served a similar function.[92] As one interview subject recalled, games were "like exercises or stunts that were for building muscles, all the muscles in our bodies had to be in shape in order for us to do the work we had to do."[93] "Target games" – marksmanship competitions involving bows and harpoons – were especially popular and useful. Inuit boys were given small bows and harpoons and encouraged to practise on birds, floating pieces of wood, images of animals, or the skull of a hare.[94] Target games equipped children with essential survival skills, but, like musketry competitions, they also provided an opportunity for adult participants to demonstrate their abilities as hunters. Interestingly, the persistence of target games after the widespread introduction of firearms in Labrador "meant that these [traditional] hunting tools stayed in use as game equipment after they had been abandoned for their original use."[95]

European games were also adopted and modified by Indigenous communities, but most popular of all was rounders. Rounders required only two pieces of equipment – a bat and a ball – that could be procured from local materials. Although rubber balls were occasionally available from trading posts or as gifts from the school or church, balls constructed of partridge feathers wrapped in sealskin were far more common.[96] The sport, widely played throughout Inuit territory, offered opportunities for communities to connect with one another as well as a means of asserting autonomy. In Hebron, for example, residents defied curfew by playing the game in complete silence, while communities well versed in rounders later organized softball teams to compete in Goose Bay, site of a massive Canadian military airport.[97] In inter-community games, rules were set by the host community, and "both young and old, male and female" played together, "helping to build a sense of community as well as tying together many of the different communities at the various regional events."[98]

THE GENTLEMEN AND THE POACHERS: SPORT VERSUS SUBSISTENCE IN NEWFOUNDLAND AND LABRADOR

The sports and games described above were largely informal, improvised, and pursued for pleasure. Sport in Newfoundland and Labrador generated little money, and only a handful of operations managed to make a business from athletics. There was one notable exception, however, and its development reflects the many overlapping borders of the colony and the Grenfell mission. In sport fishing and hunting, usually of salmon and caribou, the colonial government, the Grenfell mission, and the Reid Newfoundland Company (owner of the railway and steamship lines) recognized a lucrative tourism industry that could generate much-needed revenue outside of the fishery and increase demand for an already unprofitable railway. "Sportsmen" from New England and Britain had the necessary wealth to travel great distances, buy licences, hire guides, vessels, and other equipment, and pursue fishing and hunting in remote locations. More importantly for a government hoping to unlock the resources of the island's interior and Labrador, sport tourism offered a way of attracting potential investors, as only those with access to substantial capital could afford to hunt for pleasure.[99] The promotion of sport hunting and fishing, however, put government and other advocates of the industry into conflict with Indigenous and settler communities who depended on salmon and caribou for food. In order to ensure the continued growth of the tourism sector, these groups had to be marginalized, by force of law if necessary.

In his contribution to D.W. Prowse's *Newfoundland Guidebook*, Grenfell – who is introduced by Prowse as "surgeon, master-mariner, author and athlete"[100] – promoted Labrador as a paradise for mountaineering, salmon and trout fishing, recreational sailing, and geese and duck hunting. Labrador is a land of "unfettered freedom" where a forty-ton schooner could be hired with four hands for $100 a week.[101] The sailors, Grenfell assures the reader, are all experienced fishermen who know every part of the Labrador coast except the inside waters of fjords, where they do not go after fish: "It is here that their local knowledge comes to an end," Grenfell wrote, "and the fun of exploring for oneself begins."[102]

The sportsmen to whom Grenfell appealed were aristocratic and industrial elites, men who could afford such capital-intensive equipment as schooners, and who prized sport fishing and hunting as symbols of their social position. Since Izaac Walton published *The Compleat Angler* in 1653, a manual that "redefined angling as an art, and as an expression of the classical virtues of patience, appreciation of nature, and contemplation,"[103] hunting and fishing developed a complex set of meanings and practices that emphasized colonial control and superiority over subsistence methods. In many parts of the Victorian British Empire, foreign species were introduced both as a "method by which claims were staked upon areas of land" and to provide suitable game for colonial elites to pursue.[104] While this process occurred in Newfoundland with the introduction of moose and rainbow trout, anglers and sport hunters were also attracted by native species of salmonid and caribou that were essential components of Newfoundland and Labrador's subsistence-based communities.

With the completion of its trans-insular railway and Cabot Strait ferry service in 1898, the Reid Newfoundland Company took the lead in promoting sport tourism, targeting rich Americans who "increasingly felt that their frontier had vanished, that no longer were there vast unconquered spaces in their own country left to explore."[105] Facilitated by the railway and ferry service, the number of sportsmen and tourists grew from 1,046 in 1903 to 4,072 in 1913,[106] but in addition to increasing demand for access to caribou herds and salmon rivers, the railway also dissected the caribou's primary migratory route between the Northern Peninsula and central Newfoundland.[107] Caribou were an especially important source of food and material for both settler and Mi'kmaq communities, but their displacement from the resource was enforced with a series of acts that banned traditional methods of killing, including open pits, dogs, and traps. Closed seasons were also introduced, while killing at water crossings was prohibited in 1902. The legislation effectively made shooting with a rifle "the only legal way of killing caribou," a method that was beyond the means of many subsistence hunters.[108] In the Northern Peninsula the combined effect of the railway on migratory patterns and the imposition of new regulations left residents with "little option but to kill them in the closed season."[109]

Like caribou hunting, the promotion of sport (salmon) fishing was also detrimental to local communities. Subsistence fishers used nets to catch salmon, a practice incompatible with sport fishers, who depended on the free movement of fish and abhorred the method's lack of skill. Nevertheless, "a barrel or two of salmon to the average settler meant a great deal toward's the winter's food supply,"[110] and many settlers considered river access a birthright. As with the caribou, however, the colonial government introduced increasingly restrictive measures to protect salmon stocks from local overfishing. In 1888 it closed the season for salmon and trout from 15 September to 1 December, and in 1902 banned the use of nets in all rivers. In Labrador, where there were no wardens hired to protect salmon rivers, D.W. Prowse suggested leasing the rivers outright to sportsmen: "It becomes a serious question whether it should not be advisable, in the real interest of this important industry, to lease these Labrador and northern rivers to sportsmen. Pay the few fishermen who now obtain only a few fish by spoiling the rivers as wardens and use the rents to police the streams efficiently."[111] While the government ultimately decided against the proposition, many rivers became private property in all but name. In Hawke's Bay on the Northern Peninsula, John T. Pratt of New York, a member of the Standard Oil Company, built an elaborate salmon fishing complex that included cabins, guides' apartments, cold storage facilities, and even a purpose-built yacht constructed in Lunenburg, Nova Scotia.[112]

By the 1920s Newfoundland's caribou population was under considerable stress, and it was hoped that moose, introduced to the island in July 1904, would sustain the big-game hunting industry.[113] Salmon fishing, however, remained viable, and by the end of the Second World War the Newfoundland government and the Grenfell mission began to note America's expanding middle class, which was swelled by the huge numbers of demobilizing military personnel. In a 1946 series called Northern Pastimes, published in *ADSF* with images supplied by the Newfoundland Government Information Bureau in New York City, the reader is told, "Many returning servicemen, stationed in Newfoundland and Labrador during the war, now testify to the pleasure of the fishing there and plan to return at the first possible date."[114] Labrador is promoted for its proximity to the United States and its affordability: fishing its rivers, the piece assures its readers, requires "comparatively simple and little equipment for an unbeatable holiday in the open."[115]

Although it is commonly assumed that the more formal, organized sports that emerged in the industrial cities of the nineteenth century spread out to the hinterlands and replaced rural forms of sport, the experience on the Northern Peninsula and Labrador shows that this was not always true, even with strong metropolitan connections to Montreal, Boston, Toronto, and the United Kingdom. Informal versions of modern sports such as soccer, rugby, and hockey were played alongside older rural games, some unique to Newfoundland and the Labrador coast, and others familiar to any remote part of North America. While codified (urban) sports and what might be called physical education classes (such as Wakefield's swimming lessons) were introduced at times by Grenfell mission staff, sport and play in the mission's sphere of influence was not a simple transference of urban and elite sporting practices and values to a rural setting. The hugely successful annual sports days, for example, owed their popularity to the mission's adoption of local games, even as they sought to cultivate the same public-school values upon which so many of them had been reared. These events also provided an opportunity for local residents to pit their skills and strengths against the mission staff in an equal contest, a rare break from the patient-expert hierarchy they normally experienced.

Although the Grenfell mission tried repeatedly to engage locals in physical activity and athletic competitions, not all forms of sport were open to participation by settler and Indigenous communities. Indeed, in sport hunting and fishing, legislation was passed to discourage or forbade local access to wild game for food. In a subsistence economy, salmon and caribou were vital resources, but the methods of capture were deemed unsportsmanlike and wantonly destructive. While local peoples were forced to resort to poaching, sport hunters' observance of the laws – laws passed to protect and accommodate their specific interests – were regarded favourably as evidence of "the true spirit of sportsmanship."[116] While Grenfell actively sought the development of a sport tourism industry, the effects of sport hunting were particularly severe for the peoples under his mission's medical care.

One might imagine that if sports and games were played at all in the "remote" settlements of the Northern Peninsula and Labrador, then they would be strongly influenced by the sporting preferences of Britain, the presiding sovereign power and homeland of Sir Wilfred Grenfell. But as this chapter has demonstrated, the territory occupied by the Grenfell mission, far from being a stagnant imperial backwater, was a vibrant borderland in which sport was shaped by European, North American, and settler and Indigenous attitudes and practices.

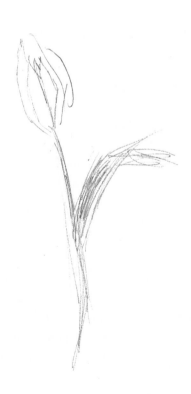

6

"Indiscriminate Bounty Makes for Pauperism": Producing Respectability through Clothing at the Grenfell Mission, 1890s–1920s

Emma Lang and Katherine Side

Clothing was a primary commodity for the Grenfell mission. Donations by member and affiliated organizations demonstrated their generosity and helpfulness, while conveying their care for people who were less fortunate than themselves. Donated clothing was distributed by Wilfred Grenfell, and by volunteers at the mission, in ways that were intended to uphold the respectability of its recipients. These ways also promoted the mission's central goals of industriousness, self-reliance, and thrift for recipients. Clothing was a visual symbol through which respectability was encoded for the inhabitants of northern Newfoundland and coastal Labrador, and through which their respectability was conveyed visually to the outside world – and in the pages of the mission's regular publications, in Grenfell's public lectures, and in photographs. In a literal sense, clothing constituted the fabric of the mission's dense networks of supporters, many of whom secured their place as benevolent benefactors through their donations.

Although clothing was central to the mission's goals and reputation, in historical accounts its role has often been eclipsed by the mission's provision of other services, notably medical care. In this chapter, we contextualize clothing and its donation first in a brief history of clothing relief, and in the import and small-scale manufacture through production in home industries in Newfoundland, to argue that clothing was integral in closing social and geographical distances between donors and recipients, as well as between the mission's northern locations and its supporters across North America, Great Britain, and Ireland. We document and analyze networks of clothing exchange and commodification in ways that attend to the special circumstances of history and place and that "respect the complexities and the inherited differences of the past."[1] We trace some of the connections from the late 1890s until the late 1920s to demonstrate the significant place that clothing occupied as a visible register of accessibility and respectability, and as a principal means through which the Grenfell mission enacted its own objectives and secured its public reputation.[2]

CLOTHING RELIEF

Clothing played a significant part in the mission, which included home-based industries (referred to by Grenfell as "fireside industries"), across northern Newfoundland and coastal Labrador.[3] Clothing exchanges existed as dedicated "clothing stores." The clothing department operated two permanent stores; one was at St Anthony, the midpoint between the winter homes of Newfoundland fishers and their summer fishing grounds, and the other at Battle Harbour, then a central activity for the seasonal Labrador fishery and trade on the Labrador coast.[4] Because of the suitability of the wharf, St Anthony was the central location for the receipt of all new, purpose-made, and second-hand clothing shipments, and the central depot from where clothing was distributed to other communities.[5] Clothing was also shipped to other mission premises at Cartwright, Flower's Cove, Forteau, Indian Harbour, St Lewis Bay, North West River, and Red Bay, and seasonally to Spotted Islands, and was carried aboard Grenfell's hospital ship, the ss *Strathcona*.[6] For example, a 1914 report on the activities of the *Strathcona* records, "Clothing to the value of $287.60 was given out this summer. Of this amount only $33.30 was wholly charity. The remainder was paid for in various ways – not in cash, but in industrial work, billets, hay, fish and labour."[7] All locations operated in the same way: new, purpose-made, and second-hand clothing was donated to the mission, which in turn exchanged it with those who needed it in return for material goods and/or labour.[8] Material goods exchanged for clothing included locally available items such as wood, fish, game birds, and berries. Local handicrafts included woodworking, and hand-hooked floor mats, which were especially encouraged as exchange items because they were sold through mission stores in the United States to generate further financial support for the mission.[9] Gendered labour could encompass roadwork, building and walkway maintenance, and services such as laundry, feeding livestock, and nursing assistance.[10]

This system of exchange was not specific to Grenfell's mission. Its origins can be traced to prominent ideas about clothing relief in England, which were also evident in the British colony of Newfoundland. Scholarly examinations of eighteenth- and nineteenth-century practices of clothing relief locate them in the UK Poor Law Amendment Act of 1834 and in processes of industrialization.[11] Prior to the Act, clothing relief for the poor and indigent was provided mainly by parishes. Vivienne Richmond argues that legal reform and industrialization shifted the prevailing charitable model of clothing relief towards an array of schemes, including sponsorship and subscription, to support those who were regarded as worthy, labouring recipients.[12] It also shifted clothing expectations for the poor towards sturdy attire that was suited to recipients' labour.[13] Richmond suggests that clothing societies "sought to promote good conduct, to check wastefulness and vice, and to restrict the types of clothing supplied."[14] She notes, "Clad in their practical garments, clothing society members were to be emblems of thrift, piety and industry, whose reward of better clothing for their exemplary conduct was to be an incentive to emulation among their peers."[15] Among mid-nineteenth-century evangelicals in England, clothing relief was also tied to religious piety, morality, and ideas about individual deservedness: "Evangelicals believed eternal salvation was available to all, but had to be earned through the constant avoidance of sin. For the poor this meant proving, again and again, that they were deserving of assistance, by being grateful and deferential, and adhering to good moral conduct and especially, by demonstrating their willingness to help themselves."[16]

Grenfell may have encountered these ideas, as he did evangelism, in his tent-site religious conversion in 1885, and during his travels with the Mission to Deep Sea Fishermen, with whom he made his first visits to Newfoundland coastal communities.[17] The provision of suitable clothing was an important aspect of this early work. From his earliest encounters, Grenfell's efforts were focused on clothing relief through exchange. In this way, biographer Ronald Rompkey's characterization of Grenfell as "a man of nineteenth-century sensibility who ... searched for a way of accommodating a nineteenth-century Christian belief to twentieth-century social change" is an apt description of the man and his efforts.[18]

Rachel Worth contends that the recent scholarly focus on clothing relief is viewed "principally, through the conduit of analyses of consumption."[19] In this case, recipients' consumption encompassed clothing, and also the moral values and religious doctrine that accompanied its exchange. Concerned that recipients recognized the importance of self-sufficiency along with their clothing, Grenfell oversaw the operation of clothing departments, which operated as their own department within the mission's structure. After 1923, it was managed by a permanent director, whose appointment expressed a preference for a background in business, and was staffed by volunteer workers.[20] The Clothing Department director reported its activities, usually briefly, in the pages of *Among the Deep Sea Fishers*, and at the Annual Meeting of the IGA Board of Directors.[21]

A magic lantern slide image shows people waiting outside the mission's clothing store in Battle Harbour and suggests their acceptance of the system of clothing exchange (figure 6.1).[22] Grenfell used images such as this one to illustrate his fundraising lectures and reinforce a need for continued clothing donations.[23] As elsewhere in Newfoundland, clothing was provided charitably only where need could be demonstrated convincingly.

CLOTHING RELIEF IN NEWFOUNDLAND AND LABRADOR

Clothing was a persistent concern in Newfoundland and Labrador because of the region's poverty and harsh climate. The provision of clothing was also shaped by prevailing concerns about the deservedness and morality of recipients. At the turn of the twentieth century, clothing needs in the region were met through small-scale home industry, merchants, and charitable organizations associated with moral reform.

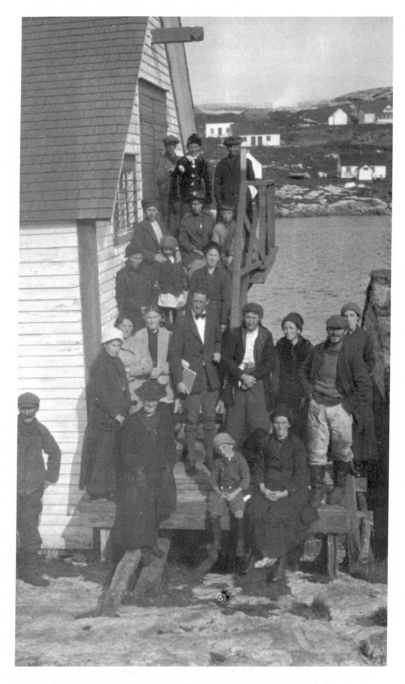

Figure 6.1 Crowd of people outside clothing store, Battle Harbour, n.d. PAD, IGA Photograph Collection, 1-226

In outport communities, families dependent on fishing acquired at least some of their clothing through the truck system as a local form of barter.[24] The extent to which households became and remained economically indebted to merchants, who extended credit to fishers in exchange for their catch, is contested.[25] For instance, Robert Sweeny's recent analysis of merchant records in Trinity, Newfoundland, demonstrates that individuals could and did opt out of this system, thereby "weakening community-based responses to merchants."[26] In his study of Battle Harbour, Sean Cadigan suggests that a majority of households "depended almost completely on fish merchants for provisions, clothing, household goods, and fishing equipment."[27] He contends, however, that not everyone was eligible to participate in the truck system, and that exclusion was exercised on the basis of moral judgments, citing two examples in 1930 of families denied credit by merchants Baine, Johnston and Company (hereafter Baine Johnston) in Battle Harbour.[28] Levi Spearing and Arch Rumbold were both denied merchant credit; the former was judged as "too lazy," and the latter was judged as unlikely to pay his debt because of his large family.[29]

A reference in the mission's quarterly, *Among the Deep Sea Fishers*, also notes that, on more than one occasion, Baine Johnston cooperated with the mission, by shipping mission goods to the Northern Peninsula and the Labrador coast aboard its ships.[30] In this way, Baine Johnston may also have used its cooperation to strengthen its own commercial interests. Through its cooperation, Baine Johnston could obtain knowledge about the goods that Grenfell could supply for those to whom they denied access. Later, allegations levelled by merchants about the mission's advantageous position in receiving and distributing clothing detrimentally affected its relationship with local merchants and resulted in a 1917 enquiry by Newfoundland's colonial government into the mission's activities and in particular, its clothing donations and exchange.[31]

Elsewhere in Newfoundland, including the city of St John's, the material needs of the poor were met primarily by charitable organizations and well-meaning reformers concerned with poverty, housing, and child welfare.[32] Led "by philanthropically minded members of the business and professional classes of St. John's,"[33] these organizations also shared

Grenfell's views about the importance of self-help and individual responsibility, as solutions to social problems, rather than an expanded role for the welfare state.

GRENFELL'S CLOTHING EXCHANGE

Clothing donations were solicited openly in several ways. Pleas for suitable clothing donations were made as a part of Grenfell's public lectures throughout Canada, the United States, and England, and through the organization's publication *Among the Deep Sea Fishers*. This request appeared on page two of its inaugural issue in 1903: "For some years past clothing and useful articles have been sent to Labrador in May for distribution. It is hoped that this year much help of this kind will be provided.... Clothing is the great need, especially clothing for men and boys. Dr Grenfell states that his stock is exhausted and that there is much need among the people. Garments need not be new, but they must be clean, in good repair (patches, of course, permissible), and suitable for the climate."[34]

Pleas for clothing donations were made consistently in an urgent but appreciative tone: "We trust that the friends of the Mission will bear in mind that we have a great need of warm, whole clothing, for men, women and children. It need not be new, but whole and clean, and if you will remember us while you are discarding a few of the winter things, and send to the office, 156 Fifth Avenue [New York], we shall be very glad to send them to most needy places. After so very cold a winter there will be much need of all sorts of clothing."[35]

The mission also printed selective requests for donations. The willingness of recipients to participate in the expected labour exchange was illustrated in their deferential language, as in this example from 1903 that reinforced need and worthiness:

To Dr Gransfield
Dear honrabel Sir,
I would wish to ask you Sir if you would be pleased to give me and my wife a little poor close [clothes]. I was going the Bay to cut

some wood. But I am all almost blind and cant Do much so if you
would spare me some Sir I should be very thankfull to you Sir.
Yours truley ——— [36]

The mission's statements of gratitude and appreciation reinforced the
importance of donors by emphasizing their roles in the system of exchange outside of charitable provision. By printing in its ADSF the quantity and dollar value of donations received, the mission encouraged subtle
comparisons and competition amongst its supporters over the quantity
and quality of donations.[37] Local branches of supporters across Canada
in Montreal, Toronto, and Ottawa, in the United States in offices based
in New York and Boston, and in Great Britain and Ireland in the London-
based office were involved in soliciting, collecting, and shipping donations of new, purpose-made, and second-hand clothing.[38] The collection
and distribution of donated second-hand clothing was the principal activity of the New England Grenfell Association's Boston-based office,
which encompassed four US states. New, purpose-made clothing was donated by at least two organizations: the Needlework Guild of America
and the Grenfell Juniors, an American youth organization.[39]

From their inception in nineteenth-century England, needlework
guilds specified the donation of "new wearing apparel or household
linen" and at least two items of clothing, one to be worn and another
to be washed.[40] Richmond suggests Needlework Guild members in England were "motivated by compassion and a general sense of duty or responsibility."[41] The provision of new, purpose-made clothing, she
argues, "gave purpose and meaning to the circumscribed lives of many
middle- and upper-class women," and "the transposition of their domestic skills to the wider community offered them participation and influence in the public sphere."[42] Likely it provided similar opportunities
for middle-class women who donated to the mission and the creation
of new garments made "good use" of their leisure time and demonstrated their concern for those whom they regarded as less fortunate.

The American-Labrador Branch of the Needlework Guild of America
began producing clothing specifically for the Grenfell mission in 1908.[43]
Although the branch's bylaws specified that no new clothing could be
sent outside the United States, they were amended to accommodate

Grenfell's plea for assistance.[44] In a single year, 1908, the American-Labrador Branch of the Needlework Guild of America provided the mission with 2,600 items of new, purpose-made clothing.[45] In addition to providing this apparel, needlework guilds also published and provided their members with patterns for embroidered and knitted apparel, perhaps to ensure that it suited the needs of recipients. Later, the mission would standardize some knitted donations by publishing knitting patterns in *ADSF*.[46] Some of this purpose-made clothing was evident at the mission. It provided mission residents with access to modern (and perhaps even fashionable) attire, and in this way connected them, despite their geographically remote location, to mainland Canada, the United States, and Great Britain.

In an image from a Grenfell album of 1912–14, four young girls at St Anthony sport large, matching, knitted tam-o'-shanters (figure 6.2).[47] Their modern hats are contrasted with their bare feet, which were not uncommon in images of children at the mission (and elsewhere in this period) and indicated the continuous need for children's footwear and the realities of its scarcity.

Targeted requests addressed the needs of a population for whom poverty was persistent. In addition to donations of new, purpose-made clothing, second-hand clothing was also welcomed. Donated clothing arrived at St Anthony in barrels, bales, and boxes.[48] Appeals were made for specific items including undergarments, woollen items, and sturdy work clothes, including overalls for men and aprons for women.[49] Durable items, such as flannel shirts and corduroy trousers for men and boys, and "stout shoes of all sizes," were particularly welcomed.[50] Sturdy, everyday clothes were desirable because they indicated active engagement in labour and emphasized the values of utility and thrift.

Clothing received at St Anthony was counted by volunteer workers, and the donor and value were recorded. Clothing was classified by type, and separate categories were maintained for men's clothing, women's clothing, boy's clothing, girl's clothing, infant's clothing, linens, and miscellaneous items. The value of each individual item was calculated by the clothing store director for the purposes of exchange. The ability to determine value permitted the mission to account for fluctuations in the availability and cost of clothing and in markets.[51] Clothing needs

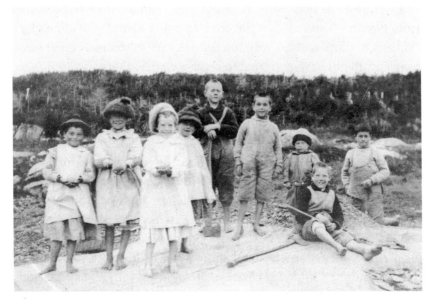

Figure 6.2 Children in tam-o'-shanters, [1914]. PAD, IGA Photograph Collection, VA 108-50.1

that could be met locally did not require the attention and resources of the colony's government. A clothing store inventory for 1924–25 provides some insight into value and exchange. New, purpose-made items were generally valued at half the purchase price in the colony's shops; second-hand items were valued according to their condition and suitability. All items were also valued according to the desirability of their material and its suitability for the climate and for labour. For instance, wool, corduroy, and flannel items were valued higher than were cotton and muslin items. A new men's woollen shirt was valued at $1.75; a second-hand woollen shirt was $0.75, which was also the same value assigned to a new cotton shirt.[52] Based on the 1924–25 inventory, the value assigned to a man's wardrobe comprising entirely new, purpose-made items was approximately $30; the purchase of the same items, second-hand, was approximately $13.[53] This difference made second-hand clothing items a necessity for many individuals and families. Bookkeeping records note the total value of clothing received in 1924–25 at

$24,841.38.[54] In that single calendar year, families received clothing from Grenfell's stores over the course of 913 visits, providing clear evidence of participation in Grenfell's system of exchange, even if some recipients might have preferred to receive clothes charitably.[55]

Clothing was shelved in the clothing store at St Anthony (figure 6.3) or was shipped along routes shared with passengers, merchant goods, and mail. A report of the Clothing Department to the IGA Board of Directors noted the laborious nature of this work: "The matter of collecting the clothing, forwarding it to St Anthony, inventorying it, pricing it, sorting it equitably for distribution, delivering it for the proper dates at the various stations and seeing that all rules are followed about its final delivery all involves great detail, infinite patience and the rigid application of the established rules."[56] Some clothing was designated specifically for use on the mission's hospital ship and in its hospitals and nursing stations and the Children's Home in St Anthony without expectations of exchange. Otherwise, clothing dispensed through the clothing stores was always exchanged; it was provided charitably only to widows, orphans, and in circumstances of "unavoidable sickness and poverty."[57]

Appeals for donated clothing reflected the historical context and pressing issues for the colony. For example, with the onset of the First World War, appeals for new, purpose-made and second-hand clothing were also accompanied by comments about the scarcity and increased cost of commodities. These increased costs resulted, in part, from conservation employed during the war, whereby manufacturers "reduced the varieties, sizes and colours of their production and even urged designers to create styles that would use less fabric and avoid needless decoration" and encouraged an economy of thrift centred upon mending, darning, and recycling.[58] The quality of knitted socks provided by the Women's Patriotic Association in Newfoundland had attracted attention among soldiers overseas. One supporter in Toronto who wrote to Grenfell hoped to "turn scores of these War Clubs into Labrador Knitting Clubs."[59]

There is little evidence of items associated with local customs of dress until later, when a 1943 knitting pattern for mittens specified trigger mittens. In the 1924–25 inventory of apparel, no distinction was drawn between knitted mittens and trigger mittens worn in Newfoundland

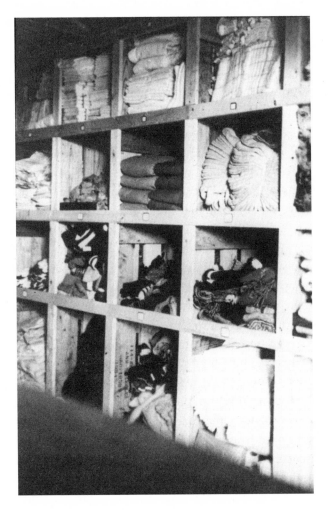

Figure 6.3 Clothing store, St Anthony, [before 1940?].
PAD, IGA Photograph Collection, 9-17

and Labrador.[60] Similarly, there is no distinction between knitted socks and locally produced vamps.[61] The endurance of these particular items into the present day was most likely the result of small-scale, home-based production that supplemented donated items available for exchange, and items available at retail shops, and were suited to local conditions and sustained local customs.

Donors were asked to send clothing that was suitable for the cold climate and/or labour. Garments were to be clean and in good repair,[62] and residents themselves asked clothing store staff for warm clothing, not thin items.[63] Writing later about New York-born, volunteer Barbara Mundy's staff position in the Battle Harbour clothing store, Anne Budgell echoes these preferences: "The clothing store staff actively discouraged donations of thin rayon socks, and sleeveless, legless summer underwear."[64] Outright criticism of donated items, however, was uncommon. Recognizing the inappropriateness of some items, volunteer staff repurposed them, adapting them to other uses: "Clothing staff found creative ways to use items that were unsuitable to wear. High heeled shoes … were cut into usable bits. 'Prize packs' might contain scraps for a quilt, or two felt hats, at least useful for stopping drafts around windows."[65] Sometimes unsuitable clothing donations were a source of entertainment: "A pink silk dress of ancient vintage was inclosed [sic], with a cap of corresponding material, and with a card attached indicating it was for the 'minister's wife.' Our minister at Battle [Harbour], a very recent arrival from the States, was quite unattached, so in order that the dress might serve the purpose for which it was intended one of the 'wops' arrayed himself in it and blushingly presented himself to the somewhat startled clergyman."[66] In telling this story, it is the unmarried status of the minister at Battle Harbour and the instance of parodistic cross-dressing that are the loci of humour, and not the inappropriateness of the gift provided by a well-meaning donor.

An individual's entitlement to clothing was indicated by a commercially printed slip that bore the name and logo of the National Mission to Deep Sea Fishermen, confirming the organization's early involvement in clothing exchange. Each slip was numbered, dated, and made out to the clothing store director. The slip included space to record the name of the recipient(s), an account number, and an amount. A perforated portion, with the slip number, date, recipient's name, account number, and dollar value was retained by the clothing store for bookkeeping. The bottom of the slip, in bold and underlined text states, "Notice – This order must be redeemed in six months, or be renewed."[67] This expiry date ensured that the mission was provided with continuous supplies of labour and the provision of services and local goods for mission staff and volunteer labourers, many of whom were unaccustomed to the local environment and its challenges.

Budgell notes that the clothing store in St Anthony, open on Tuesdays and Fridays, attracted "people [who] walked long distances from communities in the area," and "lines formed by 7:00 am and competition for certain things, like pants and shoes, was fierce."[68] The system of a non-cash exchange was, paradoxically, in opposition to the cash economy that Grenfell promoted through the establishment of co-operative stores as models of industrial capitalism throughout the region, including at Battle Harbour.[69] Grenfell introduced co-operative stores as an alternative to the truck system and offered shareholders better terms and facilitated bulk purchases through cash purchases.[70] (For discussion of Grenfell's co-operative stores, see chapters 1 and 4 in this volume.) The system of exchange for clothing, however, intentionally *excluded* cash purchases, except when accessed by mission staff and volunteers in situations of occasional need.[71] By enforcing strict oversight of the clothing exchange, the mission assured the availability of a continuous supply of labour and its gendered division.

Although Grenfell was forthright with volunteer workers, donors, and recipients about expectations of exchange, it still came as a surprise to some volunteers; Carolyn Galbraith was among them. From Springfield, Massachusetts, Galbraith spent one year, in 1926, as a mission volunteer in Forteau, Labrador. In a letter to her friend, Frances [Fran] Stilwell, Galbraith described the system of clothing exchange:

Families are almost entirely clothed by the Mission's second-hand cloths [*sic*]. We have what we call a "store." In it, a room over the shed, we have barrels of old cloths [*sic*] (coats, dresses, shoes, etc., etc.) and barrels of new-but-seconds in underwear and stockings and baby cloths [*sic*]. All of these things are gifts to the IGA. The people are never *given* anything except in very needy cases. They must work for everything. If a woman comes, asking for a dress and shoes for her little girl, we say "What can you give us for pay?" or, "What would you like to do to pay for them?"[72]

In another letter to the same friend, Galbraith details expected terms of exchange: "Perhaps she will say she can furnish us a trout once a week for a few weeks, or she may make a hooked rug for us, or wash our windows. In the way, we are kept supplies in fish, fresh birds – saltwater and partridges (we are having roast partridge this noon), cranberries, blueberries, rugs, hay for our cow, salt, caplins (fish) for the dogs' winter food and much window washing and scrubbing. Our washings are paid for in clothing."[73]

Galbraith's responsibilities at Forteau included sewing lessons for local girls as a part of the delivery of gender-appropriate, socially productive skills that enhanced girls' ability to provide for their own clothing needs. In a letter to Stilwell, Galbraith also notes the necessity of this task: "You can see that the cloths [sic] are decidedly misfits. I hope to teach the girls the making and adjusting of these otherwise very ugly and swashy-looking garments. Not a very pleasant task, but a helpful one I believe."[74] Observing that all of the ten or twelve children at Forteau were clothed by the mission store, Galbraith expressed her frustration with the lack of cloth available for sewing.[75] Local goods and labour could be exchanged at the clothing store for some supplies for home-based clothing production. In 1924–25, these items included new wool and "waste wool"; both were available by the pound.[76] Among the items recorded in the inventory of the St Anthony store were new wool, waste wool, blanket ends, waste flannel, bolts of denim, black cloth, khaki cloth, sewing needles, "common pins," thread, and buttons.[77]

Women in St Anthony, Newfoundland, and Battle Harbour and Forteau, Labrador, and women in the living rooms of middle-class homes in Boston, Ottawa, and London were connected through clothing. However, their motivations for participating in home production and the destination of garments they produced were quite different. Working women in Battle Harbour participated in home production in order to meet the subsistence needs of families; middle-class women, mostly located outside of Newfoundland and Labrador, participated in home production to further their philanthropic and reform efforts and to reproduce their abilities to determine the clothing needs of others. Clothing donated to the mission, by its supporters, also afforded some men, women, and girls at the mission with the ability to clothe families in styles that reflected the dress of staff and volunteer workers.

CLOTHING REGULATION FOR STAFF AND VOLUNTEERS

Clothing was also regulated for staff and volunteer workers, who were required to adhere to Grenfell's system of clothing exchange. A printed booklet issued to volunteers that addressed the system of exchange and the reasons for it states,

> For many years, the [International Grenfell] Association has followed the policy of giving away neither clothing or food except in rare cases of dire need; it is believed that among the people of the North as elsewhere *indiscriminate bounty makes for pauperism.* We ask that staff members do not take with them food or clothing beyond what they themselves need; that they pay cash for food or clothing they purchase; that, when they leave their stations, they turn in any food or clothing they do not wish to take back with them to the Association authorities.[78]

Staff members whose service extended beyond three years were provided with a modest clothing allowance, while volunteer workers were expected to provide their own clothing and to access the mission's clothing store only in extenuating circumstances.

Beyond this, staff members and volunteer workers were requested not to provide gifts of clothing. In at least one instance, disregard for this rule by a volunteer worker received attention from members of the IGA's Board of Management. In a report of the Clothing Department in the Minutes of the 1924 Board of Management meeting of IGA Directors, an unnamed volunteer teacher was identified as having violated the mission's clothing policy. Upon completing a summer term teaching at L'Anse au Loup, Labrador, she was said to have returned home, collected clothing, and sent it on to individuals in L'Anse au Loup without expectations of exchange.[79] Having since indicated her desire to return to teach, Board members questioned how far disciplinary actions should extend in this instance.[80] While their decision is not recorded in the minutes, discussion of this matter by IGA directors indicates the importance of this breach of mission policy.

Grenfell was also not above setting gendered guidelines on appropriate dress and behaviour for volunteers. The text in the booklet provided to volunteer workers identifies the people of Newfoundland and Labrador as "living in isolated places away from the changing fashions of the world" and notes, "These people are very conservative."[81] Gendered guidelines were intended to convey the respectability of the mission. For example, women staff and volunteers were explicitly instructed not to wear knickerbockers, and women were prohibited from smoking while travelling to and from mission locations.[82] Volunteer workers were also required to uphold the mission's policy of temperance, and while church attendance was encouraged, it was not mandated.

Staff and volunteers were likely distinguishable from mission residents by the quantity and quality of their attire. Trained staff were distinguished from other hospital workers by professional attire that included laboratory coats, nursing aprons, caps, and school pins. Volunteer workers were provided with clothing lists that emphasized suitability and practicality, and whose items were intended to prevent "actual physical discomfort" and discourage frivolity. Volunteer workers' ideas about suitability may have differed from residents' ideas.[83] For example, Jessie Luther's list notes that "one good house gown" is not to be confused with "an evening gown."

Clothing was also a means through which volunteers marked their social class connections, and in some instances, maintained volunteer workers' connections with similarly attired others. A letter from Galbraith to Stilwell thanks her for sending a tailored suit.[84] To her friend Evelyn Haviland in Northampton, Massachusetts, Galbraith wrote, "You have no idea how much I appreciate your leather coat," noting that it provides "a great comfort and convenience."[85] Volunteers' tailored suits, leather coats, and school sweaters likely distinguished them from local residents, and Millicent [Blake] Loder, a Labrador-born nurse who worked at the mission in this period, remarked on the difference in appearances between "outsiders" (mission staff and volunteers) and those who relied on the provision of mission clothing.[86] Perhaps unexpectedly, the mission also served as a source of social class difference. For example, in a letter to Lucy Clapp, Galbraith exclaims, "P.S. Miss

[Greta] Ferris has just purchased a beautiful silver fox fur for 100!!! Red foxes sell for $20 and up."[87] In these instances, travel to the mission facilitated volunteer workers' extravagant clothing purchases and perhaps also alerted others of the availability of furs.

PRODUCING RESPECTABILITY: CLOTHING RECIPIENTS, CLOTHING DONORS, AND THE MISSION

No historical records demonstrate that exchanged new, purpose-made, or second-hand clothing was denied to individuals on the basis of moral judgments or judgments about their character, as was the case among some merchants in Battle Harbour.[88] However, some individuals and families without access to goods and/or services to trade may not have participated in the mission's clothing exchange, used the truck system instead, or went without necessities. Respectability was a key concern for Grenfell, and his ideas about public respectability guided the clothing exchange, volunteers' dress codes, and expectations for their behaviour. Grenfell's ability to recruit and retain volunteer workers and to continue to receive donors' support depended heavily on the mission's favourable public reputation. (See Jennifer J. Connor's chapter 2 in this volume regarding Grenfell's efforts to convey a shared heritage and benefit among the mission's volunteer workers and recipients.)

Grenfell's system of exchange was made available, even to those who had unrealistic ideas about the value of clothing. "It [exchanging clothing] was hard work," he wrote, "and required considerable tact as some families were more needy than others and yet it was hard to draw distinctions, and it is not the policy of the Mission to appear in the light of a strictly charitable institution, except in a few extreme cases. For example, one woman came in with a slip for $10.80 to outfit for a family of eight for a year!"[89] Sometimes mission workers' assumptions were challenged by recipients' ingenuity and community resourcefulness: "One patient asked about some help in clothing for the winter. She looked so respectable it seemed hardly necessary till Dr [Cluny] McPherson recognized a dress belonging to the island. It had been lent to come to hospital in. An arrangement which we always think bespeaks those very qualities which one finds it a real privilege to be able to help."[90] In this case, respectability was understood and conveyed by members of the local community. Local residents wore their best clothing and even shared their clothing, because they wanted to appear worthy of the mission's assistance.

Grenfell staff maintained that recipients were offended by charitable provision. Maud (Alexander) Hopkins, in her role as director of the Clothing Store, exemplified the importance of individual dignity in recounting the story of a mother who chose "inside" clothing for her son, over the purchase of a hat she admired for herself:[91] "'But why didn't you give her the hat?' You just do not know our Newfoundland mothers. They are much like your own mother, and you cannot imagine her, though the family pocketbook was in desperate straits, expecting or accepting special affairs."[92]

Respectability was also important for those who lived in Newfoundland and Labrador and for its government, and Ronald Rompkey suggests there was an "ever-present nervousness" about customs privileges related to the mission's clothing donations.[93] When questioned, Grenfell invoked the Customs Act, 1924 as justification for his system of exchange: "As the Government allows his charity is free of taxation, none may be, or ever is, sold for cash. It must be given out for work, preferably freely if necessary."[94] However, local merchants' concerns about unfair competition led to a joint petition that was filed with the Colonial Government of Newfoundland in June 1917. These tensions were likely a culmination of growing distrust between the mission and merchants, arose from questions about the mission's bookkeeping practices, and were perhaps the legacy of the 1912 Karnopp scandal outlined by Heidi Coombs-Thorne in chapter 4 in this volume. Merchants asserted Grenfell had "greatly stimulated" American donors with tales of pauperism in Newfoundland, and that donors' generous clothing donations were a menace to "other mercantile concerns on that coast who have to pay duty and freight upon the material they use or vend in the prosecution of the fisheries there."[95]

The Squarey Enquiry was headed by Magistrate Richard T. Squarey. In chapter 1 in this volume, James Hiller discusses Squarey's appointment and his perceptions of the mission, which likely influenced the enquiry's findings. Squarey interrogated, among other things, the receipt and distribution of clothing in areas where the mission operated.[96] Members of the IGA's Board were also cognizant of local tension that extended beyond the findings of the enquiry. At their Annual Meeting in 1926, they addressed the issue, but stipulated that their discussion not appear in the minutes: "The Association appreciates deeply the donations of clothing, toys and so forth which are sent in by the multitude by friends. However, at times, it is greatly embarrassed by special requests to send packages or gifts to some individuals or some designated community because, under the privileges granted to the mission by the Government of Newfoundland of importing free of duty everything necessary for its work, it is not allowed to import gifts for individuals who are citizens of the country."[97]

Grenfell reportedly welcomed the Squarey Enquiry as an opportunity to clear the good name and reputation of the mission. However, others affiliated with the mission placed blame for strained relations on local officials. For example, in a confidential letter sent to Magistrate Squarey, a mission doctor who prefaced his remarks as a "man-to-man talk by one patriotic Briton to another," detailed local corruption and a lack of respectable behaviour among local officials.[98] By contrasting the morality and respectability of the mission's work and workers with less desirable influences around them, the work of the mission was upheld and its benefits to Newfoundland were highlighted.

Squarey's enquiry acknowledged "the free entry of clothing is a 'burning sore' and source of constant friction and bitterness between the [International Grenfell] Association and the businessmen of Newfoundland."[99] However, as Hiller noted, Squarey concluded that there was no evidence that Grenfell's mission exploited ideas about pauperism, or that its clothing operations competed unfairly with merchants' commercial interests. To resolve local tensions, Squarey recommended that duty be paid on imports, for which the government would provide an annual rebate, available for the amount collected, and that IGA staff and volunteers retain the right to import duty-free clothing for personal use. In this way, the Squarey Enquiry upheld the public respectability of mission staff and volunteers, and its recipients and donors.

Clothing exchanges were an early part of mission activities, including the Royal National Mission to Deep Sea Fishermen and the International Grenfell Association, and were pivotal for their operation and reputation. Through the materiality of clothing, its collection, and its exchange, the IGA's mission sought to build respectability for its recipients, for whom clothing served as tangible evidence of their industriousness, self-reliance, and productivity, and for its supporters, whose donations were evidence of caring and in some instances of their Christian faith. Clothing was also a mechanism through which Grenfell was able to extend his culture of productivity and aid. The products of this aid were made visible to donors through photographs, magic lantern slides, storytelling, public lectures, and publications. Donors were looked to for continuous support of the mission's operations and for the expansion, ideologically and geographically, of its influence. The Clothing Department and its system of exchange transcended any geographical locale and affected all of the mission's activities, including the IGA's Industrial Department, the schools and Children's Home, and nursing stations, hospitals, and hospital ship. It was also integrated, through the appointment of a director and the Clothing Department director's report, into the IGA's organization structure.[100]

Clothing constituted more than a superficial outer layer of the IGA's operations. The primary purpose of the clothing exchange was the "improvement in the social uplifting of the people" as British subjects.[101] The IGA directors' use of the term *uplift* to describe their work was an intentional effort to convey their benevolence, and to highlight the role of the mission in shaping local values that prioritized self-sufficiency, thrift, and respectability. As Jennifer Connor argues in chapter 2 in this volume, the expectations of mission staff were imbued with middle-class, Christian values. On the one hand, the provision of mission services, which included the clothing exchange, did not discriminate against individuals on the basis of religious denomination; on the other hand, this exchange relied centrally on ideas about morality for constructions of the worthy recipient. While the clothing exchange closed the gap in clothing needs between overseas donors and recipients, it also widened the gap between mission staff and local populations, the latter of whom depended on the mission to acquire suitable attire. The mission's emphasis on respectable behaviour and dress was intended to reflect positively on local residents, mission staff and volunteers, and the enterprise of the mission itself. Clothing provided a visible symbol of the mission's work, even as it made relatively few accommodations for the local customs, traditions, and dress among Newfoundland and Labrador's diverse populations.

American connections were central to the mission's clothing exchange. Community-based groups, mainly in the New England states, provided a generous and constant supply of new and second-hand clothing, much of which was shipped to St Anthony through the IGA's Boston and New York offices. American volunteers were well represented among clothing store workers, including as its successive directors. The continuous trail of new, purpose-made, and second-hand clothing and personnel closed the geographical distance between northern Newfoundland and coastal Labrador, mainly from the United States, but it also ensured the mission's reliance on American aid and influence in Newfoundland and Labrador.

7

Elizabeth Page and the White Bay Unit

Mark Graesser

In February 1921 Elizabeth Page received a letter from Ethel Gordon Muir confirming Page's appointment as a volunteer summer teacher with the Grenfell mission in Newfoundland. Page, thirty-one years of age, was unmarried, well educated, and living with her family in the affluent University Heights suburb of New York City. Muir, also single, was a sixty-four-year old professor of philosophy at Lake Erie College, Ohio. The two women played a significant role in fostering a dimension of mission work that has been mentioned rarely in Grenfell annals: the placement of volunteer teachers, mostly female and American, in tiny coastal settlements. This chapter highlights a phase of that work that took place in White Bay, Newfoundland, largely through Page's leadership, from 1921 to 1926. The "White Bay Unit" quickly evolved beyond summer teaching into a multi-dimensional program that we might now characterize as "community development" work. Although conducted under the umbrella of the IGA managers in New York and St Anthony, Page's operation was largely self-funded and was aimed explicitly at severing ties of dependency upon the charitable arm of the IGA by forging a link with the newly formed Newfoundland Outport Nursing and Industrial Association (NONIA).

ETHEL GORDON MUIR AND THE VOLUNTEER
SUMMER TEACHERS

Records are unclear about when volunteer summer teachers were first recruited by the Grenfell mission. Until around 1910, most staffing was associated with the St Anthony operation and permanent medical stations on the Labrador coast, with salaried doctors and nurses supplemented by volunteer medical personnel and untrained helpers. In 1909, however, Ethel Gordon Muir spent a summer at Red Bay, Labrador, conducting classes for a dozen children aged three to twelve years. She was accompanied to the coast by a friend who had taught in West St Modeste, Labrador, the previous summer. These two women may have been the first summer teachers; they were to be followed by dozens more over the following two decades, thanks in large part to Muir's promotional and organizing efforts. Muir herself spent twenty years of summer teaching in the settlements.

Muir was born in Halifax, Nova Scotia, in 1857, the daughter of a prosperous merchant.[1] The family heritage was Scottish and Presbyterian. After high school she taught for several years at the Cambridge House, "our aristocratic Halifax Boarding School." Apparently still living at home, she entered Dalhousie University, completing her BL and ML degrees in philosophy at the age of thirty-five. She went on to study for a PhD at the Sage School of Philosophy, Cornell University. Muir completed that degree in 1896 and in 1898 published her dissertation, "The Ethical System of Adam Smith."[2] A significant number of women's colleges in the United States were established before the turn of the twentieth century, and others, such as Briarcliff, were being founded at about this time. At the age of thirty-nine, Muir embarked upon a fully fledged academic career in a succession of these institutions: Mount Holyoke in Massachusetts, Pennsylvania College for Women in Pittsburgh, Briarcliff in Westchester County, New York, and finally Lake Erie College in Ohio. At Lake Erie she was professor of philosophy from 1919 until her retirement in 1937 at the age of eighty. She lived her final years near Halifax and died in 1940. Muir never married. This was not unusual for a woman of her background and achievements. A study of Dalhousie coeds between 1881 and 1921 found that at least 41 per cent did not marry, and many pursued higher degrees and academic careers.[3]

How did a fifty-two-year-old woman whose life to that point had apparently been led in the cloistered surroundings of academe choose to go "north" in 1909 to embed herself in a remote Labrador village, to conduct summer school classes? She offered this explanation:

> Before going to Red Bay last year I had often wondered at the great fascination that work on the Labrador coast seemed to possess for many people. I did not start with a very enthusiastic frame of mind. When my friends and family asked me, as they frequently did, "What in the world are you going for?" I replied somewhat lamely that my friend Miss Dwight, who had been teaching in West St Modeste the previous year, thought that there was important work in the way of teaching to be done on the coast, and that I wanted to try and do some of it.[4]

We must bear in mind that there was virtually no precedent for Grenfell workers to live and work away from one of the medical stations, dependent solely on the hospitality of the local community for accommodation, and upon their own resources for direction in defining and carrying out their duties.

Muir published two accounts of her Red Bay summer in *Among the Deep Sea Fishers.*[5] One of these articles had been an address to the American-Labrador Branch of the Needlework Guild of America, an established benefactor of the mission. She gave several other talks to church societies describing her summer and promoting the work of the mission. The story she told set a sort of pattern for the chronicles of the many other summer teachers to follow. She had been told (probably by Wilfred Grenfell) that she would be staying with the Pike family, who managed the co-operative store. This proved to be a satisfactory arrangement. The thirteen children in her charge gathered for daily school sessions in a "mission house" or parsonage, while a new school building was being constructed. Nothing more is said of the provision of regular schooling by the responsible Church of England authorities. However, for their ages she found the children generally wanting in academic attainment. As to her own contributions in that regard, "while I cannot truthfully describe their educational advance as proceeding by leaps and bounds, I am truly thankful that I have made their acquaintance, and many incidents in which they figure prominently are likely to remain a permanent part of my store of memories." Certain children who endeared themselves to her are mentioned, and she provides examples of distinctive local expressions and pronunciations. She had brought a supply of yarn and taught the older girls to knit socks. She conducted Sunday church services and a men's Bible class. Muir repeatedly compliments the people of Red Bay for their moral character and resilience as they coped with isolation, privation, and "the poorest fishery that the people have ever known." Outlining the needs of the people of Labrador to which volunteers might respond, Muir offered a modest list beyond the teaching and amateur preaching: supplying clothing and footwear to some of the poorest; bringing wool and teaching rudimentary knitting; assisting with medical problems, for which she readily acknowledged she was ill-equipped; and reading and writing letters for illiterate adults. She thoroughly enjoyed the experience, to her surprise, and readily acknowledged the rewards to herself: "One requires only to spend a few weeks among [the people of Red Bay] to realize to the full the fascination and the enjoyment of the work. Their simple lives, their unaffected kindliness and hospitality, their manly courage and earnest faith in God, seem to bring one in touch with the realities of life, and I do not think anyone can live among such a people without feeling that he has received from them far more than he can in any way have bestowed."

Muir returned to Red Bay in 1910 and over the next twenty years spent summers in other settlements. After a summer in Eddies Cove, on the Northern Peninsula, she wrote, "More and more I feel the great need there is for educational work among the people. As a means of elevating them and leading to a higher type of civilization, I do not think that this school yields in importance to any of the wonderful industries and enterprises that the Mission is carrying on the Labrador and in Newfoundland."[6] In April 1914 she made a focused appeal for teachers to meet requests from four coastal villages. "Schools are badly needed in all these places, and volunteer teachers will be warmly welcomed."

In the event, six volunteers, including herself, served that summer. In October, a note in the mission magazine invited interested readers to contact Miss Muir directly at Briarcliff Manor.

From 1915 to 1920 an average of eight teachers per year were posted. Table 7.1 presents a statistical and geographical overview of this dimension of the Grenfell mission project from 1908 to 1920. At least seventy-one volunteers were placed in thirty-nine settlements.[7] These communities were widely scattered along the coast of the Northern Peninsula, and on the Labrador coast as far north as Rigolet and even Turnavik (near Hopedale). There appears to be no geographical focus or pattern to the location of volunteers. Half the communities hosted just one volunteer; only five benefited from more than three visits. With the exception of several male students from the Columbia University Medical School and Amherst College, who from 1909 to 1914 taught school at Spotted Islands and the Horse Islands, all but two volunteers were female. All were unmarried, and unlike Ethel Muir, most were probably quite young. Their addresses were primarily in the northeastern United States, with a few coming from Canada, and one from St John's.

From 1916 onward, *Among the Deep Sea Fishers* published reports from the summer teachers under the heading "The Educational Department," and this category was used in the annual list of staff and volunteer workers. As of 1920, Ethel Muir was styled "Superintendent of the Education Department," a position paralleling the superintendents of the Children's Home and the Industrial Department. Unlike those officials, however, Muir remained a part-time volunteer and attended to recruiting and assigning volunteers from her base at Lake Erie College. The minutes of the IGA Board of Directors from 1914 to 1927 do not mention the summer teachers. Ethel Muir is mentioned just once, in 1916, when she was permitted to erect a cottage in St Anthony at her own expense, "provided she limit her activities by the direction of the Superintendent in connection with teachers."[8] (It is not known whether she actually built this house or used it; normally she spent her summers in one of the coastal villages, and the remainder of the year in Ohio.)

In 1920, fifteen female volunteer teachers were assigned to settlements along the coast, a number which may be compared with about thirty male college students placed in St Anthony and three other hospital sta-

Table 7.1
Grenfell mission summer teachers, 1908–1920

Labrador	Placements		Newfoundland	Placements
Bolster's Rock	1		Bellburns	1
Cartwright	1		Black Duck Cove	1
Deep Water Creek	1		Brig Bay	2
East St Modeste	1		Cremaillere	2
English Point	1		Eddies Cove	5
Henley Harbour	3		Graufer's Cove	1
Indian Cove	4		Green Point	1
L'Anse au Loup	2		Green Island Brook	4
Muddy Bay	1		Green Island Point	1
Red Bay	2		Horse Islands	3
Rigolet	1		King's Cove	1
Seal Islands	1		Old Ferolle	2
Snag Cove	1		Parson's Pond	1
*Spirit Cove	1		Quirpon	2
Spotted Islands	3		River of Ponds	1
*St Paul's Island	1		Sally's Cove	1
Trap Cove	2		St John's Island	2
Turnavik	2		St Paul's	4
Venison Island	4			
West St Modeste	1			
William's Harbour	2			

*Location not verified.
All placements were single females appointed to settlements that were not established medical stations, with the exception of Horse Islands and Spotted Islands, where male students from Amherst College and the Columbia College of Physicians and Surgeons were appointed from 1909 to 1914. The placements do not include postings to the Grenfell School in St Anthony. Derived from ADSF annual staff reports (1914 onward) and occasional articles and notes.

tions as "other volunteers." However, despite their swelling numbers, it is not clear that the summer teachers fulfilled a purpose in the mission program beyond modestly supplementing the hit-and-miss schooling provided by Newfoundland church authorities. Perhaps more important, having experienced "the coast," the volunteers would return home as useful emissaries for the mission in its constant quest for donations and professionally qualified volunteers. In 1920, Kathleen Ewing of Enfield, Massachusetts, summed up her summer in Venison Tickle: "I often wonder how a trained teacher would have handled my school," she began; nonetheless,

> I honestly think that Miss Muir's summer schools are accomplishing a tremendous amount of good. Such children, as the ten year old girl who came to me every evening for extra spelling words ... are at least given a chance; and the benefit to a little isolated fishing village of having some one of them from the outside world with new ideas and an entirely different point of view ... is very real, I think, to people who are grateful for new ideas.

And the benefit is not one-sided. I remember the man on the Labrador boat who remarked, "A lot of you come down here every year. I don't see why you do it, but then Americans is queer." He ignored the fact, possibly he did not know it, that the teacher receives quite as much as she gives.[9]

ENTER ELIZABETH PAGE

Likely it was articles such as this, as well as contact with Grenfell alumnae, that piqued the interest of Elizabeth Page in 1921. Page was born in 1889 in Vermont and raised in Manhattan. Her father, Alfred R. Page, was a lawyer, a member of the state senate, and a judge on the New York State Supreme Court from 1910 to 1923.[10] Her mother, Elizabeth Roe Page, was on the Women's Executive Committee of the Reformed Church in America and was a leader of church missionary work.[11] During her high school years Elizabeth spent summers as a volunteer worker at the Reformed Church Indian mission station in Colony, Oklahoma, under the auspices of her aunt and uncle. She received her BA from Vassar College in 1912, and an MA in history at Columbia University in 1914. Vassar friends and connections were to remain significant for the rest of her life. For several years she taught English and history at Walnut School, a private institution in Massachusetts aimed at preparing girls for attendance at Wellesley College. In 1918 she joined several other Vassar alumnae in operating a YMCA canteen in France for American soldiers.[12] That year her younger sister, Marjorie, worked as a summer volunteer in the Grenfell mission hospital at St Anthony. The record is unclear about Page's activities in the years just before her first summer with the Grenfell mission. In the 1920 census, she is described as a social worker for the Red Cross, possibly on the basis of volunteer work. She remained at home with her family, now living in the University Heights area of the Bronx. While not wealthy, Page evidently had sufficient family resources to permit her to pursue her personal, altruistic interests without need for gainful employment or a supportive husband.

In February 1921 Page and a friend had written to Muir applying for a summer teaching positions.[13] There ensued a series of letters to establish that Page would serve in a new field of activity, White Bay, along with two other volunteers.[14] Muir wrote, "All my usual hamlets" already had volunteer workers assigned, but she had new settlements in urgent need. "Being pioneer places, I know absolutely nothing but their names, Sops Island and Beaches." She described the duties of volunteer teachers: "Do any and everything for the physical, mental and moral uplift of the people in the hamlet to which you are sent. We teach five days in the week, hold Sunday School or church service or both on Sunday, help people to better methods of housekeeping, gardening, teach knitting, sewing, etc., according to the attainments of the volunteer. Above all we try to induce in the people cleanliness as regards both their homes and their persons and teach the children to play."

Likely the request for Grenfell volunteers had come from the local Church of England "missionary," Rev. J.A. Meadon in Jackson's Arm. Page was urged to write directly to him for more information, and she was told that the church Board of Education in St John's would pay $20 per month for board, which was to be paid to a local host. Meadon wrote to Page with details of the communities to be served: Sops Island, Bear Cove, and Beaches. Host families were identified in the former two, but he suggested that tents would be required for both the school and the teacher's accommodation in Beaches. He advised that all religious instruction should be from the "point of view of the C. of E. [Church of England] (or Episcopal, the American equivalent)," and the hymnal was specified. Finally, he explained how to reach White Bay by sailing on the ss *Rosalind* from New York and the ss *Prospero* from St John's. Page apparently had little direct contact with the IGA offices in New York or in St Anthony and was expected to be quite self-reliant in getting established in her post in remote White Bay.

In its evolution over the previous two decades the Grenfell mission had been active in communities along the west coast of the Northern Peninsula as far south as Sally's Cove, but never further into White Bay than Canada Bay. (Grenfell's hospital ship, the *Strathcona*, occasionally called in to some of the settlements during its summer rounds).[15] From the perspective of Newfoundland settlement history, White Bay was among the most remote and underdeveloped regions.[16] The inner reaches of the bay provided little reward for either French or Newfoundland fishers. Steep, heavily forested, or rocky cliffs bordered much of the bay, punctuated by isolated coves offering little shelter or arable land. By the end of the nineteenth century, a dozen settlements had formed, supported by a tenuous mixture of inshore fishing and logging. In 1921 about 1,200 people lived in some fifteen settlements around the bay. The largest of these were Jackson's Arm and Westport (figure 7.1.) To a degree, they were "out of sight, out of mind" to both government and church authorities in St John's and equally neglected by the nearby Grenfell mission, which had seized the challenge of serving similar places further north.

After several potential volunteers had dropped out and communities were reassigned, Page and two others (also Vassarites) made their way to Bear Cove, Brown's Cove, and Sops Island in early July. After her summer's work, Muir had requested that Page send a report on conditions in these hitherto unknown places. This Page did in November 1921.[17] The early pages of the letter resembled reports by summer teachers previously published in ADSF but were more detailed. The trip to White Bay on the *Prospero* was eventful and fascinating, and White Bay stunningly beautiful, all icebergs, densely wooded mountains, and red-brown cliffs. Her companions were deposited in Bear Cove and Sops Island Upper, in accordance with arrangements made by Rev. Meadon. Page was placed in Brown's Cove. She describes the community in some detail as "a patriarchal group of five households." Economically,

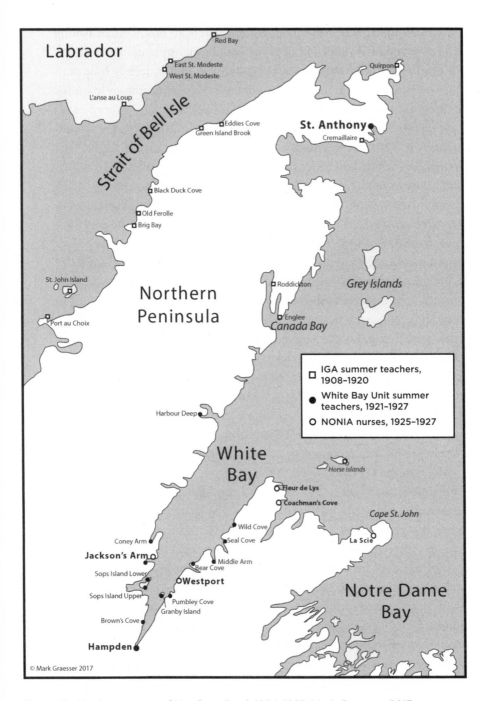

Figure 7.1 Northeast coast of Newfoundland, 1924–1925. Mark Graesser, 2017

times were hard. Skipper Langford had given up commercial fishing after several failed years and operated a sawmill but had no market for his product. As a result, there was virtually no money to buy food supplies beyond flour and tea. Page conducted classes for nine children for six weeks. "There had been a Newfoundland teacher ... for short periods of time twice before," so some of the older children displayed a rudimentary level of literacy. Such was thought to be the case with all of the settlements in the bay other than Jackson's Arm and Westport, which had full-time teachers each winter. Besides reading and arithmetic, Page taught history, geography, handwork, hygiene, and "their catechism in preparation for the Bishop's visit." In August an itinerant nutrition team from St Anthony arrived, Dr Wilshusen and Miss Blayney.[18] They found most of the children seriously underweight and left a supply of supplementary foods – dried milk, cocoa, prunes, and tomatoes. This diet, together with prescribed naps twice a day, seemed to work wonders, according to Page, with weight gains being recorded within weeks. Page attempted to foster better health conditions in the village by giving daily talks on hygiene. The children were given toothbrushes and instructions for their use and coached on the importance of cleanliness, fresh air, correct posture, "and such-like elementals." She treated "a regular epidemic of boils and infections" with a kit of supplies she had obtained from New York Presbyterian Hospital but readily acknowledged that she was in no way qualified as a "district nurse."

  After six weeks, Brown's Cove fell victim to "a mild form of the flu." The *Strathcona* happened to call, and Grenfell urged Page to withdraw to St Anthony for her own health. However, he also wanted her to explore the possibility of introducing the IGA industrial program into Brown's Cove and the neighbouring communities. This department was well established in St Anthony and the communities of the Labrador and western Newfoundland coasts. It was a cottage industry whereby women utilized traditional skills to make hooked mats and knitted goods to IGA designs and standards to earn much-needed cash. After scouting for potential craft workers, Page repaired to St Anthony, where she spent several weeks thoroughly familiarizing herself with the industrial work – product designs, standards, pricing, and marketing. On her way back to New York, she stopped again at Brown's Cove to leave a sample Grenfell mat and materials with Mrs Langford, whom she envisioned as a leader of the initiative in the area.

The remainder of Page's report went well beyond the accounts of previous teachers, who generally described their contributions as modest, and the experience personally rewarding, and left it at that. They had done their bit, enjoyed it, and encouraged others to do the same. Page, on the other hand, was determined to return and undertake a multifaceted program to address what she identified as the "three great needs" of the fifteen settlements in White Bay: education, nutrition, and dependable employment. To meet these needs a staff of six or seven workers and one or two motorboats would be required. There would be teachers posted again to Bear Cove, Brown's Cove, and Sops Island, but they should also receive some preliminary training in nutrition work. In addition, there would be a trained nutrition supervisor. She would be assisted by a doctor to examine all the children in the bay at the beginning and end of the summer. Through the summer she would travel from village to village monitoring child health (especially weight gain), distributing food supplements, and supervising this aspect of the teachers' duties.[19] To address the economic need, there would be a full-time industrial worker "to introduce, supervise and standardize work which can be marketed through St Anthony." This work would focus on the most impoverished communities in the bottom of the bay. Finally, the boat would require an operator, either a summer volunteer or a local man hired for the purpose. (Implicitly, all the other workers were to be volunteers.) Page offered herself as the industrial worker and suggested that her fellow 1921 volunteers would return to their respective schools. However, more volunteers would have to be recruited and funds raised to fill out her design.

THE WHITE BAY UNIT TAKES SHAPE

It is evident that Page's plan was a projection of the larger Grenfell mission, which by this point had education, nutrition, and industrial "departments" to supplement the core medical operations. It went well beyond the scope of Ethel Muir's ongoing summer teacher program and also seemed intent on operating with relatively little direct involvement by the full-time staff in St Anthony. As such, its approval required the consent of Wilfred Grenfell and the involvement of a number of operational leaders in the mission, and its implementation required the mobilization of resources by Page herself. She was later to write to a friend and co-worker, Mary Card, "When the work in White Bay was first projected, the Mission was having difficulty in carrying the stations already instituted, and the Board of Directors allowed us to enter the new field only with the understanding that we would assume the full financial responsibility ourselves."[20] She had lunch with Grenfell in December, during which she laid out her plans and reported that she had a personal commitment of $500 from the girls of Briarcliff School (Muir's former institution) to fund a motorboat for the summer, and another $100 from "a lady" for additional expenses.[21] Grenfell gave his blessing to her plans in a letter on 31 March 1922 and offered her the use of a mission-owned motorboat in St Anthony, which would be re-christened the *Briarcliff*, provided that Page stood the expense of refitting and fuelling the boat for the season. He assured her that a WOP qualified to operate the boat could easily be found through the general recruitment of college boys for the summer.[22]

There ensued a flurry of correspondence.[23] Dorothy MacAusland in Boston, secretary of the all-powerful Staff Selection Committee, chaired by her husband, wrote, "At the request of Mrs Grenfell, we are placing you in charge of a Unit" (a novel entity in the organization). Marion Moseley, head of the nascent IGA child welfare initiative, wrote, "It is simply great that you are to be head of the White Bay Unit." She made suggestions regarding plans to get milk to the White Bay children and urged Page personally to recruit a dedicated doctor and dentist for her unit, rather than relying on those in St Anthony. Ethel Muir placed the appointment of White Bay teachers in Page's hands, subject to vetting with the Church of England Board of Education. Page strenuously resisted the idea, attributed to Mrs Anne Grenfell, of sending industrial workers not of her choosing to White Bay, insisting that she alone would take on those duties; indeed, this dimension seemed to have assumed first priority in her plans to uplift White Bay.

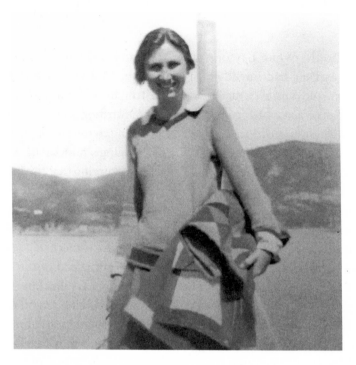

Figure 7.2 Elizabeth Page in White Bay, ca 1924. EPHP, box 70, folder 1488, White Bay photo album

Ultimately, MacAusland wrote that Page (figure 7.2) had the full confidence of the committee to staff and organize the unit exactly as she preferred. Page was to be the industrial worker as well as secretary of the unit, making her rounds in the *Briarcliff*, which was to be operated by Charles Drummond, a University of Toronto student. She would be accompanied by Beulah Clap as nutrition worker, a Vassar student who had taught in Sops Island the previous year. Elinor Goodnow would return to teach in Bear Cove, and Alice Burrows, also of Vassar, would teach in Brown's Cove. During the first two weeks Dr William Emerson toured the bay with Page, Clap, and an assistant (also from Vassar) to examine and assess all the children, mainly noting those deemed to be "underweight," and leave instructions for their dietary improvement and continued monitoring. Thereafter, members of the Vassar group busied themselves in their respective stations and roles for some six weeks.[24]

And so the White Bay operation was implemented in its first year, largely as Page had intended. In November, Charles Watson, general secretary and business manager of the IGA in St John's, sent Page a statement of account for the "White Bay Nutrition Fund." It showed total expenditures of $1,224, with $175 owing to the IGA. Page replied with a detailed statement of her own, challenging a number of Watson's entries on both the debit and credit sides and claiming that the fund was in fact owed $45.29 by the IGA. In no uncertain terms, she also corrected Watson's name for the fund, which was to be "the White Bay Fund," not limited to "nutrition" as he had implied. This exchange confirmed both the financial and policy autonomy of Page's project.[25]

A potentially disruptive development arose at the end of the season. Before leaving St Anthony, Page had been told by Mrs Blackburn, head of the Industrial Department, that Mrs Anne Grenfell had gotten wind of certain unspecified "indiscretions" committed by two or three Vassar girls on the coastal boat earlier in the summer and that Mrs Grenfell had therefore decided that Vassar girls would not be accepted as volunteers on the coast for one or two years. Page wrote to Mrs Grenfell, vigorously arguing the unfairness of punishing all Vassar girls for the offensive behaviour of just two of their unnamed compatriots. As a practical matter, she was obviously alarmed because she counted on Vassar as a principal source of volunteers and funding for her White Bay project. She pointed out that fifteen of the thirty-four girls on the coast in 1922 came from Vassar. She signed her letter "for the Vassar girls working in White Bay." Anne Grenfell replied, in effect, that this was a tempest in a teapot. It seemed that two girls (whose names she did not know) had indeed smoked on deck, after being asked not to do so by the captain because the local people found this objectionable. Miss Muir had been quite disturbed and wrote to Mrs Grenfell at the end of the season. Mrs Grenfell said that she really had no authority in such matters and would turn Muir's concerns over to the Staff Selection Committee. But she accepted Page's argument that the best response was simply to delegate a rigorous screening role to committees at the various colleges to weed out in advance those prone to irresponsible behaviour. Since the advent of student volunteers on the coast, the mission had been sensitive to what it perceived as "very conservative" sensibilities of the local people. A set of instructions issued to staff members in the late 1920s included an injunction: "We ask women staff members not to smoke either at their stations or while travelling on the coast."[26] Apparently the matter was laid to rest, because several of the White Bay volunteers in 1923 were Vassar students or alumnae.

THE WORKERS AND THEIR ROLES[27]

The White Bay Unit was most active in the summers of 1923 to 1925. During these years, the staff complement ranged from twelve to sixteen, including an average of five teachers, two nutrition workers, two industrial workers (including Page), up to four medical personnel (doctor, dentist, and assistants), and several crew to operate two motorboats. The unit remained off the main IGA financial books but was incorporated in the annual staff reports published in the July issues of *Among the Deep Sea Fishers*. Accounts for the separate White Bay Fund were maintained by Page as well as the IGA office. Most of the staff were volunteers, but some were paid for their work (notably some of the medical staff and the Newfoundland boat skippers), and others their expenses. An idea of the way in which Page balanced these resources is indicated in her provisional staff list for 1924[28] (see table 7.2).

The recruitment and deployment of the White Bay staff required a great deal of work by Page during the winter and spring. In 1923 Harriet Houghteling, a volunteer from Chicago, became chairman of the Staff Selection Committee, which she ran in a much more systematic fashion than previously. The two women worked closely, with Houghteling requesting from Page a list of her requirements for the upcoming season, and Page referring recruits to Houghteling for the completion of application forms. Formal appointments were in Houghteling's hands, but she invariably deferred to Page's choices. Travel arrangements to "the Coast" were then handled by the New York office.

Most of the teachers were recruited by Page, most being Vassar College students or alumnae. Others were drawn from the pool of those who applied to the IGA directly; of these, Houghteling seemingly offered Page "first pick." Page made one or more visits each year to Vassar to

Table 7.2
White Bay Unit provisional staff list, 1924

Teachers	5 "full volunteers" and 1 "half volunteer" with expenses paid by the Vassar Christians Association
Nutrition workers	1 "full volunteer"
Industrial workers	2, expenses paid by White Bay Fund
Trained nurse	1 "full volunteer"
Doctors*	1 "part volunteer" with expenses, and $100 honorarium paid by the IGA Child Welfare Department, 1 "full volunteer"
Dentist	1, expenses paid, $100 from Child Welfare Department and $150 by White Bay Fund
Engineer (wop)	1 "full volunteer"
Sailor (wop)	1, expenses paid by special gift
Nfld skippers	2, expenses paid by White Bay Fund

*The "doctors" were normally second- or third-year medical students on their summer vacation.

speak and raise funds for the Grenfell mission and the White Bay Unit. She then relied on her network of previous volunteers at Vassar to find and assess new recruits. Some of the volunteers were of Page's own generation (in their thirties) and had teaching experience. Each year, one was designated as the "educational supervisor" for the unit, and these individuals developed a set of guidelines for daily work in the classroom and a teaching plan for the season. The general advice was, "Don't expect too much." While this advice was no doubt helpful to the young women with no teacher training or knowledge of outport life in Newfoundland, once installed in their posts they seem to have been left largely on their own, although in regular contact with Page as she made her rounds by motorboat. With one exception, all of the teachers were female, and all were Americans. As we shall see, the latter fact was a matter of concern to Page.

The experience of Florence "Fliss" Clothier illustrates the White Bay teachers' role. She was recruited as a twenty-year-old Vassar sophomore and spent the summers of 1924 and 1925 in Sops Island Upper, population about thirty. This was a typical post, being one of the smallest and poorest settlements in the bay, without the regular services of a Newfoundland teacher. Clothier wrote detailed letters to her wealthy Philadelphia family, describing day-to-day life with her host family, the Gales, and the eight or nine children in her charge.[29] She took her teaching duties seriously, keeping strict hours. (The children often clamoured for more.) She also conducted Sunday services, offered night classes for the women, and doled out nutritional supplements and medical advice for the children on behalf of the travelling nutrition worker. In all of this, she expressed appropriate skepticism about her qualifications, but this did not dampen her enthusiasm. She was happy to assist Mrs Gale's efforts to garden in the rocky soil (the IGA volunteers were provided with a supply of seeds as part of the nutrition program); she joined the family at fishing, haying, berrying, and socializing in other communities. When the Gales became embroiled in a serious dispute with another community over rights to cut hay on common land, Clothier became an active advocate, assisting in writing up their legal case and presenting it to the magistrate. In 1925, she became involved in the contentious process of setting up local committees to raise funds for NONIA district nurses.

Clothier's experience was probably not unlike that of most of the teachers, although none left so vivid an account. Some formed strong and lasting bonds with the families they lived with. A baby was named after Florence, and later Florence named her own firstborn after Johanna Gale, her host. However, in Page's larger scheme for fostering improvements in White Bay, the summer teachers were incidental. Clearly, they were not going to remedy the fundamental deficiencies in schooling for children in tiny and isolated outports; this was a long-term problem that only the government and churches could address. Rather, Page saw the teachers as "propagandizing" agents, cultivating greater community awareness of the possibilities for achieving better health and desperately needed income through the nutrition counselling and industrial work, which were the more important arms of her project.

The Grenfell mission had for some years taken an interest in promoting better nutrition as an essential component of healthful living.[30] In 1923, sporadic efforts to this end were supplanted by the formal establishment of a Child Welfare Department directed by Marion Moseley.[31]

A budget of $1,500 was allocated, and Moseley created summer "Nutrition and Child Welfare Units" for the Labrador and West coasts, each with a doctor, dentist, and one or more "nutrition workers." These travelling teams examined all children in each village for evidence of nutritional deficiencies and disease, conducted classes for mothers and children, and dispensed food supplements considered beneficial, especially for vitamin deficiencies. The most notable indicator of child health was "underweight," by which children were classified against American norms using a simple scheme devised by Dr Emerson. The White Bay Unit, already established, was folded into this program but remained Page's responsibility, with a small amount of supplementary funding. Page expanded the geographical reach of the unit, primarily for nutritional work purposes, to include an eastern section comprising communities from Fleur de Lys to La Scie on the Notre Dame Peninsula. One nutritional worker was posted in Jackson's Arm and another in La Scie. Motorboats were required in both areas to facilitate travel by these workers, as well as a doctor, dentist, and dental assistant or nurse (the exact complement varying from year to year). The nutritional worker maintained records and encouraged summer teachers to reinforce the educational work. Children were given food supplements such as powdered milk, cocoa, sugar, and molasses, generally encouraged not to drink tea (a local dietary staple), to take rest periods during the day, to get fresh air at night, and to use the toothbrushes issued by the IGA. Progress in the form of weight gains was carefully noted on charts posted in each village.[32]

As noted above, at the end of her first summer in White Bay, Page had spent time in St Anthony familiarizing herself with the IGA industrial department in St Anthony. Women in White Bay had expressed interest in participating in this scheme. Thereafter, as the industrial worker for the White Bay Unit, Page took a particular interest in this work. It was her role to find capable women in each settlement to lead by example and then to pass out "work" – materials and designs from which women working on their own over the winter would produce the products that the IGA would market, primarily in the United States. Although requiring just one or two staff, this dimension of the White Bay project within a few years laid the economic foundation for introducing the "self-help" NONIA model of rural health care.[33]

THE ORGANIZATIONAL EFFORT

Throughout its relatively brief period of intense activity, the White Bay Unit was the product of extraordinary drive and acumen by Elizabeth Page. The IGA leadership was content to leave her to carry on in an auxiliary fashion, so long as there was no financial demand on general mission funds and relatively little management responsibility. Page seemed to be quite happy with the autonomy this arrangement allowed her to run things in her own way, ultimately with goals rather different from those of the Grenfell establishment. This entailed managing relationships, often rather delicate, in several spheres: the American field of fundraising and volunteer recruitment; the IGA operational bureaucracy; potential allies among Newfoundland elites; and ultimately with families and leaders in the two dozen villages of White Bay. Hundreds of letters and documents carefully preserved among her papers attest to the professional efficiency with which she personally orchestrated all of this.[34]

To raise funds, she cultivated a number of donors in the New York area who probably began with her parents' connections. There were regular gifts from a number of Presbyterian and Reformed Church groups. Briarcliff Manor and Knox School were each good for as much as $500 per year, and in one year her acolytes at Vassar raised more than $1,200. In all, her fundraising had increased to about $7,400 per year by 1925.[35] To achieve this she kept up a busy schedule of speaking engagements, much in the manner of Grenfell. These ranged as far afield as Detroit, Ohio, and Chicago.

An extraordinary challenge was met over the winter of 1924–25. For three years Page had operated with motorboats supplied by the mission in St Anthony. These had regularly broken down, despite the best efforts of her Newfoundland skippers and WOP "engineers." So she determined that the only solution was to buy and fit out her own boat. This entailed shopping at boat auctions and salvage yards on the upper east coast of the United States. Ultimately she purchased a surplus forty-foot steel hull from the US Navy and had it re-fitted with a two-masted sailing rig and a powerful used motor. All of this cost more than $5,000. The hull was paid for by a special fundraising effort at Vassar, led by Florence Clothier, and much of the difference by a Mr A.D. Baldwin and the "town of Cleveland through the efforts of Mrs Tillinghast."[36] To ship the boat to Newfoundland, she prevailed upon Eric Bowering, president of the Red Cross Line, to provide free passage on the deck of the weekly steamer from New York. Since the boat was too large to sit on the deck of the *Prospero* on its coastal voyage to White Bay, Page arranged for her skipper, Patrick Lewis of Fleur de Lys, to meet her in St John's with a crewman. The trio sailed happily to White Bay, where the newly christened *Loon* performed splendidly for the White Bay Unit.[37]

Although her unit had great autonomy, Page operated within the IGA structure for the management of personnel and financial records, arranging logistics, and so forth. In this regard, Page corresponded actively with Harriet Houghteling, and they became close friends and confidants. In addition, two of the three fields of endeavour – nutrition and industrial – were intended to conform to the policies being developed by the operational heads in St Anthony.[38] This meant that Page would work closely with Marion Moseley and Elizabeth Criswell, successive heads of the Child Welfare Department, and with Catherine "K" Cleveland of "the Industrial." Like Page, these were all highly committed and accomplished single, professional women; their correspondence was very business-like but was also marked by cordiality and affection. Only rarely did Page have any dealings with Dr Charles Curtis, the crusty supreme official in St Anthony. None of the White Bay activities came under his purview as chief medical officer, and he seems to have been happy to let Page go her own way as long as she did not do anything to put the mission in a bad light. With Grenfell, Page seems to have enjoyed a pleasant relationship, as when they conducted joint speaking events, but beyond obtaining his blessing for her grand plan in 1921, there is no record of any practical interaction.

In addition to her dealings with Eric Bowering, Page cultivated links with other influential Newfoundlanders such as Harry Crowe, a colourful and successful logging and lumber promoter originally from Nova

Scotia. In 1924 Crowe had obtained timber-cutting leases in White Bay and was building a mill in Hampden. With the mill he built a company town for his workers and their families, instantly making Hampden the largest community in the bay. He had a reputation as a relatively beneficent magnate in the timber industry, and in that light he installed a doctor, nurse, and social worker in Hampden. Page made Crowe's acquaintance by chance but moved quickly to secure agreements from him to release his doctor for a month of work with her summer program. ("Doctor" Louis Conroy, from St John's, was a McGill University medical student at the time, and later became a noted orthopaedic surgeon in Newfoundland. He was a popular weekend friend to the Vassar students in the bay.) Crowe was generous and supportive in other small ways, and his mill created desperately needed jobs and marked a turning point in the economy of White Bay. But Page privately hoped that he "would not cut all the trees," and Clothier observed that conditions in Hampden and the logging camps were far less healthy than the village fishing life.[39]

Schooling in White Bay, as elsewhere in Newfoundland, was exclusively provided by the major religious denominations, under their respective Boards of Education in St John's. Direct responsibility was in the hands of the local ministers, such as Rev. Meadon. In the case of White Bay, most communities and schools were deemed to be Church of England, while a few came under Methodist jurisdiction. Therefore, in making her annual teacher appointments, after refining her detailed plans with Houghteling, Page submitted the names of her proposed appointees and their stations to the respective superintendents of education, Dr W.W. Blackall, Church of England, and Dr Levi Curtis, Methodist. With Blackall, in particular, there typically ensued detailed correspondence, further involving the local minister, before appointments were settled. Page also met with him while stopping over in St John's en route to White Bay, to iron out final details and resolve issues. Mostly this seemed to be a matter of courtesy, because Blackall invariably expressed gratitude for the work Page and her group were doing in White Bay and confidence in her choices, but he also proffered advice and preferences. For example, one year he noted that the local minister, a rather difficult man, insisted that the volunteers be Church of England adherents. Page was discreetly mum on this topic, religion not being a criterion in her selection, but in relaying her names to the White Bay minister, Blackall bridged the gap by simply noting "Episcopalian" after each name.[40]

A consideration of greater concern to Page was that all of her teachers were Americans. In 1924 she wrote to Blackall, "As I wrote to you last year I am very anxious to have at least two Newfoundland teachers on the White Bay staff. I feel that we Americans need such an influence." She suggested that she might speak to students at the "girl's school or college in St John's ... if by so doing I can get the opportunity to see any girls that you think might be available for the summer. I cannot tell you how strongly I feel that we need the inside help of the Newfoundland point of view. Please do all that you can to save us from the mistakes that we as outsiders are undoubtedly making." Blackall responded that he would undertake to provide Newfoundland summer teachers, but that they would not be found in St John's, where the school girls were too young for such an experience. In the end, through the local minister, he asked a young woman from White Bay, who was already teaching in the winter, to spend her summer at Granby Island as part of Page's program, but paid a regular salary from Church of England funds. The woman declined, preferring to spend her summer at home with her family in nearby Westport. However, lurking behind this polite set of negotiations was a view by Page and her colleagues and volunteers that better-off Newfoundlanders in St John's – the equivalents of themselves – ought to "do their bit" to help their less fortunate "brothers and sisters" in the impoverished North.[41] Page was later to make a similar overture to Lady Allardyce, who had recently founded the Girl Guide movement in Newfoundland, to send a couple of young leaders from St John's to spend a summer in White Bay with her teachers setting up Girl Guide troops.[42] She saw this, again, as a cultural bridge between the extremes of Newfoundland society. In the event, nothing came of this proposal.

Page's dealings with the Newfoundland educational hierarchy took an interesting turn in 1926. Late in 1925, illness had forced Page to withdraw totally from her usual winter cycle of raising funds and recruiting volunteers. Florence Clothier, now a Vassar senior, partly filled the breach by working with the IGA office to complete the summer appointments. She wrote to Page,

> Miss Fowler [the new Staff Selection Committee chair] showed me a letter of yours requesting that the appointments for White Bay be confirmed by Mr Blackall. Miss Fowler does not feel that she can do this, because Dr Grenfell seems to think that that makes it look as though Mr Blackall and not the Grenfell Assoc. were making the appointments. Of course your policy of cooperating with Mr Blackall is wise but since the Grenfell Assoc does not usually ask for these confirmations, Miss Fowler feels that it would be better for her not to do so in her official capacity, especially since Dr Grenfell is against it. They evidently think it right for you to do just as you please about it, as head of the White Bay Unit. Do you want me to write Mr Blackall telling him of the appointments?[43]

This suggests that the scores of summer teachers appointed over years to other IGA districts had not been vetted with the Newfoundland educational authorities and that Page's practice was exceptional. However, in 1922 Ethel Muir stated that in her view the appointment of a teacher to any particular place in White Bay required the consent of Dr Blackall.[44]

TRANSITION AND EXIT: THE NONIA CONNECTION

In late 1925, Elizabeth Page became severely debilitated with heart failure, forcing her to suspend most of her White Bay work. Over the winter, Clothier and other supporters at Vassar organized fundraising and recruitment of five teachers and two WOPs along lines Page had previously established. Edith Tallant, who had been Page's assistant on the *Loon* in 1925, assumed management of the industrial work and of the White Bay Unit as a whole. A volunteer dentist and dental assistant were found by the IGA office, and the nutrition and child welfare duties were carried out by the two NONIA district nurses, as in 1925. Thus, apart from the absence of Page pulling all the strings, the White Bay

Unit in 1926 appeared on paper to be operating at the same level as in
the previous three years. Meanwhile, plans had been afoot, probably
led by Houghteling, for Page to be offered a new position as executive
secretary of the Staff Selection Committee and industrial secretary in
charge of sales promotion. It would be a senior position based either in
New York or Boston, at a salary of $2,500 per year. It would relieve
Page of the rigours of summer work in White Bay. But this left the question of what was to become of the White Bay Unit. For example, would
the IGA take it over, formally adding it to the operations managed from
St Anthony? This might include establishing one or more nursing stations. There is no suggestion that this was contemplated in a period
when the association was constantly struggling to meet the expenses
of its existing establishment. White Bay was never recognized as "IGA
territory" by Grenfell or others speaking of the broader mission and
achievements. From this perspective, the project might simply have been
left quietly to wither away. Indeed, the 1927 and 1928 staff reports
identify just two summer teachers in White Bay locations, with no mention of a "White Bay Unit." After that, White Bay disappears altogether
from the records.

   However, this was not entirely to do with Page's departure or incon-
sistent with her own plans. In her annual report to the IGA in late 1925,
Page wrote, "In the fall of 1924 it appeared to those of us working in
White Bay that the time had come to place some of the responsibility
of the welfare work on the shoulders of the people themselves. By the
advice of Doctor Grenfell a consistent propaganda to arouse individual
initiative had been carried on for five years, and increasing prosperity
gave the hope that the means were now at hand."[45] The "means" she
had in mind was the introduction of the Newfoundland Outport Nursing and Industrial Association to the bay. Page had always felt that the
central goal of her project was to establish better health-care facilities,
sustained largely or entirely by the people themselves. And, although
she made the obligatory nod to Grenfell in the statement above, she did
not see an extension of the IGA model into White Bay as the best way
to accomplish this. As Page wrote to Mary Card early in 1925, "If we
can raise the money that we need this year to establish permanent nursing stations that we are striving for [using the NONIA scheme], the dis-

trict will be practically self-supporting, or carried by Newfoundland charity. For thirty years such assistance as the [IGA] general fund could afford was only palliative, but five years of this intensive work has brought about this constructive result."[46] In the same vein, she wrote to Elizabeth Criswell,

> I wish to correct what seems like a misunderstanding on your part of my position in regard to encouraging the people of the coast to pay for what they get. I have stood for that principle in White Bay against considerable opposition not only in the Bay but from others of the Mission Staff ... *White Bay had been thoroughly pauperized by more than half a century of Government doles and by Mission policy before I went in,* and if the results I have to show after five years are not as great as elsewhere, please remember the handicap under which we have worked. Part of the hostility that Mary Card reports is undoubtedly due to the unrelenting stand that I have taken on this matter. I have opposed the establishment of [an IGA] nursing station in White Bay, badly as it may be needed, and frequently as it has been urged by members of the summer staff, because I could see no way in which it could be made self-supporting; and I am backing Lady Allardyce's project solely because it does give such a program of self support.[47] (emphasis added)

NONIA was recreated in 1924 under the vigorous leadership of Lady Elsie Allardyce, wife of the newly arrived governor, after a similar organization started by her predecessor in 1921 had faltered.[48] The object of the organization was to place fully trained nurses in rural locations supported largely with funds raised by the sale of knitted goods produced by local women and marketed through a St John's depot. The women would earn cash from their work, some of which would go to local committees that would pool the funds to pay the salary and expenses of the nurse. Twenty-five per cent of costs would be supplemented by a government grant. Critical elements of the scheme were the production of high-quality, attractive products and the formation of effective local committees. The nurses were recruited primarily from Great Britain through Lady Allardyce's connections. The production and marketing sides resembled the IGA industrial scheme, but the idea of deriving funds through community committees was novel. That aspect particularly appealed to Page. She contacted Allardyce in the summer of 1924, and arrangements were made for a meeting when the governor and his wife visited White Bay in September.[49]

The two women evidently agreed in principle that their respective enterprises could be combined with the appointment of two NONIA district nurses in Jackson's Arm and Fleur de Lys. The exact terms of the partnership, however, took some delicate negotiations by Page. First she met with Dr Curtis in St Anthony, who endorsed Page's terms. NONIA would recruit and appoint two highly qualified district nurses from Britain. In addition to their regular duties, the nurses would carry on with the IGA nutrition and child welfare work under the direction of the IGA. The White Bay Unit would organize the NONIA committees in each village during the summer of 1925. On a one-year basis the unit would commit $1,500 to cover shortfalls in the community contributions as the committees began raising local funds. The unit's industrial worker would assist with distribution of NONIA wool and patterns to women in the bay (apparently alongside their continued work on IGA products, notably hooked mats).

However, Page later received a letter from Catherine Cleveland, IGA industrial director, who had apparently been in contact with Allardyce, implying a misunderstanding about the marketing side. Page replied,

I told Lady Allardyce that I would be very glad to do all that I personally could to get to a permanent market for her goods by seeing if certain stores in New York might not carry her things, but I intended to make it clear that I was merely offering to assist her to set up her own market. The whole point of appealing to the Newfoundland Nurses Association at all was to place the burden for the medical work in White Bay where it belongs on the shoulders of the Newfoundlanders. The district is potentially self-supporting and the Newfoundland Association offered what seemed to be the quickest means of securing that self-support. We are interested in seeing the district succeed in this experiment and I am willing to work hard to help them on their feet. But I do wish to be certain that it is their feet that I am assisting them to stand on. I do not wish to find at the end of the extra effort that they are still leaning on us. For that reason, although I asked Lady Allardyce to send me samples of her things that I might peddle them around, I am willing to do so only if I am assisting her to an independent market. I am absolutely averse to the Mission attempting to market her things. There is room to spare for both of us. But we should be absolutely independent.[50]

In April 1925 Allardyce wrote that she was pleased that Page had committed to the support of two nurses, whom she would soon be bringing from England. But then she raised another matter of concern: she was pleased that "you'll have a band of workers to supervise the work in White Bay; they had better put in a few days at least in St John's to see our method of work and the standard [for Shetland garments] ... Would it be wise to have one of your voluntary workers to work with ours, dispatching and receiving work for White Bay (I might be able to count on her, as I cannot always do on my own!)."[51] This suggestion raised alarm bells with Houghteling:

It does seem to me that we are stepping on very delicate ground to send a young American to St John's to take the place of their own people. How is this enterprise ever going to be put on a sound basis if the local people of St John's cannot carry it on *now* under the most auspicious circumstances with Lady Allardyce on the spot with all her enthusiasm and charm? ... As far as proving "that the Mission is willing to help with a strictly Newfoundland enterprise if asked to do so" – would not this assignment stir up anew all the antagonism to the Mission work South of St John's? Of course you know the situation much better than I do and I would abide absolutely by your judgement.[52]

Page apparently smoothed all of this over. She did not place an American volunteer in the NONIA depot. She reported from White Bay in July 1925 that an excellent English nurse had arrived, with a second expected soon; community committees were organized throughout the bay and had $1,400 pledged, plus $250 from Harry Crowe; and "the women" were eagerly awaiting their wool, patterns, and needles.[53]

It was on this basis that Page charted the path toward progress in White Bay in her 1925 report, and more fully in her valedictory report in December 1926, when she was very ill. As she summarized the benefits of the IGA-NONIA alliance, "This plan at once secured unification of work by placing general oversight in the hands of workers resident winter and summer, removed a large burden of medical care from St Anthony, and realized to a considerable extent the original purpose of the White Bay work through the voluntary assumption by the people themselves of a considerable measure of executive and financial responsibility, and by providing a common basis of effort which should consolidate the interests of the bay."[54] Without herself as director, she proposed that the essential components of the White Bay Unit program could nonetheless be carried forward:

• *Medical and child welfare work* would be entirely in the hands of the NONIA nurses, supported by local fundraising. Dental work would continue to be provided by volunteers under the IGA Child Welfare Department. (As she recommended, a third nurse was appointed to Westport in 1927. White Bay thus became host to about one-third of all NONIA nurses for several years, before the Newfoundland government took over the nursing function in 1934.)[55]

• *Industrial work* could be managed by an IGA volunteer based in St Anthony, making one or two tours of the bay each year in the *Loon*, and linked to commitments by the women to contribute part of their earnings to the NONIA committees. (Edith Tallant carried on in this manner as a "travelling assistant" until at least 1929.)[56]

• *Summer teaching* could continue with volunteers from Vassar College, with the hope that Newfoundland teachers could also be supplied by Dr Blackall. It was hoped that this might lead to building an interdenominational boarding school in the bay. Page acknowledged that this was a faint hope, given the strength of "denominational feeling ... on the part of both the resident missionaries and the people." (In the event, the last two summer teachers in White Bay were appointed in 1927, and they did not come from Vassar.)

• *Funding* would be required only for the operational expenses of the *Loon* and the industrial work, about $1,600. Reliable sources of revenue were Briarcliff School, Knox School, and Baldwin School (Clothier's old high school). For any shortfall, Page would turn over to the IGA her list of White Bay donors, worth several thousand dollars per year, to be added to general Grenfell funds.

• *Management* of White Bay might be taken up either by the IGA or by NONIA. However, Page expressed doubt that NONIA was sufficiently well established to take on this responsibility.

And so ended an unusual episode in the history of the Grenfell mission. It is beyond the scope of this chapter to assess the results of Page's intervention in the longer term.[57] However, the immediate experience suggests that by the 1920s strong-minded and capable American women had begun to question the paternalistic "permanent mission" model that was Wilfred Grenfell's legacy.

Elizabeth Page's ill health prevented her from taking up the executive position with the IGA. After a lengthy convalescence, she moved to live with relatives in Wyoming for several years. While there, she was briefly in contact with Martha Beckwith and Elisabeth Greenleaf of the Vassar Folklore Foundation and Maud Karpeles, a British folklorist, about their respective plans to collect Newfoundland folk songs. (Page's skipper Patrick Lewis of Fleur de Lys was a source of several songs in Greenleaf's *Ballads and Sea Songs from Newfoundland*.) During the 1930s she wrote several novels based on western pioneering themes, and then a major bestseller, *The Tree of Liberty*, which also became a successful Hollywood film. Thus becoming independently wealthy, she devoted the rest of her life to humanitarian causes. She became a Quaker and ardent pacifist and in the 1940s was a rare advocate for the rights and welfare of interned Japanese Americans. At the age of sixty-five she married an aged, long-term friend, Herbert Harris. Following Page's death in 1969, her sister Marjorie wrote to friends from her years in Newfoundland, "Her thoughts were often of White Bay friends and it was the greatest pleasure for her to have the news items which you often sent."[58]

8

Education at the Grenfell Mission in the 1920s

Helen Woodrow

Organized educational opportunities were extremely rare for working-class individuals from coastal regions in Newfoundland and Labrador in the early years of the twentieth century. Throughout the colony, most children might have access to a few years of schooling, and then they apprenticed within families. The overwhelming majority lived their adult lives as their parents had: they fished, trapped, and raised their families, moving between their inland and coastal homes as work and weather demanded. Wilfred Grenfell had such a dim view of this nebulous education structure that he designed a private education system. This chapter examines the educational work of his mission until the 1930s, which involved some mission schools in northern Newfoundland and Labrador and access to further education and training outside the region. Philanthropists began sponsoring young men and women around 1908, with the New York training of Ted McNeill from Island Harbour and Archie Ash of Red Bay, Labrador; in the 1920s, a scholarship grant was made available to the IGA by the Carnegie Corporation of New York, and in that same decade, an important relationship was established with Berea College in Kentucky.[1]

The concept of capital forms developed by Pierre Bourdieu informs this analysis. Bourdieu maintained that cultural, economic, social, and symbolic capital have exchange values and operate as markers of distinction in society. Culture is integral to the social organization of class domination. Schools help reproduce class inequality by transforming social class distinctions into educational distinctions. Education is a form of cultural capital, as it harnesses the knowledge and skills that people draw upon as they engage in social life. Bourdieu identified three types of cultural capital: embodied, objectified, and institutionalized. The last consists of institutional recognition, usually in the form of academic credentials or qualifications. It is the means by which cultural capital is converted to economic capital. Objectified cultural capital refers to physical objects such as works of art, scientific instruments, or individual libraries. Such objects can be sold, but the transaction does not include the conceptual capital that enabled the seller to fully appreciate and understand the object. Embodied cultural capital is consciously and unconsciously acquired through socialization within families. Bourdieu concluded that all groups do not have knowledge of what is valued and considered appropriate within the dominant culture, and this inequality is maintained through the education system and other social institutions.[2]

In the period to the 1930s, the dominant society viewed residents of northern Newfoundland and Labrador as having extremely limited or no embodied cultural capital. Yet the residents were endowed with an abundance of embodied local cultural capital. I use this term to refer to the knowledge accumulated by coastal dwellers from their life experience. It was given less value because it was not extracted from formal education settings or associated and controlled by upper-class interests. However, what northern people knew about numerous subjects was critical for the survival of their families and for the Grenfell mission staff. Grenfell's reforms sought to make education more available in the North and to provide access to further training in the dominant society so residents could help the mission achieve its goals. Some recipients might have wanted to use education as institutional cultural capital, a marker of social difference. Others sought to transform mission philosophy so that local cultural capital was valued. I argue that some mission educators believed the people of northern Newfoundland and Labrador needed social uplift and that the training of young men and women was designed to produce a mission workforce that would have a greater impact on local residents.

Some students selected for training saw it as the fulfillment of a long-cherished hope for the future and shaped the opportunity to meet their needs. Others were thrilled to open up a new possibility in their life and were less interested in their suitability for the trade or occupation they were encouraged to study. A portion of those who were trained found opportunities that were better suited to their career or personal interests outside the North. Others made important contributions to their homeland that many still remember.

After considering the state of education in Newfoundland and the United States, the chapter explores the contributions and tensions of this educational work with an American foundation funder, a bureaucratic representative of the colonial government, and the principal of Memorial University College. As the human agency of seemingly ordinary, everyday people often remains unheard and invisible in the dominant culture, the discussion includes the voices of four people who were trained outside the dominion with the support of the IGA.[3]

STATE OF EDUCATION IN NEWFOUNDLAND AND THE UNITED STATES BEFORE THE 1920S

Increased awareness of the importance of education arose in the colony of Newfoundland, where education was nominally controlled by the state, in the same period as significant changes were being made to formal education in the United States.[4] During the Progressive Era, schools became important institutions, as many Americans believed that formal education would meet the needs of their changing nation. In 1900, people typically had only a primary school education. John Rury identifies two groups of progressives who offered solutions for the education system.[5] The pedagogical progressives, such as John Dewey, wanted change in classroom practice: they maintained that education should be more responsive to children's needs and sought closer relationships between school and community. The administrative progressives focused on efficiency, differentiation, vocationalism, and management; it was a form of applied Taylorism, the system of scientific management advocated by Frederick W. Taylor through his time-motion studies.

The growth of the secondary school system in the United States between 1890 and 1920 enabled the administrative progressives to create pathways for the future for their students. Several trade schools were opened in the 1880s, and by 1910 many educators were calling for vocational training in high schools. Private commercial schools were replaced with similar programs inside public high schools. The development of home economics, introduced as a field of study in the schools in the first decade of the twentieth century, led to a movement that organized an entire discipline around the experiences of women in their roles as mothers and housekeepers. Karen Graves has pointed out the negative consequences of such changes: a differentiated curriculum restricted women's knowledge, particularly in mathematics and science. The public school was expected to restore traditional images of women and offer sex-specific training for boys and girls in their roles as workers and citizens.[6] Claude Fischer and Michael Hout noted as well that the introduction of mandatory high school attendance captured "unruly" youth, usually thought to be the children of immigrants, and trained them for a changing economy.[7]

New educational programs and approaches were also organized for rural areas and the teaching profession. In 1890 the second Morrill Act gave more federal funds to agricultural and mechanical colleges to expand instruction in agriculture, the mechanical arts, and economic science. Research from the emerging social sciences and psychology was being applied to learning settings, and teachers were being trained in increasing numbers: by 1892 a teachers' college opened and within a year became part of Columbia University.

In Newfoundland, James Murray, a member of the House of Assembly, submitted a resolution to the House in 1890 calling for a public commission to establish an improved school system in language that reflected these trends in the United States. "The cause of education is of supreme importance in the estimation of every civilized and enlightened country at the present time," the resolution stated, "and especially so in the estimation of all communities of a progressive tendency ... Newfoundland is singularly backward as regards its educational facilities."[8] In fact, the educational system in both Newfoundland and the United States reflected class interests for decades to come. Vincent Burke, a superintendent of education who had been educated at Columbia University in New York, wrote in his 1917 report that "until recently,

school education [in Newfoundland] was planned to serve one class
only, that is those who would not have to work with their hands and
who would pass their lives in pursuits of a more or less intellectual nature."[9] His view accords with a contemporary study by George Counts,
an American educator and sociologist, which concluded that high school
education had been limited to a select group of adolescent children
privileged by race, class, and ethnicity.[10] By the 1920s, the Methodist
superintendent of education in Newfoundland offered further condem-
nation of the educational system: it failed to reflect the fishery, the
colony's primary occupation. "It must be admitted that the contribution
made by the schools to that great enterprise is almost negligible. It is
true, of course, that the young people learn to read and are in this way
enabled to obtain for themselves any information made public; but for
a fishing country that should not be deemed sufficient."[11] The education
system failed to recognize the way in which wealth was generated in the
colony and did not address who benefited from the labours of fishermen.
Many families could not afford to have their male children engage in
more than a few years of education.

Furthermore, a religious denominational education system had been
formally enshrined in the colony long before the passage of its 1874 Education Act, which provided a further division of the Protestant grant.
Among other things, the research of educational historian Phillip Mc-
Cann concluded that the "strength of the [denominational] system to a
large extent mirrored the weakness of the state insofar as the latter was
unwilling to undertake the direction and planning of education and
many of the other functions normally undertaken by a secular bureaucracy."[12] Denominational competition in the colony's education system
led to increased duplication and a waste of scarce resources. The best
of the system was reserved for the St John's secondary colleges whose
students, in the majority, represented the privileged classes. Most fishing
families, on the other hand, were scattered over 6,000 miles of coastline
where settlement reflected the patterns of work.

In most of Labrador and northern Newfoundland, there were only
rudimentary educational services in this period. On the north coast of
Labrador, the Moravian missionaries provided elementary schooling
(essentially freeing the colony from responsibility), but the educational

needs of the children on Labrador's "forgotten coast," from Cape
Charles to Sandwich Bay, received less attention.[13] In 1905 William
MacGregor was the first governor to visit the region; he recommended
more schools and teachers for the Europeans and settlers in southern
Labrador.[14] That year there were 425 students in eighteen communities
from Blanc Sablon to Cartwright.[15] By 1921, the census for the colony
determined that the average population of Labrador's 103 settlements
was twenty-six residents. Yet the Department of Education then maintained schools only for four or five months where there was a population
of thirty people. Schools were therefore available in only 16 of the
larger settlements, or 16 per cent of Labrador communities.[16] An itinerant teacher with the Methodist Board in Labrador in the 1920s, for
example, was at "North West River for four months, travelled to Butter
and Snow for three weeks, Grand Lake for two weeks, Kenemich for
three or four weeks, and Sebaskachu and perhaps Mulligan too."[17]
Maud Chaulk lived at Mulligan, and she remembered "the teacher
would come from Newfoundland for six weeks of the year."[18]

In 1903, an Education Act allowed for the creation of "amalgamated
schools in sparsely populated settlements where the number of children
will not warrant the establishment of separate schools."[19] Such schools
would be established on the recommendation of the denominational
Boards of Education and with the approval of their superintendents.
The first amalgamated school was built in 1908 in the industrial town
of Grand Falls, a sign that denominationalism was irrelevant to the new
capitalists. One of the original promoters of the school was Thomas
Judge, an American from Maine who sought to replicate the American
public education system at Grand Falls. By 1927–28 the Bureau of Education reported the Grenfell mission was operating amalgamated
schools at St Anthony and North West River: they were two of nine
amalgamated schools under the jurisdiction of the Bureau of Education
at that time.[20]

Henry Gordon, the Church of England minister at Cartwright, was
to launch an effort to build the first public school in Labrador.[21] One
of the men Gordon relied on in his discussions about education was
Charlie Bird, a Labradorian who shared Gordon's vision for an improved system of education in Labrador.[22] However, some Labradorians

later recalled the role of the Grenfell mission in education in terms that point to differing notions of cultural capital. Ben Best, born at Mud Lake in 1923, offered a succinct analysis of the value of institutional cultural capital in those days: "There was nothing to do if you did get an education. Like the boys they'd go and start workin' in the woods and the girls would go and try to get jobs as servant girls, maybe with the Grenfell Mission."[23] Fellow Labradorian Ben Powell, on the other hand, placed a priority on institutional capital and the availability of schooling for the development of the coast. "Our greatest problem," he wrote, "was education. We didn't have the benefit or the opportunity that some people had ... where the Grenfell Mission, in the early days, done that spading that resulted in schools."[24]

Indeed, Grenfell was harshly critical of the education system, and he was not alone. Newfoundland native Arthur Barnes, who was to become the first minister of education in the colony, concluded in 1917 – echoing Superintendent Vincent Burke – that Newfoundland was "non-progressive" in education and depended on the philanthropy of religious and secular organizations such as the Newfoundland School Society, the Society for the Propagation of the Gospel, and the Benevolent IrishSociety.[25] According to historian William Hamilton, Grenfell was an articulate critic of the denominational education system as being inefficiently organized, fostering ignorance, and diminishing the students' interest in continued learning.[26] Not only did Grenfell view sectarianism as one of Newfoundland's three great evils, James Hiller noted, but he also thought the colonial denominational education was "medieval."[27]

Grenfell's beliefs about education initially reflected his muscular Christianity, a source of athleticism, anti-intellectualism, and esprit de corps that permeated the British public schools and was a leading propaganda tool for British imperialism.[28] "Education as we see it," he wrote, "means the training that enables one most completely to correspond to one's environment, together with the development of a healthy body, and primarily of a spirit which makes living to serve the world the first objective."[29] Subsequently, the Grenfell mission adopted a broad definition of education. It held summer schools in coastal communities; circulated travelling libraries; organized socials and formed Boy Scout and Girl Guide troops;

arranged adult classes; opened non-denominational schools; and co-ordinated participation by young men and women from the North in training and career programs in the United States, Canada, and Great Britain. General studies of education in the region do not discuss all these IGA efforts but do acknowledge the full-time IGA schools. George Hickman stated that there were four schools under the direction of the IGA, and that the association largely financed the educational effort.[30]

On one occasion, Grenfell attempted to intervene on behalf of the non-denominational approach of his mission. Ruth Keese, a young teacher from Massachusetts, had come north in 1910 to introduce kindergarten methods at St Anthony but encountered difficulties with the government. Grenfell wrote Prime Minister E.P. Morris about the status of Miss Keese's teaching certificate. William Blackall, the super-intendent of the Church of England schools, investigated the matter on behalf of the prime minister and noted that Miss Keese had not declared her denomination. "Until the Education Act is amended," Blackall wrote, "it will be impossible for anyone to obtain an undemoninational certificate."[31] It was not until the next year that a two-room schoolhouse was built in St Anthony. By 1917, when Magistrate Squarey filed a re-port on complaints against the IGA (as discussed in chapters 1 and 6 in this volume), he offered a short description of the "splendid," "unde-nominational" school at St Anthony that 100 children attended at the time of his visit to the North. Squarey wrote that the Newfoundland government did not subsidize the school, and the local inn boarded the children who attended from outlying communities. Crafts were also taught at the mission industrial school. He observed that the Agricultural Department was similar to the Mount Cashel Institute, an industrial school for orphaned boys in St John's operated by the Christian Brothers of Ireland.[32]

For many years the IGA attracted well-educated and experienced professional women from the United Kingdom and Canada, and the largest group of teachers came from the United States. Some came as full-time staff members, and others volunteered their services. Higher education prepared the young women to devote at least some portion of their lives to service, and that provided them with the opportunity to move beyond traditional gender roles.[33] Elizabeth Criswell was the

principal of the Gordon School in Cartwright and outlined the purpose
of the mission school in a society where work appeared more important
than education:[34] "We hope to teach the children how to read for enjoyment and to know enough arithmetic to take care of their accounts
... but principally we want to teach the children of Labrador to love
their own country and to be ready to do their part to develop its vast
resources when the opportunity comes."[35] Research on the experiences
and views of Grenfell mission classroom teachers is beyond the scope
of this chapter; however, these educational objectives are reminiscent
of other missionary ventures in North America. In eastern Kentucky,
young Protestant women in missions to the mountain white people of
Appalachia were known as "fotched-on" women, or women from afar.
Appalachian scholar David Whisnant claims they were motivated by
cultural and revivalist values to bring mainstream middle-class American civilization to their mountain pupils, and fictional works depicted
the fotched-on women as "virtuous, high principled, Christian, altruistic, steadfast servants of mountain people – bringers of culture, morality, table manners, book-larnin'."[36]

    Katherine Reynolds and Susan Schram identified social uplift as the
focus of activities pursued by many such socially conscious outsiders,
activities that were usually located inside traditional school settings.
Religious piety, personal hygiene, morality, and basic academic subjects
were central to the uplift curriculum.[37] Historians of Appalachian mission education also use many of the same arguments as those writing
about similar efforts with Aboriginal peoples. Both recognize the sense
of cultural superiority in some of the missionaries, although one was
founded in race and the other in social class. Whether examining government and church policies or individual reformers, historians agree
that missionaries considered both Aboriginal people and Appalachian
mountaineers deficient in particular skills, including some that were
taught in their home settings. The embodied cultural capital of their
families was not recognized by the dominant culture. Given the perspective of some Grenfell mission staff, the people of the North might
be added to that list. In the opinion of Grenfell and some of his volunteers, the population of the regions was one that needed some "civiliza-

tion." Residents were therefore given instruction appropriate to a Western capitalist economy and the mores of that society.

This approach was also evident in accounts of some of the non-formal education programs in Labrador. Anthropologist John Kennedy's analysis revealed the cultural capital at play in the interactions between mission staff and local people. His informants noted that the mission "had the rule of the place," and local people were expected to obey its laws. Kennedy noted that mission staff with responsibility for social programs even imposed class-based notions of appropriate recreational activities. Staff commented that local people had no idea of party games such as "Throw the Towel" or "Going to Jerusalem," but when they were "allowed" their traditional dances at the end of the social evenings, everything changed dramatically:[38] forty-eight shuffling feet belonging to reticent party-game players rocked the floor.

Grenfell wrote in the fall of 1926 to Canon Nathaniel Noel, the Church of England clergyman at St Anthony. His letter captured the philosophies underlying the educational work at the mission and the Church of England schools.[39] He understood that Noel was telling people the quality of the Church of England one-room school in St Anthony, with a single charge teacher, far exceeded that of the Grenfell school with five teachers. If this was correct information, his critique seemed to focus on the Council of Higher Education (CHE) certification process. Noel had been heard saying, "The CHE prepares people better for fishing and domestic lives." Grenfell challenged the claim that French, algebra, and geometry fitted people for those occupations as well as did the domestic science, music, and manual training offered at the IGA school. Noel referred to only one "successful" case from the Grenfell school in St Anthony, but Grenfell named fourteen people who subsequently held positions as engineers, teachers, businessmen, industrialists, and other occupations. He also acknowledged former students who fished. Clearly, the mission provided new career opportunities for technical education: as Frederick Rowe indicated in his study, it "emphasized mechanical and manual training, particularly for Eskimo children."[40] In contrast, Canon Noel apparently sought to reproduce traditional occupational lives, claiming that was best done through a classical curriculum.

There were also residential schools in Labrador. The first one located at Muddy Bay was a project of Henry Gordon, the Anglican minister at Cartwright who wanted a public boarding school so itinerant teachers could provide children of all faiths with more than a few weeks' education each year. Dr Harry Paddon, described by Ronald Rompkey as Labrador's first nationalist, joined Gordon in his fundraising efforts.[41] Before the school opened in 1919, the region lost 23 per cent of its population during the Spanish influenza epidemic of 1918–19.[42] Some fifty children were left homeless.[43] Consequently, the building was opened as a home and boarding school. In October 1926, the Yale School opened at North West River and had between sixty and seventy scholars in 1928; in 1931, the IGA doctor in charge of Battle Harbour district, Herman Moret, established the St Mary's River (now called Mary's Harbour) Boarding School.[44]

IGA members maintained that these boarding schools were philanthropic institutions that ensured that children in the region could attend school year round, but they also reflected the sentiments heard from other North American advocates of residential schools.[45] In Paddon's view, "One hope for many of these children was to get them away from home, sad as such a conclusion was and great as were the responsibilities that went with it."[46] Janet Stewart, the housemother at Cartwright, suggested to the school's benefactor in 1933 about four children who had come to the school the previous winter, "I was anxious to keep them away from their home environment as much as possible for a few years. I am sure they will then be able to improve conditions in their own homes without much urging from us. They will be so used to living a clean, healthy life that our training is bound to tell in the long run."[47] Writing about missionaries to American Indian people, feminist historian Carol Devens argued that the Victorian standards of the missionaries similarly led them to view Aboriginal women as lazy, careless, and dirty. The residential school program indoctrinated Indian girls with the ideals of Christian womanhood: piety, domesticity, submissiveness, and purity.[48] Girls were expected to take responsibility for the cleaning, cooking, sewing, washing, and serving of food, and Devens argued that the curriculum placed greater emphasis on vocational instruction for girls than for boys. Many of the skills were useless for families who lived in tipis or lodges and would find application only for young women who worked for mission or local white families. She concluded that the underlying principle of the curriculum was that Anglo-American history, morality, and health practices were inherently superior and should replace those of the students' culture.

Residents have memories of the IGA schools that they subsequently shared in *Them Days*, a periodical of oral histories and other primary sources from Labrador. For example, although Jean Crane's family lived at North West River, and she could see her family home from the Yale School, it was expected that she would board at the dormitory when she studied there during the Second World War.[49] Finley Lemare described how Rev. Henry Gordon chastised the nurse at the Muddy Bay School for rationing out such little food that the children were often hungry: "Miss Ashbury was nice," reported Lemare, "but she didn't know any better, being from England."[50] Millicent Blake Loder left her home at Rigolet to complete her elementary schooling at the Muddy Bay School in the 1920s: "No one could understand how you could miss your family and home so much but would tell you how lucky that you were to be in a place where you could get better food and nice clothes."[51] Blanche Williams was sent by the IGA for education to the United States and later worked for the mission at the Cartwright School; when she died of pneumonia in 1934, leaving five children ranging in age from two to eleven, her last wishes were that her husband would keep the family together and not send them to a boarding school.[52] Many Labradorians offered similar insightful critiques of the embodied cultural capital of mission staff and volunteers.

In sum, in the period up to the 1920s, the government depended on the churches and missions to deliver education in the North: the Moravians took responsibility for the education of the Inuit; the churches established school services on the Northern Peninsula and the Labrador Straits. The Grenfell mission built a school at its headquarters at St Anthony, and one school board shared a portion of its school grant with the mission rather than compete with it.[53] On the south coast of Labrador, from Cape Charles to Sandwich Bay, the small, shifting populations made delivery of educational services extremely difficult. Rev. Henry Gordon's success with the first non-denominational school in

Labrador set the path for other residential schools in the region, though it would be some years before students could complete secondary schooling in Labrador.

EDUCATIONAL BROKERING AT THE MISSION

As indicated by Frederick Rowe, the IGA attempted to provide training opportunities to promising people from the North. After attracting Grenfell's attention when he offered to exchange an hour of learning for a day of work at the mission, Edgar ("Ted") McNeill of Island Harbour, Labrador, became one of the first young men from the North (and one of the most well known in the organization) to be offered free tuition at the Pratt Institute in Brooklyn, New York. The institute had been established in 1887 by Charles Pratt, an early pioneer of the natural oil industry, who recognized the growing need for trained industrial workers in a changing economy.[54] The Pratt family had supplied an electricity plant for the mission hospital at St Anthony and offered free tuition to students from the North. Other philanthropic friends of the mission supported students' transportation and living costs. Ted McNeill travelled to Brooklyn around 1908 to spend the year studying machine construction and later became the superintendent of the mission buildings.[55] He also joined the first municipal council at St Anthony in 1945 and served as a council member, chair, and vice chair. Other men and women were educated at Pratt in those early years and returned to serve at the mission. Wilfred Mesher graduated in machine construction in 1916 and then went on to receive his certificate for the electrical construction course at New York Trade School; in New York he also received advanced training in X-ray photography at St Luke's Hospital and later built a portable X-ray machine for diagnostic use on the wards of St Anthony Hospital.[56] Like Ted McNeill, Mesher would become invaluable to the mission, not only because of the high standards each man set for his own labour but also for both their efforts to support other mission programs. John Newell took courses in chemistry, soapmaking, skin tanning and dyeing, and Archie Ash took a course in electricity.[57] Wilson Jacques took a sheet metal course, and Emmie Roberts completed a dressmaking program. Ted McNeill's sister, May (McNeill) Pardy, was working at the St Anthony orphanage when the mission registered her for a domestic science course at Nasson Institute in Springvale, Maine; she returned to work for two years at the St Anthony orphanage "teaching the girls in the kitchen."[58]

In the 1920s, other coastal women studied at hospital nursing schools in the northeastern United States, including Mary Fletcher Hospital in Burlington, Vermont; Mary Hitchcock Memorial Hospital in Hanover, New Hampshire; Brightlook Hospital in St Johnsbury, Vermont; and Brooklyn Hospital in New York. Admittance to nursing schools and other education programs required high school graduation, and at that time there were no senior high school grades available in the North. These students had to complete their secondary schooling in the United States before beginning their training programs.

In 1917 Reuben Patey and Edward Green were sent to Bishop Feild College in St John's, a school operated by the Church of England, to prepare for courses at Wentworth Institute in Boston.[59] It was extremely rare for the IGA to place students in denominational schools, and records available on Patey indicate he did not stay in St John's for high school completion (see "Life Story 2" below). These are the only records found for students who went to the capital of the colony in those early years.

As the mission grew and expanded its programs, young men and women were sent out for training that would support the work at the offices, in the gardens, at the Industrial Department, and in the boarding schools, hospitals, and orphanage. Grenfell wrote that the primary objective of the supplementary technical training branch was "to use the more able young men and women as instruments for the betterment of their own land and people ... they are expected to return to the country in some capacity for two years at least, and disseminate the knowledge they have gained."[60] At the 6 May 1920 board meeting of the IGA, he reported that fourteen people had received scholarships during the past year.[61] These scholarships came from individual IGA supporters, but the next year the mission was to receive a special grant from the Carnegie Corporation of New York to support participation in education and training programs offered in the United States. Created in 1911, the CCNY was the largest of philanthropic trusts established in Andrew

Carnegie's name. Carnegie was a steel magnate with an abiding concern for "education and improvement of the poorer classes." One of his most well-known contributions to learning was the development of community libraries. He provided more than $56 million over the years to build 2,509 libraries in the United States, Canada, Great Britain, Ireland, and other British Commonwealth countries.[62] Barbara Howe argues that the overall thrust of Carnegie's philanthropy was designed to ameliorate the problems of industrial capitalism. The CCNY's main mission was "to promote the advancement and diffusion of knowledge and understanding ... by aiding technical schools, institutions of higher learning, libraries ... and by such other agencies and means as shall from time to time be found appropriate therefore."[63] The CCNY offered the IGA up to $5,000 per year for seven years beginning 1 July 1921 for scholarships for study in the United States. The selection of students would be the responsibility of the IGA Board.[64] A proviso stated that each year the IGA Board would match the funds provided by the Carnegie Corporation.

In anticipation of its success, the IGA Board decided at its 21 May 1921 meeting that organizations affiliated with the IGA would remit to the treasurer of the New England Grenfell Association any invoices or funds received for education purposes.[65] The NEGA would be responsible for bookkeeping and forwarding reports to the CCNY. By the end of that year, Anne Grenfell, Wilfred Grenfell's wife, was appointed chair of the United States Educational Committee, expanding her service to the world. Other committee members included Grenfell and Charles Watson, the business manager of the IGA. The board asked the committee to keep a register and include details about the students and their training programs in the United States, as this information would be required by the CCNY. They were also to keep records for students studying in Canada.[66]

The conditional support of matching funds posed a problem for the IGA, and on 17 December 1921 Wilfred Grenfell wrote to Dr Angell, CCNY president, indicating that at least $5,000 was already spent on education in the United States, and that the IGA would not be able to raise new funds. As evidence Grenfell attached a list of four boys and fifteen girls studying at that time and their costs.[67] He wrote, "The friends donating to the students, either for board, lodging, tuition, clothing or incidentals make it their form of contribution to the work of the IGA. The individual student is not educated for his own sake but that he may return to his country better fitted to aid in the work of bettering the conditions of his people."[68] The CCNY accepted Grenfell's proposal and agreed to make payments twice a year, up to a total of $5,000, to match the total expenditures of IGA friends, staff, students, and family members. Grenfell wrote about the "great offer" of the CCNY in the July 1922 issue of *Among the Deep Sea Fishers*.[69] This article obviously had an impact on Newfoundland readers, as Grenfell soon received correspondence from a minister at Curling, Newfoundland, who asked if the mission had a way to help finance the education of the sons of clergymen.[70]

The CCNY funding necessitated a change in the IGA managerial role. Often individual sponsors had taken responsibility for a young man or woman, providing support. Now Anne Grenfell co-ordinated the movement, registrations, reimbursements for living expenses, and perhaps even the program choices of some students. The committee requested nominations of those who should receive scholarships from a variety of individuals including Dr Paddon, Rev. Gordon, Rev. Richards of Flower's Cove, Mr LeGallais, Miss Edwards, and others.[71] Yet mission teaching staff questioned how individuals were chosen for the program. Clara McLeod first came to St Anthony as a volunteer and spent three years teaching at the Grenfell school. In the fall of 1922 she wrote to Wilfred Grenfell expressing her regret that three particular female students had not been selected for the program. They were "as capable as others who have been given the chance to get into other schools ... they have proved themselves studious and diligent."[72]

The Carnegie grant expanded the number of students who could engage in education and training programs. Every student covered by the grant was bound by a contract with the IGA. In consideration of the chance of supplementary education in the United States, the student would "return and work for his own people for a minimum of two years."[73] IGA insiders such as Charles Curtis, the medical officer in charge at St Anthony Hospital and later the superintendent of the IGA, lauded Anne's work. "She wrote hundreds of letters, begged for scholarships, studied catalogues ... No one ever worked harder for the education of the young people of the northern Newfoundland and Labrador coast than Anne Grenfell."[74] Others might debate whether the mission could represent the people of northern Newfoundland and Labrador, as Anne Grenfell proposed.

In 1923, Anne Grenfell wrote to the CCNY about those who returned to the coast from their training program in 1921–22. Her report included people now working at the hospital as nurses, aides, teachers, and an individual who established a shoemaking and cobbling business. The head of the Dietetics Department and the assistant cook at the St Anthony Hospital had also been sent for training. Grenfell was very aware of her cultural capital, and at times her correspondence seemed to victimize local people for the failures of the colonial government. "There is no compulsory education in this country and the effect of this on the young people has in too many cases been to leave them very lazy in regard to such matters, as even the simplest rudiments of education."[75]

By 1924, the IGA had created an education department on the recommendation of Harriet Houghteling,[76] who had first come to the mission in 1911 at the urging of Anne Grenfell, her childhood friend from Chicago. She worked as a volunteer for many summers, was the orphanage superintendent in the winter of 1921, and the director of staff selection in 1923. Houghteling married Dr Charles Curtis in 1929 and spent most of her years at the mission involved in education.[77] When Anne Grenfell was abroad, Harriet took on her responsibilities. On at least one occasion, she joined Anne for a meeting with officials of the CCNY.

The report prepared for the CCNY in 1926–27 listed twenty-seven students who were engaged in training programs in the United States. Most studied in institutional settings, though there were some exceptions. After completing a year of study in the plumbing course at Wentworth Technical Institute in 1925–26, a student returned to the United States to apprentice for a year with a master plumber. Dr Joel Goldthwait, a long-time supporter of the mission, organized a splint and appliance-making course for one of the students at a Boston hospital. Nursing training occurred at various hospitals on the eastern seaboard.

Fourteen (52 per cent) of the students were male and thirteen (48 per cent) were female. Though it may appear that the leadership of Anne

Grenfell and Harriet Houghteling ensured a near-equal representation of each gender, many essential jobs at the mission were considered women's work at that time. That year, the largest numbers of female students were engaged in nursing programs, and high school completion attracted the most male students. Students also trained as missionaries, at schools of domestic science, agriculture, occupational therapy, and in business colleges. Twenty-six per cent of the group were from Labrador, and the remainder were from mission communities on the Northern Peninsula. Eleven per cent resided full-time at the St Anthony Orphanage. The institution that attracted the largest group of students was Berea College, with 19 per cent of the students attending the college that year. More discussion of Berea College appears later in this chapter.

Payments from the Carnegie grant started in 1921–22 when Wilfred Grenfell presented the CCNY with the list of students then studying in the United States. The seventh and last year of the grant was 1927–28. According to the report filed at the CCNY, thirty-one students engaged in education programs that year. Sixty-five per cent of that group had been involved in training in 1926–27. They continued their course of study or entered a new program. Ten per cent of the students in 1927–28 resided at the St Anthony orphanage. Just over 50 per cent were from the island. Twenty (65 per cent) of the students were female and eleven (35 per cent) were male. The largest occupational training group for women was still nursing, which represented 25 per cent of registrations. There was less concentration in specific occupational groups for men, although 18 per cent were involved in training for religious life (see table 8.1).

The final report provided Anne Grenfell with an opportunity to reflect on the benefits of the CCNY program for a country with an "antiquated" system of denominational education. She felt the training programs had a modernizing influence on the students and made them more useful to the mission: "They have brought home very different standards and ideals of living than they could have acquired otherwise, and their own people would naturally be more influenced by their report and their teaching than they could be by that of the staff of the Grenfell Association, who are after all in most cases not of their own country."[78] Her assessment of the impact of the educational intervention was favourable.

The evaluation distinguishes between those staff who had come to serve the mission, and those the mission trained to serve.

In 1927–28, Anne Grenfell noted that eighty-nine students had benefited from the fund and eighty had returned. Students had achieved senior high school grades and trained as teachers, nurses, in domestic science, trade, and technical programs. Using language reminiscent of her father's Civil War battle experiences, she wrote that one encouraging aspect of the education work "has been the almost negligible number of young people who have deserted their own country, even if they have received a training which would enable them to make much more money in the US or Canada than they can ever hope to do in Newfoundland."[79] She believed the IGA had instilled their philosophy of service to the world, particularly in the students' own communities.

Since most of the educational institutions that the students from northern Newfoundland and Labrador attended were located on the eastern seaboard of the United States, students were placed in close proximity to friends of the mission, and those studying in the New York or Boston area could access the offices of the Grenfell Association of America and the New England Grenfell Association. In 1920 Wilfred Grenfell was to discover Berea College, located at the foot of the Appalachian Mountains in Berea, Kentucky. The college was founded in 1855 as the first interracial college in America, but by the turn of the century there was a growing hostility towards social equality of the races and decreasing philanthropic interest in interracial education.[80] Berea consequently amended its constitution and made Appalachia its sole field of service. By 1913, five distinct departments had been established at the college under the leadership of President William Frost: the College; Normal School; Academy; Vocational School; and Foundation School. These departments took students at various points in their learning, from the elementary grades to a four-year college degree.

Fireside Industries at Berea College did work similar to that of the Industrial Department of the IGA, and the *Berea Citizen* reported that Grenfell had come to Berea in the "interest of the weaving industry which he is establishing among his people."[81] Minnie Pike of the Industrial Department at Red Bay, Labrador, spent a year at Berea studying

Table 8.1

Educational activity supported by CCNY by educational program/
institutional setting and gender, 1926-1928

Program type	Male	Female	Total for 1926–27	Male	Female	Total for 1927–28	Grand total 1926–28
Secondary school	5	2	7	2	2	4	11
Trades and technical schools / programs	3	1	4	3	1	4	8
Nursing school		5	5		5	5	10
Business college					3	3	3
Domestic science programs		1	1		3	3	4
School of occupational therapy		1	1		1	1	2
Seminaries / missionary training	3		3	2		2	5
Hospital training – splint and appliance making	1		1				1
Berea – industrial programs		2	2		1	1	3
Berea – academic programs	2	1	3	3	4	7	10
University				1		1	1
TOTAL*	14	13	27	11	20	31	58

*Actual registrations, not individuals. Derived from BCHL student registration records, Education Committee reports to IGA Board of Directors; CCNY, IGA reports.

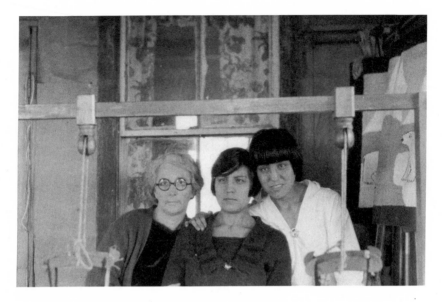

Figure 8.1 Minnie Pike and the "blind twins" Clara and Marnie Morris.
PAD, IGA Photograph Collection, VA 118-240

weaving with Anna Ernberg, the director of Fireside Industries (figure 8.1). In 1921, J. Ed Davis of Berea went north at Grenfell's request to make new looms, alter old ones, and assist in the industrial program in the community houses.[82] Edith Tallant, an industrial worker with the White Bay Unit, described the women of Kentucky and the North as "sister spinners" for "their use of old English words and songs retained from common Anglo-Saxon forbears, their handicap in book learning, their absolutely selfless devotion and sacrifice for their large families, their easy going way of granting supremacy to the man of the household."[83] This was how the dominant culture viewed the women. Like Labrador, Appalachia also was perceived as a strange land whose residents included a Protestant, Anglo-Saxon, native-born population. Grenfell described the college as "a wonderful uplifting machine."[84] He wasn't just building a relationship with an educational provider. At Berea, he found men and women who shared his ideology.

In this period, the IGA registered twenty students in formal programs at Berea (table 8.2). At the time of entry, the youngest student to register at Berea was 14, and the oldest was 33. The average age was 20.5. *Them*

Table 8.2
Berea College, 1920–1930: Educational level at program exit

Program	Male	Female	Total
Foundation (elementary/junior high)	2	5	7
Academy (high school)	4	3	7
Vocational programs		3	3
Normal school			
College	1	2	3
Non-formal programs at Fireside		4	4
Industries (no registration record)			
Total	7	17	24

BCHL Newfoundland student registration records

Days and *Among the Deep Sea Fishers* provided the names of other people who attended the college. At least three of these women were active with the Industrial Department at Red Bay. The fourth had written a letter from Berea to her brother in Labrador.[85] Not all of the Newfoundland students at Berea were from the North. A woman from Pool's Cove, Newfoundland, completed normal school and a year of college at Berea as a result of her involvement with the Newfoundland Outport Nursing and Industrial Association in Fortune Bay.[86] A woman from Westport, White Bay South, also registered for a one-year vocational program in 1924. It is possible she was affiliated with the hospital at Pilley's Island.

Eighteen registered students were sent to Berea from the North, one third from Labrador. The majority of the students were working towards their high school completion. Rhoda Dawson, a painter from Britain who came as a volunteer with the Industrial in December 1930, described one of the women who participated in the Foundation program at Berea "as a true artist. Her taste was impeccable – far too good for the tourist trade on which the Mission depended."[87] One of the college students, Horace McNeill, was to become an integral part of the mission in his role as assistant superintendent.[88] Another graduate of the academy was on the honour role at Berea and the recipient of a number of scholastic awards. A review of staff lists published in *Among the Deep Sea Fishers* for this period suggests that at least 44 per cent of the Northern students at Berea returned to work with the mission (figure 8.2).

The IGA had always hoped the CCNY scholarship would be renewed. Anne Grenfell raised the possibility of a grant from Carnegie that might support younger students and discussed future funding possibilities with President Frederick P. Keppel at a 13 December 1927 meeting at the CCNY offices. Keppel's notes on the meeting indicate that Lady Grenfell had stated that there was "a real cleavage between north and south in Newfoundland, and that St John's was completely apathetic to the needs of the north." These dismissals led to a firm response from Keppel. He asked if the IGA was prepared to recognize the existing machinery of government and to work with them towards a common end. In that instance, two Americans were debating the role of government in a British dominion. The potential plan was not developed, although Anne did continue the program in 1928–29. She forwarded a copy of the annual report to Keppel in 1929.[89] At that time, twenty-two students were "under the care of the Education Department."[90] In May of that same year, Anne resigned from her position with the Education Committee.

At the beginning of the relationship between the organizations, the IGA might have been seen as embodying Carnegie's philosophy. James Angell, president of the CCNY from 1920 to 1921, believed a "giving corporation" should be "a human agency seeking out the great and significant causes."[91] Some tensions arose over the course of the grant about personalities and institutional interests in Newfoundland and New York. Keppel, CCNY president from 1923 to 1941, was known to prefer alliances with groups dominated and controlled by men, who in his view were more likely than women to hold professional status.[92] Other tensions were revealed between educational officials in Newfoundland and the mission. In fact, Keppel had already decided the next step would involve the colonial government.

Vincent Burke, the first deputy minister of the Department of Education, was no stranger to the CCNY. He had been involved in negotiations for funding of a new college in Newfoundland for a few years. In fact, Burke travelled to the mainland and New York so often that the college principal, John Lewis Paton, jokingly wrote to Burke that an Order of the British Empire in his name would mean "Out by Express."[93]

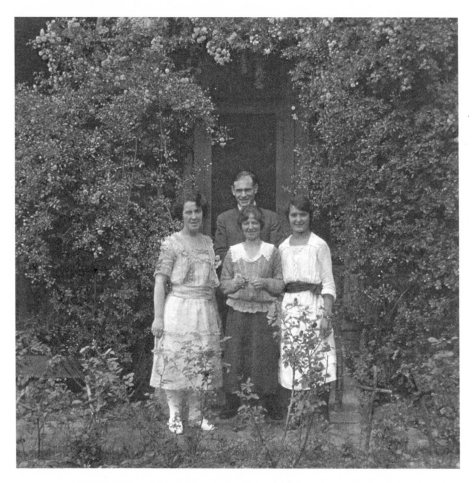

Figure 8.2 Students at Berea College, Kentucky, 1922: Ethel Pye, Susan Crombie, Phyllis Blake, William Clark. PAD, IGA Photograph Collection, 1-412

Burke became more focused on the educational work of the Grenfell mission, particularly after he became chair of the Board of Trustees at Memorial University College in 1925. His interest may have been prompted by philosophical differences between the more traditional classical education system in the colony and that of American progressive educators, such as John Dewey, who placed student experience at the core of the pedagogy. Dewey's thinking influenced the American teachers at the mission schools. Burke's widening institutional gaze might also have revealed a desire to harness the resources that the mission had been able to attract.

In an interview with Keppel on 15 November 1927 about the Memorial University College grant, Burke outlined the difficulties they were experiencing in raising the sum required by the CCNY. Keppel spoke about the IGA grant and asked Burke if he thought that money might be diverted to adult education work at Memorial University College. He also asked about feelings between the "natives and Grenfell Commission." Burke replied, "While there had been somewhat of a rift, since the knighting of Grenfell and subsequent support of newspapers of Newfoundland, this had lessened."[94] The next day Burke spoke to CCNY staff member Robert Lester and proposed alternative scenarios for the $5,000 annual grant that had been given to the IGA. It is not clear that Burke had the Northern population in mind when he suggested that the money could be used to establish short courses for fishermen and scholarships for top-notch Memorial University College students. There was no clear explanation of how short courses could be delivered in scattered coastal communities or how many students were at the college from Labrador at that time.[95] In February 1928 Keppel indicated that his Board would be interested in a joint proposal from the government and the IGA for $35,000 in the interest of education in Labrador.[96] This proposal was never written but, with the support of the CCNY, Burke began a new career in adult education with the Department of Education and was to obtain Carnegie grants for that work on the island.

In the summer of 1928, with the knowledge of the IGA Board, Memorial University College President Paton undertook a study of the IGA's educational work during a northern field trip that was financed by the CCNY. He visited mission operations at Spotted Islands, Indian Harbour, Battle Harbour, and the headquarters at St Anthony. He spoke with medical staff, mission WOPs and volunteers, and teachers in both the Grenfell and public education system. One objective was to obtain information on the administration of the Carnegie grant. He was unable to obtain written reports, as Anne Grenfell was not on the coast, but was told of several cases of returned students who "were making a splendid contribution to the life of the community from which they had sprang" since returning from the United States.[97] However, Paton was unwilling to write any report based on "hearsay evidence." Over the fall and in the winter of 1929, he gathered the information he needed, much of it from the staff of the IGA schools.

By May 1929 Paton's report "Education on the Labrador" had been sent to the CCNY.[98] At that time, there were three agencies engaged in educational provision: the Bureau of Education, through the Denominational School Boards; the Moravian mission; and the International Grenfell Association. There was no history of liaison or co-operation between the groups, but Paton did not see that as serious problem for the Moravians, who were dealing with a racially distinct and geographically separate population. "South of Hopedale," wrote Paton, the lack of co-operation could lead to waste and ignorance of each other's work, and both sides recognized that the current situation was undesirable and were willing to co-operate.

In his report, Paton called for a special curriculum for Labrador. The schools would supply knowledge related to and growing out of the immediate environment while providing opportunities to enlarge the students' outlook on the world. According to Paton, the curriculum developed by the CHE reflected the perspective of urban males and was designed for those who sought professional careers or commercial lives. The IGA schools, Paton noted, had not sacrificed the practical interests of the community and placed emphasis on community gardens, woodwork, domestic science, crafts, and nature work. Paton recommended that five large residential schools be located at St Anthony, Forteau, Cartwright, North West River, and St Mary's River. The schools would serve all denominations and hire teachers who represented those faiths. Students from eleven to fifteen years of age would attend from October to June, and children from seven to eleven years would be schooled from June to September. The girls would "render service in the houses, and make and mend their own dresses." The boys would "chop wood ... manage cattle, mend boots and generally be 'handy men.'"[99] The children would also receive training in arts and crafts, which Paton identified as a strength of the IGA system, which at that time generated $49,000 in business.[100] Such a system would provide continuous training in health habits, manners, morals, and religion. It was a social uplift curriculum, reminiscent of the work of the lay missionaries of Appalachia. Though the report does not comment on the proposed balance between work and study, Michael Coleman and other historians have documented the "half-and-half" model of the Indian residential school system. Half of the day was spent on academic instruction, which included the 3 Rs, history, geography, and religion, and the other half was spent on labour.[101]

In a section of the report on scholarships, Paton reviewed Anne Grenfell's work with the recent grant from the Carnegie Corporation. He understood that the mission had trained foremen of masonry work, plumbing, electrical fitting, and agriculture; a teacher and the heads of the Martha Gibbs and Willis Wood Home at the Yale School at North West River; and the forewoman of the Industrial work. Paton suggested, however, that scholarships might have also supported education and training for doctors, fishermen, clergy, foresters, and surveyors, and in rope and sail making. He also indicated that without an Intermediate Honours diploma or its equivalent, teachers returning from Berea qualified only for the lowest grade of certificate under the Education Act of 1927. Should the Northerners come to the normal school at St John's, a grant of $360 per annum for two years would enable a student to pass the junior matriculation and then attend normal school, which at that time consisted of six months of training. A grant of $440 per year would enable a student to take the first two years of a university course in science or arts, which would also qualify the candidate for a teacher's certificate with university grade. Students could also attend such sites as Truro Agricultural College in Nova Scotia or other Canadian technical institutes. Paton investigated fisheries training as well. "As for a young fisherman, I do not know of any place which provides a suitable course … on this continent, except Halifax, NS."[102]

The report also covered adult education, a subject of increasing interest to the CCNY, and libraries, the legacy of Andrew Carnegie. Paton ended by praising the Grenfell workers. He shared Grenfell's view that Labrador "needs the helping hand from without to enable it to fulfil itself."[103] At times, Paton's report reads like a testimony to the mission, and at others as a bid to educate the Northern students.

By the late 1920s, Wilfred Grenfell had suffered his first heart attack. He seemed more motivated to co-operate with the St John's authorities, which would result in more state funds for education in the North. Yet the mission did not have a long history of working with a single institution like Memorial University College, which focused on a classical curriculum. Students commonly studied in the home communities of mission supporters or in institutions that forged relationships with the mission by offering free tuition or scholarships. Paton's allusion to the Truro Agricultural College is undoubtedly a reference to James Tucker of St Anthony, who was a 1928 graduate of its two-year program; however, it would not have been covered by the CCNY grant, which was given to support study at American institutions.[104] In separate correspondence, Paton addressed the question of why the mission was sending students to Berea College. Lady Grenfell had told Paton that the mission valued the tone of the institution, the practical training, and the students it served. The cost at $150 per annum for board and tuition also made it more economical than St John's.[105] With these explanations, Paton supported her choice. By the end of the 1920s, therefore, internal changes, external pressures, and changing personnel pushed the IGA toward more cooperation with colonial authorities.

LIFE HISTORIES

The experiences of a few of the men and women who trained in occupations with the support of the IGA have been published in their own accounts or documented in other sources. These accounts allow a fuller understanding of students' career paths and provide important reflections on their relationships with the IGA. A significant example was Millicent Blake Loder, who trained to be a nurse. The following description, distilled from two of her autobiographical publications, reveal a lifetime connection to the IGA that provided her with particular insights into the nature of class relationships that characterized mission interactions with local people.[106]

Millicent Blake Loder was born in Labrador in 1915 to John and Jemima (Oliver) Blake. In the summer, the family lived at Rigolet and in the winter moved to Double Mer, close to John Blake's traplines. Millicent first went to school at about eight years old, studying with a

Newfoundland teacher who came to Rigolet to teach for a few weeks with the Church of England School Board. The next year she wintered with family friends so she could attend full-time school at Rigolet. At the age of ten, she travelled to the boarding school at Muddy Bay. On arrival, the head mistress instructed that Millicent be inspected for head lice, bathed, and dressed in decent clothing. Millicent was saddened, knowing that her family was not poor and that her mother had insisted she take the best clothing the family had. From the perspective of Bourdieu's framework, her family lacked the cultural capital of the dominant society, an attitude noted by Loder: "The staff were good to us, but always let us know that we were not their equals. The staff came from abroad and felt themselves to be missionaries, trying to bring a bit of England to the Labrador world."[107] Her happiest hours at the Muddy Bay School were spent in the library.

After completing Grade 6, Millicent went to the school at St Anthony, which offered the highest level of schooling available in the North at that time. It was a welcoming environment, and Millicent felt like she was with family. Students who boarded at the orphanage sat at the dining table with Miss Karpick, the superintendent, and her helpers – quite a different arrangement from the one Millicent had experienced at Muddy Bay. The principal of the school and Millicent's teacher was Miss Frances Baiers, an American whom Millicent remembered with love and affection, an outsider she could relate to as a friend. The next year Millicent was sick with typhoid fever and spent a long time as a hospital patient. Miss Baiers worked with her on Saturdays to catch up on the school material she had missed; when the CHE results were announced, Millicent had passed with honours.

Millicent was fourteen years old when she left St Anthony and took a position in 1929 as a servant girl at the IGA Hospital in North West River for fifty cents a month. There she saw many displays of class privilege: "There was one other job for the staff girls, making butter balls. There were two little paddles with grooves in them and a pattern on one side. You dipped the paddles in ice water and placed a blob of butter on them, then rolled it around to form little balls with a pattern on them. I bit my tongue to keep from asking what difference it would make. For supper the staff would dress and the staff girl would have to wear a black dress with a frilly apron and a little white headdress."[108] She had many occasions to observe how staff worked in the hospital, and Dr Paddon told her the mission would help to train her as a nurse in America. By that time she was eighteen, making $5.00 a month, and knew it would be impossible to finance her own education. In 1933, Millicent was offered living space by a nurse at the North West River Hospital who was heading home to Madison, Wisconsin. She studied in Madison for her secondary school diploma and surpassed her own expectations by being inducted into the National Honours Society.

Millicent was accepted at St Luke's Hospital School for Nurses in Duluth, Minnesota, for January 1937. She paid for her own tuition from her earnings as a hospital cleaner that previous fall, and for the next three years she worked twelve-hour shifts every day for six days a week. One doctor who recognized the realities of Millicent's future practice had her help with all his deliveries so that she would have experience with difficult births. In the spring of her final year, Millicent wrote to the IGA in New York about her interest in returning to work with the IGA in Labrador after her graduation. She accepted a position at Cartwright for a salary of $315 and was later posted to the hospital at St Anthony.

As the only nurse from either Newfoundland or Labrador on staff at that time, Millicent noticed how differently outsiders treated her. In Bourdieu's formulation, she now had institutionalized capital and was seen by other IGA staff as a member of the dominant society, while some of her relatives or friends "were looked down upon." Millicent reflected on this situation: "I soon concluded that the Mission was missing a golden opportunity by sticking to their own group ... The IGA did not make the most of their opportunities to educate the people about health matters."[109] She clearly knew the value of the local cultural capital that the outsiders ignored. She would continue to provide nursing services in Labrador, either as a volunteer or paid staff member until her retirement in 1980.

The life stories of Nathan Budgell, Reuben Patey, and Hazel Hart afford additional perspectives on the role of the IGA in their education and training, and again most importantly, on the impact of the IGA in cultural capital and social interactions with local residents. In each case, the IGA appears at times in a somewhat negative light: one person was dismissed, apparently with little cause or empathy; another decided not to study at the school for which he had been selected; and another was badly treated by a teacher associated with the IGA in Ontario. At the same time, these life stories demonstrate the resilience, talents, and achievements of those whom the IGA aided in achieving their educational and career goals. (See Life Stories 1 to 3 below.)

Though the life stories of Millicent Blake Loder, Nathan Budgell, Reuben Patey, and Hazel Compton Hart do not represent the experiences of all of those trained by the IGA, they demonstrate how individual interests, families, and significant role models helped shape the long-term occupational and career interests of some children who resided in the North. All took advantage of further education, and this experience included both great hardship and instances of kindness and support. Most afterward pursued their lives in the locations they called home. While likely grateful for the opportunities provided by the IGA and other outsiders, many probably shared Hazel Compton's appreciation for the "really grand" people of their own communities and the local cultural capital prevalent in the region.

EDUCATION AT THE IGA

There has been limited scholarly work on the education efforts of the IGA in the first decades of the twentieth century. At that time, northern Newfoundland and Labrador was squeezed between the Old World imperialism of Grenfell and the modern imperialist notions of mission supporters in the United States. Lennox Kerr, a Grenfell biographer, wrote, "It was fascinating that the people of the United States responded to appeals by an Englishman for the benefit of the people of an English colony."[110] Even the *New York Times* regarded the mission as an American institution and characterized the work as one of the great adventures of the twentieth century.[111]

Exploring the contributions and tensions of the educational work with an American foundation funder, a bureaucratic representative of the government, and some recipients of programs inside and outside

LIFE STORY 1

A Northern Farmer: Nathan Budgell

Nathan Budgell was born in Brown's Cove, White Bay, in 1912 to Peter and Susan (Langford) Budgell. In those years, Nathan wrote, "education, as we view it today was considered unnecessary, as hard work requiring only physical effort provided the necessities of life."[a] The family moved to Springdale when his father began work for a contractor supplying wood to the Grand Falls paper mill. Peter died after contracting pneumonia in the woods camp, an indication that the jobs of the new industrial economy were no less hazardous than the fishing boat.

In the fall of 1915 Nathan was brought to the orphanage at St Anthony with his brothers, Peter and George. There he would eventually meet Christine Fellows, a horticulturist from England. She travelled to St Anthony in 1921, 1923, and 1924 to initiate and develop the mission's agriculture program. Nathan spent those summers weeding, hoeing, and harvesting the crops. He wrote that many of the residents of the orphanage received technical training in the United States, but in 1924 Fellows asked Nathan if he would like to go to England. He attended school there and continued his interest in agriculture through school programs, summer work on local farms and estates, and touring the Continent with Miss Fellows. In 1928, he began a program at Chadacre Agricultural Institute in Bury St Edmunds, Suffolk. Endowed by the Earl of Iveagh, the institute provided free agricultural education that combined lectures on agricultural science and manual instruction in farming practices.[b] Nathan wrote Dr Grenfell from Chadacre Hall, describing the farm and the program, which included "milking, butter making, dairying, veterinary work, horse shoeing, harness mending ... we have lectures on soils and manures, poultry keeping and dairying, implements, farm accounts, mensuration and surveying, the chemistry of science and medicines for sick cattle."[c] He graduated from the institute in the spring of 1930.

Nathan then went to the IGA office in London, where he met Sir Wilfred, William Job, who was retired from the Job Brothers firm and living in England, and Katie Spalding, the IGA office manager. Nathan was offered a job at North West River at $500 a year, a reasonably good salary at that time. After his arrival in Labrador, he wondered why the farm had not been established at Mud Lake. Fifty acres of land were cleared at that location, and the microclimate registered high temperatures for growing. In his first year at North West River, Nathan cleared four acres of land with the assistance of the Aboriginal people who camped in the area in the summer months. This was planted for animal fodder, and the grass at Mud Lake was cut for hay. He also planted a vegetable garden for winter use containing potatoes, turnip, and cabbage. Three milking cows were forwarded from St Anthony, and Nathan requested that a bull be sent before freeze-up. It was landed at Rigolet but lost overboard on the trip to North West River. Another disaster occurred when huskies gnawed their way through the barn and killed one of the station's five pigs. Though pesticides had been ordered in the fall of 1930, they did not arrive, and Nathan was hesitant to plant cabbages in the spring. He began by transplanting 200 seedlings and, seeing no damage, planted 300 more ten days later. Only fifty plants would survive the infestation of grubs after three weeks. Though other seasonal plans were on schedule, Paddon fired Nathan. Devastated, Nathan wrote Grenfell, who responded with a note that God had work for him in St Anthony. Nathan received Grenfell's correspondence around freeze-up, and as it was too late in the season to travel to the Northern Peninsula, he trapped that winter. He later travelled overland to St Mary's, boarded the SS *Sagona* for the trip to Flower's Cove, and walked most of the journey to St Anthony in the spring of 1932.

Nathan would work at the St Anthony mission garden and farm from 7 a.m. to 6 p.m. each day. The pay was $1.80 a day until the mission scaled back and paid for labour with a voucher from the IGA's Spot Cash Store. Nathan had no money, not even enough to purchase a postage stamp for a card to Miss Fellows. Charles Curtis, physician to the St Anthony Hospital, provided him with a small cash allowance but with the worsening effects of the Depression advised him that he might be better off in Canada.

Nathan followed his advice and in the spring of 1933 found his way to Ontario and worked at various jobs. In 1935, using an inheritance gift he received from Miss Fellows's estate, he registered at the Ontario Veterinary College and graduated in 1939 as a doctor of veterinary medicine.

It is unclear why Paddon dismissed Budgell, but his case demonstrates that the mission did not have an effective operational plan for graduates of the technical program. Paddon had an intense interest in his "sub-artic Garden Of Eden" and may have resented Grenfell's intrusion in the mission farm and the salary paid to Budgell.[e] By that point, American agronomist Fred Sears was the chief advisor for the IGA agriculture program and spent extensive time at North West River. Jim Tucker had been trained at Truro Agricultural College for the farm at St Anthony, and Jacob Compton, also a graduate from Truro, was at St Mary's River. Finally, increased financial pressure in the 1930s may have made IGA officials less patient with slow progress. Curtis's encouragement to Nathan to leave Labrador was certainly a departure from earlier IGA policy that urged northern men and women to use their education in their own country.

NOTES

[a] Budgell, *Newfoundland Son*.

[b] Chadacre Agricultural Trust.

[c] Budgell, "From a Newfoundland Agricultural Student."

[d] Budgell, *Newfoundland Son*, 50.

[e] Harry Paddon was raised by his grandfather Van Sommer to tend and nurture plants. He was particularly interested in producing food for the mission: Paddon, *Labrador Memoir*, 213.

LIFE STORY 2

I Aim Higher Than a Narrow Education: Reuben Patey

Reuben Patey was born in St Anthony in 1899 and grew up in a family of five boys. Patey's schooling plans changed when he enlisted in the Newfoundland Regiment. While he was training at Aldershot, England, he contracted pneumonia and was unable to travel to Sulva Bay to engage in the Gallipoli Campaign.[a] Returning to Newfoundland, he worked at the mission offices and along with Edward Green went to Bishop Feild College in St John's for the 1916–17 school year.[b] Reuben and Edward were two of the rare northerners who were sent out by the mission for training at a denominational school in St John's.

In October 1919 Reuben registered at Tilton School in New Hampshire, graduating from the program in June 1921.[c] The institution was founded as a secondary school for boys and girls in 1845 and now functions as an independent college preparatory school serving students from the ninth to the twelfth grade. There were four choices available in the differentiated curriculum at the time Reuben attended the school: Classical, Latin Scientific, English Scientific, and Business.[d] Like many other of the northern students, Reuben did well at Tilton, not only academically, but also socially. He held many leadership positions with a secret society known as the United Knights Panoplian, served as the vice president of the YMCA, and was a member of the Boys Student Council.

Even outside his own environment, Reuben already displayed the kind of leadership abilities the IGA favoured. Perhaps this trait, likely an example of embodied local cultural capital, singled him out for further training. IGA teachers and administrators may have recognized a young man with the ability and personality to serve the world well. In fact, Reuben had developed a strong sense of his own abilities and, while accepting much of the Grenfell ideology, was determined to have a say in the type of education he wanted and how it would be used.

In 1922 he wrote to Wilfred Grenfell explaining that he would not be registering for the educational program that the mission had selected for him that fall.

I carefully considered my situation, the possibilities of serving the world, and the time and money involved at Burdett
College and thought I could do better. I came to the conclusion that it would be more profitable for me if I worked for a
year or two during the days and studied during the evenings.
By doing that I could save some money and also prepare
myself to enter some larger college ... I think a good solid
general education ... will be better for me in the long run
than business training ... I think a person at my age ... should
aim higher than a narrow education.[e]

It was an independent decision, Reuben wrote, and he hoped
Grenfell would understand and approve of his action. He then went
to work with the Vacuum Oil Company in New York for two years,
returned home to St Anthony to work with his family for a year,
and in 1926 entered Columbia University. That same year he began
his long career with the New York Trust Company.

Reuben served as a director of the Grenfell Association of
America and was on their executive committee for more than
thirty years. He wrote a few articles for *Among the Deep Sea Fishers,* and Elizabeth, his American wife, acted as a Grenfell representative and hostess on a cruise on the Northern *Voyager* in 1936.
Grenfell often visited the Patey family at their home in White
Fields, New York.

In January 1939 Reuben wrote to Grenfell proposing a business
venture that would involve fishermen at St Anthony.[f] He developed
a comprehensive business plan to produce a top-quality cured
fish product for sale on the New York market at almost twice the
price the fishermen would receive locally.[g] While he pursued his
own career ambitions, he did not forget his home. Reuben Patey's
service to the world included this effort to double the income
of fishers at St Anthony and promote Newfoundland in the
United States.

NOTES

[a] Delatour, "Reuben Henry Patey."

[b] "Notes and Comments," *ADSF* 5 (April 1917): 23.

[c] PAD, IGA Collection MG 63.2088, Sixth Annual Report of the IGA 1919, 5. Patey's graduation was confirmed by the author with the Tilton School Alumni Office.

[d] Didsbury, "In the Shadow of the Tower Clock" (unpublished), 22.

[e] PAD, William Thomason Grenfell Association Collection, MG 327, reel 114, Reuben Patey to Wilfred Grenfell, 20 September 1922.

[f] PAD, William Thomason Grenfell Association Collection, MG 327, reel 114, Reuben Patey to Wilfred Grenfell, 6 January 1939.

[g] PAD, William Thomason Grenfell Association Collection, MG 327, reel 114, Reuben Patey to Wilfred Grenfell, 27 October 1939.

LIFE STORY 3
Really Grand People: Hazel Hart

Hazel (Compton) Hart lost her father at sea in 1920 when she was ten years old and was one of three children placed in the St Anthony Orphanage. Harriet Compton was deeply saddened by the loss of her husband and what she hoped would be the temporary break-up of her family. She kept Hazel's baby brother and found work in St Anthony as a cook. Hazel reminded her mother that they would get a good education at the orphanage and that was what her father had wanted for his children.

In response to an offer that Miss Karpick, head of the orphanage, had made to all the children, Hazel moved to Brockville, Ontario, to live with Annie, a teacher active with a local Grenfell Association who had asked for a child from the orphanage. Annie would dress Hazel up and take her around the community. When the ladies commented that she must be glad to be out of the orphanage, Hazel responded, "My most wonderful friends and family are in St Anthony. My friends can't wait for me to return home. No, they don't dress grand, not like this dress, which is very fancy, but the people are really grand."[a] Annie physically and psychologically abused Hazel, and after some harrowing months Hazel devised a strategy to leave Annie's care.

Hazel returned to St Anthony in January 1922, and in 1924 her mother remarried. By that time, Hazel was fourteen and had been selected for industrial training in Boston. As she prepared for her departure, Dr Grenfell embraced her and said, "We have a responsibility to make our fellow man glad that we were born."[b] Hazel completed the Industrial Arts Training program and then attended Burdett Business College. She was encouraged to apply for a nursing program and received her acceptance from Brightlook Hospital for the class of 1929. She graduated as a registered nurse in 1932.

Miss Carlson, head nurse at St Anthony, had made Hazel aware that many Newfoundlanders had been sent to the United States for their education and had not lived up to expectations. Hazel began working at St Anthony Hospital in 1932 and, after a number of years on the job, applied for the midwifery program at Liverpool Maternity Hospital in England. She wrote her certification exams in November 1937 and the next year left the mission to serve with the Frontier Nursing Association in Kentucky. This association had advertised for trained midwives who would be willing to provide service throughout the mountains, where transportation was on horseback. In 1939 she returned to Labrador, to work with Dr Forsyth at the Cartwright Hospital.

Hazel married in 1943, raised her family, and returned to nursing in St John's in 1958. In 1965, she began a ten-year career of providing services to special needs children.

NOTES

[a] Power, *Hazel Compton-Hart*, 20.

[b] Power, *Hazel Compton-Hart*, 33.

Newfoundland and Labrador demonstrates that the system of education developed by the Grenfell mission was distinct from that developed by the Department of Education. Students in the North attended private mission schools that were vastly different from those that served other coastal dwellers in the colony. The mission schools attracted more qualified teachers, had more teaching rooms and resources, and employed a curriculum that was infused by everyday life. I placed the school program of the mission against the progressive reforms of the American education system. Many American teachers came north to fulfill their desire to serve the world, and for some this meant a focus on social uplift: personal hygiene, morality, and religious piety were central to the schooling experience. Both the volunteers of the North and the "fotched-on women" of the American South focused their attentions on "worthy" Anglo-Saxon populations. At the request of the Carnegie Corporation of New York, John Paton, principal of Memorial University College, became involved in defining the shape and function of the Labrador schools in particular. He supported the mission's view that the people of the North were in need of a helping hand. Certainly there had not been many helping hands or support from the colonial government. At the end of the 1920s, the administration of the programs changed when the residential schools shifted under the administration of the Bureau of Education. This process would intensify under the Commission of Government.

Some young men and women were provided with access to further training at universities, colleges, technical institutes, and other post-secondary sites, but many students had to complete secondary schooling first. The program was designed to fulfill the mission's desire to equip the medical, educational, industrial, and agricultural programs with a local workforce. In exchange for financial support from the mission, a bond requirement stipulated that students were required to return to work for two years in the North. There is no evidence of any penalty for those who failed to return.

Students who studied in Canada attended such prestigious institutions as the University of Toronto and Upper Canada College. Most of the training, however, took place in applied or technical schools and institutes in the United States, and in addition to individual philanthropists, the CCNY provided a grant to support the work. Berea College in Kentucky became an ideological partner of the mission, and some students continued to be educated at this college after the 1920s. Children living in the St Anthony orphanage and mission communities had access to these training opportunities. In most cases, they increased their cultural capital, served others, and became instruments for social change. Many of those students made significant contributions to their northern homeland. Teaching these young people the value of serving the world, starting with their own communities, was probably the easiest of the lessons they were expected to learn.

9

Behind the Scenes at the Grenfell Mission: Edgar "Ted" McNeill and Counter-Biography as Material Agency

Rafico Ruiz

On 25 July 1927, St Anthony's new hospital was officially inaugurated. With all the pomp and circumstance befitting the achievement, Charles Curtis, the medical officer in charge of the Grenfell mission's St Anthony station, presided over a carefully planned ceremony. The first to speak from the stage erected adjacent to the hospital was Rev. John T. Richards, rural dean of the Church of England parishes in northern Newfoundland, who blessed the new hospital in the name of Christ:

And now, O Son of God, we dedicate to Thee this monument of love and labor and we sign it with the sign of Thy wondrous cross, that emblem of our redemption, and of all true sacrifice, in token that in the years to come, when the hearts and hands that fashioned it have ceased to function in their mortal bodies, and the voices of all in this august assembly have been hushed in the peace of Paradise, there shall not be wanting hearts and hands ready to offer themselves and theirs, full of the love similar of God and of mankind to carry on the great and Christ-like work of Dr Grenfell and his co-workers. In the name of the Father and of the Son and of the Holy Spirit. Amen.[1]

Rev. Richards's blessing refers to the "hearts and hands" that were instrumental in the material and symbolic building of the St Anthony hospital. Its opening marked an important stage in the mission's evolution. The sense of generational passing implicit in the blessing, that subsequent set of "hearts and hands" ready to sustain the mission's real and imagined purposes, was part of that evolution, with Grenfell's central place in the mission's activities moving towards its "last lap."[2] Grenfell's very tangible "lifetime" had enabled the cultivation of a whole series of generational "hearts and hands" who both believed in the mission's work and also laboured, voluntarily and for a wage, to achieve its aims of social reform. As a material embodiment of the Grenfell mission, as an institutional reality and a more distributed ethos of humanitarian, inter-denominational medical relief, the new St Anthony hospital was perhaps the privileged site of the mission's otherwise difficult-to-grasp, contested, and dispersed self-identity as an international and regional philanthropic institutional actor.

The story of the building of the mission's 1927 hospital, while not widely known in its details, reflects broader perceptions of the mission as an institution defined by its metropolitan philanthropic networks. More specifically, this network's prime representatives came from New York's Fifth Avenue liberal elites and included the New York architect in charge of the hospital project, William Adams Delano, a vice-president of the Grenfell Association of America in the 1940s and 1950s. Yet, underlying this metropolitan narrative of fundraising and philanthropic concern was the actual labour involved in erecting the hospital: coordinating the collection of materials, their arrival in St Anthony, and then contending with local building technologies and practices in order to build what was, according to Wilfred Grenfell, the most modern hospital in the British Empire.

Edgar "Ted" McNeill would prove to be one of the mission's most adept builders and the foreman in charge of the 1927 hospital project. McNeill, a Labrador-born ward of the mission, would be sent to the Pratt Institute in New York to receive instruction within its School of Science and Technology, that at the time granted certificates in Steam and Machine Design, Applied Electricity, Applied Chemistry, Machine Construction, and Carpentry and Building. What I set out to accomplish in this chapter is a counter-biographical sketch of Edgar McNeill that, for the purposes of this volume, will assess how he was part of a broader network of fisherfolk manual labourers involved in erecting the St Anthony hospital that could provide a "made-in-Newfoundland" authenticity to the northerly modernity of the institution. In the process, McNeill would prove how this seemingly alien building type was co-produced by both off- and on-island institutional, material, and human components, capital and equipment from New York, as well as a local labouring population with newly acquired skills, construction mettle, and a long-standing work ethic.

McNeill could be portrayed by the mission, perhaps truthfully, as a ready-to-hand problem solver, who was Pratt-educated by the mission's practical, longevity-driven social philanthropy. In making McNeill's work public, largely through publication in *Among the Deep Sea Fishers*, the mission was highlighting the expanded sense of situated agency that the fisherfolk had started to attain. Thus, while McNeill may have been "behind the scenes," he was nonetheless worthy of being brought forward for both display and recognition as a practical, human symbol of the mission's work of social reform. By way of contrast, this chapter attempts to show how, by reassembling McNeill's role in the construction of the 1927 hospital, the architectural histories of both McNeill and the building itself can be rewritten against the prevailing biographical norms surrounding the mission and its emblematic collection of male, largely British and American doctors. As such, in the case of McNeill and the Grenfell mission, I understand "counter-biography" to mean a genre of writing that "talks back" to the established biographical lives that defined the mission for much of the twentieth century. The somewhat nebulous field of auto/biography studies has begun to question how the medium-specific properties of the materials that go into the narrative "making" of such textual lives can co-shape those narratives themselves. "As methods of media production and consumption continue to evolve," Ken Cormier writes, "so must our conceptions of narrative and our assumptions about how lives can and should be represented."[3] It is in this sense that I am pursuing a method that privileges what could be thought of as the media traces of McNeill's role in the building of the 1927 hospital and one that can start to inform how a Grenfell mission-specific biographical counter-narrative can emerge through archival media such as letters, newsletters, and construction reports; the recollections and voice of his daughter, Dorothy; and a scattered photographic record dating from the 1920s to today. To some extent, there is a certain inadequacy in the very term "biography" for what follows. Perhaps a more apt characterization would be that of a modified form of "media life writing" that concedes its partiality and the ways in which it tries to run counter to the scale and scope of the narrative figureheads in the Grenfell mission story. This chapter is nonetheless a contribution to the project of expanding the "definition of what constitutes biographical expression,"[4] particularly through the recognition that, as Harold Innis and others have noted, the historical record is made up of its own media. In a narrower, disciplinary sense, my investment in this chapter lies in its ability to signal how biography studies can be informed by media studies' understanding of historiographical agency, equally in its conceptions of the material and symbolic registers of recording media.

The chapter draws on archival research, as well as on an interview with Dorothy McNeill, McNeill's daughter and a long-time resident of St Anthony.[5] It will combine two narrative registers, the analytical-historical and the oral, in order to reassess the role a foreman such as McNeill played in the institutional identity of the mission, and to demonstrate how counter-biography has the potential of expanding what sorts of documentary evidence can count in the assembling of a difficult-to-locate life. In this sense, as I noted above, I am attempting to foreground the various media of communication through which McNeill's life still retains a degree of "material agency": the words of his daughter, Dorothy, his dispersed appearances in the records of the International Grenfell Association, the symbolic and concrete remnants of the 1927 hospital, that still stands in St Anthony, and, finally, his influence on the mid-century building practices prevalent on the Northern Peninsula. Edgar McNeill's life is still very much the agential "material" of all of these elements, and as such he stands in for a broader network of anonymous and difficult-to-trace fisherfolk manual labourers involved in the construction of the mission's vast medical and philanthropic infrastructure.

* * * * *

We weren't isolated.

First of all, my father, in 1928, I'm pretty sure Marconi sent some-one out here and he was trained. The mission was given a call num-ber and my father was trained to do the radio operating.... He would be the one communicating with the Boston office and New York. I remember when he first started he'd just send out a "CQ," I suppose that's what you'd call it, that's when you call out and anybody can answer you, and eventually some man in Boston said, "Look, we'll have a regular schedule, really early every morning," and any mes-sages would be passed along. If you had staff here from the States, they'd go over and give Daddy a message or something, and he would send it off by talking to this man in Boston by voice or Morse code.... Daddy did it for the Mission up until the War.

...

To get down to Mom's home [by boat], in St Lunaire, for me in the summer that would be really thrilling. I grew up here, and it's kinda a different place, just walk down the road to this Grenfell school and back, the hospital was sort of right there, the focus. In those days it was only that blue one [*points out the window*], it didn't have that facade then. It was an architect from New York who donated the design, and my father put it up. It was a really big do. This was 1925. That's when he went out to New York for the winter. He went over to the firm of Delano and Aldrich. The Rockefellers' house on the Hudson was built by them. Anyway, he went over there every day for about three months to learn how to construct the hospital, 'cause it was steel beam. That had never been done, especially in northern Newfoundland. One fellow from here told me that the way the beams were put together was very advanced, even for Canada at the time. I don't know. There are two ways to do steel beams. That's all I know, really. I don't know what the two ways are. I got pictures of this. They dug the base, the foundations by hand. By horse and buggy. I think my father rigged up things like elevators and stuff like that, for lifting things once they started on the second floor. Then they eventually had a humungous boiler come, and he figured out, with a pulley system, how to tug it up. But in the pictures it's a stone-coloured brick facade, and some man did all that by hand. And then it was done to the specifications of Delano and Aldrich. Somewhere around the windows there was this pattern. So that's all covered in now.... The back part was built in the early 1950s. It was a TB san.... My father drew up the plans for that. That part that's attached [to the original hospital].

I never knew anything about this, but my half-brother told me, in more recent years, that when Daddy was there in New York they wanted him, once he finished that project, to come back and work for them, 'cause he picked up things very fast. A very quick learner. And he refused. He was very much a perfectionist ... in building. Some man I met on a ferry once, who came from somewhere else in Newfoundland, before the war, this was the late thirties, he said he'd been at school with my father, and he said he could look up at a ceiling and see if it was half an inch off.

So anyway, Daddy drew the plans for the san. Basic drawing he could do, and carpentry. That furniture there, the table, and those over there [*points to side tables*], he did. The bookcases. That thing the TV is on.

* * * * *

It was in the April 1925 issue of *Among the Deep Sea Fishers* that Arthur Cosby, the executive officer of the IGA, announced that the mission would be building a new hospital in St Anthony.[6] With work slated to begin in the summer of that same year, Cosby cited both the fire at the North West River hospital in 1924 and the fact that the current hospital was simply worn out and thoroughly on its last legs as the principal reasons for going ahead with the costly project. With plans donated by William Adams Delano, most often referred to in the magazine as "the New York architect," the hospital was also devised in consultation with Charles Curtis, the medical officer in charge of St Anthony (figure 9.1).

The building was to be a substantial improvement over the mission's current hospital. Built in 1903, its third hospital, coming after those at Battle Harbour and Indian Harbour, it was also expanded numerous times over its twenty-four-year history. Its genesis story, as told by Grenfell, has the doctor and a group of a hundred men and three times as

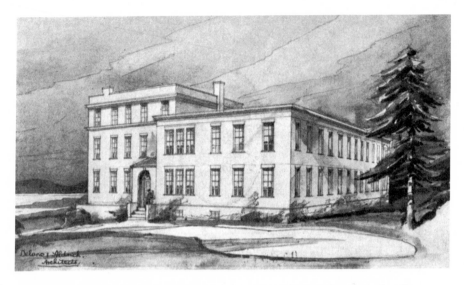

Figure 9.1 New St Anthony Hospital: from architects' drawing. "Frontispiece,"
ADSF 23 (April 1925): 2

many dogs heading out by sled into the outport's adjacent wilderness
for a fortnight in early spring and coming back with the raw materials
for a hospital thirty-six feet square.[7] As rudimentary as it was, the hospital nonetheless served, by the beginning of the 1920s, roughly nine
thousand patient days of care per year.[8] As Dr Curtis would put it,
albeit with the prospect of the new hospital on a very near horizon, "I
do not believe there is a hospital in the world that cost so little, and has
accomplished so much."[9]

Some of this perception of accomplishment, as Curtis acknowledges,
was bolstered by the fact that many nursing stations, in particular the
station in Flower's Cove, took on much of the patient load from the regions surrounding St Anthony that were more difficult to access. For
instance, in 1925, Nurse Amie Futter, in charge of the Flower's Cove
station, was responsible for a population of two thousand people, all
of whom fell within her station's district. By dog team and on foot, she
would cover hundreds of kilometres over the course of a medical season.
As such, this itinerant work would act as a stopgap to keep an adequate

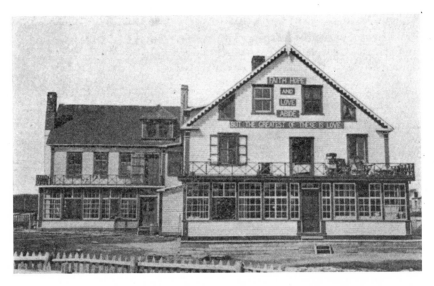

Figure 9.2 The enlarged hospital, St Anthony. Emma Demarest, "History of St Anthony Hospital," *ADSF* 23 (October 1925): 104

number of patients away from the operations of the hospital at St Anthony, hence allowing the small hospital to be only intermittently overwhelmed by patient demand (usually during the summer months and its bringing of facilitated means of transportation).

The first major improvement to the building came in 1908 when the Pratt Institute of Brooklyn sent a student volunteer to St Anthony to install an electric lighting plant. Grenfell had lectured at Pratt in 1907 and had sparked an interest in the mission.[10] As the Pratt's philanthropic logic went, and as they were searching for some practical way in which to aid Grenfell with his missionary work, they came upon the idea of providing an electric lighting plant to the outport, as its shorter winter days implied a greater reliance on artificial light, especially for the mission's hospital work. Drawing on a sketch plan of St Anthony provided by Grenfell, Pratt's electrical department sent one student volunteer, Frank Hause, to St Anthony in the summer of 1908 to install the system. As Hause writes, "Mr Edgar McNeil [*sic*], one of Dr. Grenfell's wards, and one of the two selected to be given a scholarship at Pratt, was there to help me in all of my work and it was largely due to his quick adaptability to new conditions that I was able to make a success of the installation"[11] (figure 9.2).

* * * * *

I remember one Christmas. We had an office in the house, it wasn't this house. I can remember him at the drawing board table. Always at the drawing board. So he got his plans approved when he was in Ottawa. Dr Curtis was there, fussing and worried he wouldn't get funding for it. Or his plans weren't good enough. Or whatever. Anyway, they were fine. And so they got funding for the TB san ...

People assume how isolated we were. But, as I told you yesterday, Daddy was born in 1884, between Makkovik and Hopedale in a place called Island Harbour. It's the family homestead. When he was a child, in the summertime they went out to some islands offshore, the Turnavik Islands, and so they could send the fish directly to the Bartletts' because they were the ones who had the fishing premises. And so Grenfell came there in 1892. He stopped at Turnavik. Daddy would have only been about eight or something. I think he was there when Grenfell first came by. But Bob Bartlett ... you really should read the famous story of his walking across to Siberia, but I won't get into that ... there's so many stories. Bob was about sixteen to Daddy's eight. So he was around. And I told you Daddy would remember loading fish on the boats going to Spain, and I don't know if they were Newfoundland companies, I think they were. I don't know if the Bartletts had their own boat, schooners that took salt cod directly to Spain or Italy, I'm not sure, it could have been both. So here you are with boats going back and forth to Europe, and then the Moravians were there. So you were exposed to the world through them.

My great-grandfather was living in St John's. Some summers he'd come down from St John's, give them news, and bring things for them that they couldn't get ordinarily. But there was always the Moravian, the German connection. Somewhere there was news getting around about what was happening in the world.

* * * * *

The summer of 1925 saw the launch of the new St Anthony hospital project in earnest. With a strong contingent of WOPs on hand for the good summer months of construction, it was hoped that they would complete the foundation work and possibly erect the steel skeleton of the building prior to their return to their respective colleges in the fall. McNeill, the foreman of the project and at the time superintendent of construction for the mission as a whole, spent two months in the spring of that same year in New York learning about the methods and processes of steel construction that would be necessary for work on the St Anthony hospital.[12] With the steel construction of the hospital as a flagship example (figure 9.3), it drove much of Grenfell's touting of the hospital as the most "modern" in the entire British Empire: it would be the most northerly orthopaedic clinic "this side of the North Pole," and already possessed the only radium north of Halifax (donated by the female members of the Twentieth-Century Club of Pittsburgh), and the only concrete structure at such a northerly latitude.[13] This relationship between northernness and architectural, engineering, and medical accomplishment was one that the mission allied to its emphasis on the Anglo-Saxon heritage of its resident population (as Jennifer Connor describes in chapter 2 in this volume). Taken as a representable whole to donors, volunteers, and the resident fisherfolk themselves, this relationship was predicated on the unlikely work that had to be done amongst a resident colonial population that was eminently available for a race-based sense of philanthropic affiliation in metropolitan centres across Canada, the United States, and Great Britain.

The fact that the mission could realize such unlikely accomplishments, and, as the St Anthony hospital project demonstrates, with the cooperation and labour of local fishers and women, this sense of mutual aid defined the sort of philanthropy the mission wanted to foster and also provided assurance to donors that the Grenfell mission cause was worthy of international finance and concern. In both of Grenfell's 1925 fundraising efforts in *Among the Deep Sea Fishers*, he mentions having visited the Rockefeller Hospital and Peking Union Medical College over the course of his travels. The Peking Union Medical College is a large medical complex in Beijing, completed in 1921, and designed by the firm founded by architect Henry Hobson Richardson,

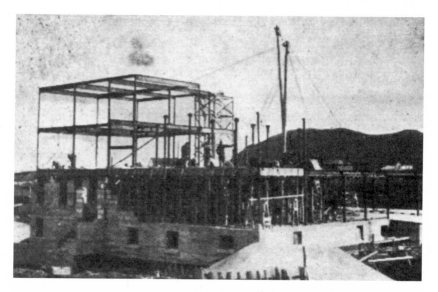

Figure 9.3 The steel frame goes up. Charles Curtis, "The Year's Work at
St Anthony Hospital," *ADSF* 23 (January 1926): 148

comprising some fourteen hospital, medical school, and laboratory
buildings. With yet another former Grenfell mission volunteer, Dr
George Van Gorder, as professor of orthopaedics at the Rockefeller
Hospital, establishing a direct connection with the mission's network
of medical professionals, Grenfell tangentially introduces to his readers
the presence of orthopaedic care in such a seemingly remote location
as Peking.[14] As such, the St Anthony hospital project was framed as
simply keeping up with an international standard of care, one set by
such philanthropists as the Rockefellers. In Grenfell's logic, it was also
all the more deserving of both moral and financial support, given the
racial and colonial ties at play.

By the end of the summer of 1925, McNeill's workmen, including
both WOPs and local fishermen, had all the steel in place, had put in the
basement walls, and completed the pouring of the first floor slab and
half of the second. In addition, they had produced 3900 concrete blocks
to be used for the hospital's walls, largely through the continuous (and
noisy) work of an on-site stone crusher. According to Dr Curtis, they
regularly worked from 8 a.m. to 10 p.m., often staying on until the

early hours of the morning when the concrete was being poured.[15] Word of the mission's success, both of the undertaking and of the construction itself, began to circulate to other parts of the colony. The St John's *Daily News* ran a laudatory article, dated 9 September 1925, that was reprinted in *Among the Deep Sea Fishers*. The article praised the hospital's use of local labour, particularly McNeill's ability to keep the project on time and budget, given that "every part of the structure is the handiwork of men, most of whom have been more accustomed to the fishing boat and cod trap skiff than to the plane and saw."[16] With stern pride, if a bit of confusion, the *Daily News* mentioned how "except for the steel, cement, and some of the fixtures, which were brought from the United States, everything is being finished or made in Newfoundland."[17] With the concrete blocks indeed "made" in St Anthony, the concept of "finishing" was also a powerful one to invoke. The northerly modernity of the hospital, a seemingly alien institutional building type in the region, could thus be co-produced by the aforementioned off- and on-island institutional, material, and human components, capital and equipment from New York, and a local labouring population with newly acquired skills, construction mettle, and a long-standing work ethic. McNeill, the "master-of-works" and "a man of exceptional ability,"[18] along with Wilfred Mesher, who is also mentioned, could, according to the *Daily News* reading of the situation, play a leading role in the St Anthony hospital project.

McNeill and Mesher would also be acknowledged in the July 1927 issue of *Among the Deep Sea Fishers*. With the newly completed hospital on the cusp of its official inauguration, the mission magazine strung together a revealing sequence of articles that explore the central actors behind the project. As its frontispiece, the issue opens with a photograph of William Adams Delano, "architect of the new hospital at St Anthony," as the caption reads.[19] It is followed by seven articles: "The New Medical Era in St Anthony," by Herbert Threlkeld-Edwards, offers a detailed description of the new building; "Let Us Do Good to All Men" is another Grenfell New Testament homily on the pleasures of service; "The Year's Work in Review," is a recapitulation of the IGA's annual activities, its various stations on the coasts and the financial reports of its local associations; "A Great Acquisition," by Harry Paddon, informs readers of the gift by an anonymous donor of an oil cruiser, *Maraval*, for the mission's activities; "William Adams Delano," a portrait of the "mind and hand and heart" who shaped the new hospital building, is written by Theodore Ainsworth Greene;[20] "How Stores and Supplies Are Handled at St Anthony," by A.C. Blackburn, highlights the importance of the department of stores and supplies in the functioning of the mission; and, finally, "The Men behind the Scenes," records and recognizes McNeill and Mesher's work on the hospital (figure 9.4). The narrative across this first half of the magazine exposes the many actors who came together to assure successful completion of the hospital. While the question of hierarchical arrangement is of importance (one could simply compare the portrait of Delano to the photographs of McNeill and Mesher in the issue), the sequence of articles also shows the disjuncture between an architect's plans and their practical implementation. In this reading, Delano is a polished figurehead, an archetypal WOP as a Yale alumnus, fellow of the American Institute of Architects, and member of the federal Fine Arts Commission, for the IGA's metropolitan donors; an eminent someone from the appropriate class doing the "right thing" for an Anglo-Saxon population in need.

Greene notes how Delano has two "hobbies." The first involves making old-fashioned furniture, with a set of Stanley tools, in an old greenhouse on his Long Island property. The second, "as you may have guessed already, is his very great interest in helping to advance the Grenfell Mission's program in Newfoundland and Labrador."[21] By contrast, McNeill, Mesher, and their workmen are presented as the supplement to the mere execution of "building" as verb and "the building" as noun: "But there is more to a building than pouring concrete and placing blocks. What would have been the use of a steamer-load of materials, carefully drawn plans, and even the most willing workmen, if there had been no one to interpret the plans, direct the workmen, and solve the thousand and one problems?"[22] For the readers of the magazine, McNeill and Mesher could be portrayed as those ready-to-hand problem solvers who were both Pratt-educated by the mission's practical, longevity-driven social philanthropy. "The many daily problems were too numerous to mention," the article asserts, "but it was always the same story of 'Work it out yourself,' and both Ted McNeill and Wilfred

THE MEN BEHIND THE SCENES

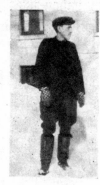

WILFRED MESHER
SUPERINTENDENT OF
ELECTRICAL, STEAM
PLUMBING INSTAL-
LATION

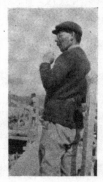

TED MC NEIL
GENERAL SUPERIN-
TENDENT OF ALL
CONSTRUCTION

THERE are always men "behind the scenes" who construct and prepare the stage for others, never appearing themselves in the final production. Their work is quite as important to the finished performance as that of the people who speak the lines, in fact, it is in a way more so, because without them the others would have found it difficult to appear in any capacity. have been the use of a steamer-load of materials, carefully drawn plans, and even the most willing workmen, if there had been no one to interpret the plans, direct the workmen, and solve the thousand and one problems? These problems were often very real ones which would have taxed the skill of the most expert contractor, and they were problems which the average builder never has to face. If mistakes had been

Figure 9.4 The men behind the scenes. *ADSF* 25 (July 1927): 66

Mesher deserve the highest credit for this, the crowning achievement of the long records of their useful and indispensable activities for the Mission."[23] As I noted above, in making McNeill and Mesher's work public, the mission was highlighting the expanded sense of situated agency that the fisherfolk had started to attain. While McNeill and Mesher may have been "the men behind the scenes," they were nonetheless worthy of being brought forward for display and recognition as practical, material symbols of the mission's work of social reform; in their cases, through education at such institutions as the Pratt, and, in Mesher's case, also the New York Trade School where he studied practical electricity.[24]

* * * *

We had a visitor one day when I was about seventeen. He was Daddy's age. He was a great friend of Grenfell's. He was Grenfell's best man at Grenfell's wedding in 1901 in Chicago. And he married Woodrow Wilson's daughter in 1912, and Grenfell was his best man at the White House. My half-brother again told me, this was so long

ago, that Daddy apparently had an invitation to that wedding, but ...
I didn't pay attention, like I say, when I was a kid, I wasn't one bit interested in all this ... romanticism to me was living in France or England or Europe somewhere ... it certainly wasn't this. I was like an
only child, 'cause my brother was so much older, and he was never
home. So anyway ... I just immersed myself in escapism ... books.
On the radio we'd hear good stories.

...

In one sense they weren't mentally isolated. And they always sort
of knew where was what in the world. It hadn't been long before,
when Daddy was a little boy, his great-grandmother was still alive,
her husband was the one who came from Scotland ... So he had people coming, immediately, not that long ago from Scotland. It was not
like a hundred years ago. And then on Daddy's mother's side, his
grandfather came from Norway. And he lived in Makkovik. He was
alive until Daddy was twenty. Daddy would have known somebody
in his family who was from Norway. So you had that outside world
connection. So you knew your basic geography, right.

Those Moravian missionaries had often been in South Africa.
Daddy's teacher, I think that's where he met his wife. I think he
was in South Africa as a child.

...

Here's when I was seventeen in our house. Daddy was an old man,
retired, and not very well. Here was this visitor in the house. I'm
going back somewhere else now, back to the White House connection. A president's son-in-law coming in to visit ... the same guy
had set up the constitution, or helped do it, or drew it up for ... the
constitution or body of laws for Thailand. I got his book here somewhere. He ended up being a lawyer. He was a law professor at Harvard. I don't know if it was the prince or king of Thailand, it must
have been his father, he went to the States and lived with this family.
Anyway, after that this man was also high commissioner to the
Philippines when war broke out, and that was McArthur, the general,
they had to escape in a submarine from this place down the bay from
Manila called Corregidor ... Now Wilson's daughter died, then he

remarried, this man. He helped draw up things for the United
Nations. His name is Francis Sayre.

* * * * *

With McNeill, Mesher, and their work crew having taken advantage of
the summer months of 1926, the new hospital was able to accommodate
patients by January 1927, prior to its official inauguration in July.[25] On
the 27th of the month, with the thermometer marking -25°F yet planned
with apparent military precision by Dr Curtis, the new hospital was occupied by the mission's staff and patients. "The general exodus of the
thirty patients started at one o'clock, some few walking, the others well
bundled up and carried," mission volunteer Herbert Threlkeld-Edwards
relates. "Stretcher followed stretcher, komatik followed komatik between the two buildings, and barely an hour later every patient had
been moved and was safely in bed!"[26] Over the course of the fall, prepa-
rations for the move had been ongoing, with painting, the installation
of equipment, and the completion of the lighting system, all necessitating
additional work by not only the fisherfolk volunteer labourers, but also
by the hospital's staff of nurses and doctors. The patients were installed
in their new wards, "a patient's world" according to Threlkeld-Edwards,
and one made up of grey and buff stucco walls, ample corridors, and
waxed linoleum floors.[27] On the day itself, hospital staff also had to
move their own furnishings, the equipment from the operating and dispensary rooms, as well as the kitchen range.

The new hospital, begun in May 1925, was completed, save for cos-
metic painting, on 1 January 1927 (figure 9.5). Work had been continuous, with, as noted above, that first summer seeing the excavation of
the basement, the erection of the steel frame, and the walls and floor
slabs poured. With gravel produced on site by the aforementioned stone
crusher, sand had to be brought in from North West River and Forteau
by specially chartered steamers from Twillingate – a costly if necessary
method to produce the hospital's concrete. Over the course of the building process, in addition to the local labour supplied by the residents of
St Anthony and White Bay, plasterers and carpenters were brought in

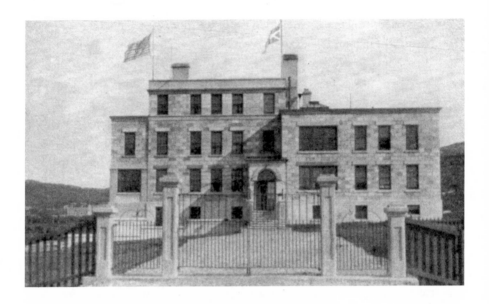

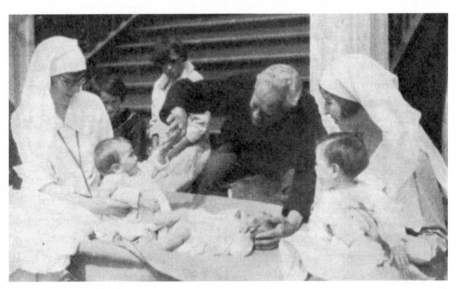

Figure 9.5 New St Anthony hospital, with patients and Wilfred Grenfell.
"Frontispiece," *ADSF* 25 (October 1927): 98

from such southern locales as St John's, Bay Roberts, and Twillingate. During the winter of 1926, the water and steam pipes were installed, and the mission's local machine shop set about manufacturing the necessary windows and doors. In the spring, a steamer from New York was chartered to bring the remainder of the supplies and equipment, including two eight-ton boilers that would cement McNeill's reputation as an ingenious problem solver, as he managed to bring them from the deck of the schooner onto the wharf via a runway, and then had a thousand-yard wooden road built from the wharf to the site of the new hospital by means of a movable block and tackle, with the mission's Ford truck and tractor pulling the boilers along with ropes (figure 9.6).[28]

Threlkeld-Edwards's thorough description of the new hospital was, in part, meant to bring it and its ideal functioning to life for the IGA's network of donors. Attention to detail and soundness of both design and construction seem to be assured through the interplay of American manufacturing and the integrities of materials that seem to speak for themselves. As Threlkeld-Edwards reiterates near the end of his article, "The building is entirely fire and water proof. The exterior walls are of eight inch concrete blocks made on the site. The steel frame was made in New York by the National Bridge Company and bolted on the site. The Lally columns and steel beams are encased in cement, the stairways are of concrete. Floors are of six-inch reinforced concrete with grey Holland linoleum cemented to slab and waxed; the walls are cement plaster, while the ceilings are calcium plaster."[29]

Design, manufacturing, and assembly had to proceed hand-in-hand in order for the building to materialize. To some extent this explains the crucial role McNeill would take on, not only in the actual erection of the building, but also more indirectly in the new hospital's discursive deployment by mission doctors, nurses, and other volunteer chroniclers. McNeill could circulate between these three realms, being at once, as Threlkeld-Edwards notes in one of his final paragraphs, a pupil of Pratt, Delano, and the National Bridge Company in the matter of steel frame construction, a foreman with knowledge of the necessary coordination of ordering, transport, storage, and use of the appropriate materials, and, finally, a symbolic local labourer, in charge and on the site for the entirety of the building's construction period. It was McNeill who would

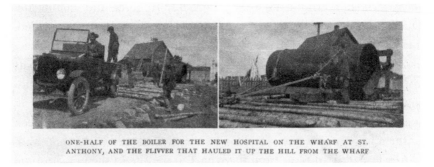

ONE-HALF OF THE BOILER FOR THE NEW HOSPITAL ON THE WHARF AT ST.
ANTHONY, AND THE FLIVVER THAT HAULED IT UP THE HILL FROM THE WHARF

Figure 9.6 One-half of the boiler for the new hospital. "The Men behind the
Scenes," *ADSF* 25 (July 1927): 67

devise "a hand built crane operated by a steam hoist" in order to solve
the major problem of raising and placing the steel girders in position.[30]
And it was Mesher, working from plans donated by the firm of French
and Hubbard of Boston (as, like Delano, Hollis French was the vice-
president of the New England Grenfell Association), who would successfully install the electrical, plumbing, and water systems for the
hospital. "It is a testimony to the detailed care with which [the plans]
were prepared and to the skill of Wilfred Mesher who superintended
the installation," as Threlkeld-Edwards writes, "that when the boilers
were started not a joint in the building leaked."[31] This period, from 1
January to 25 July 1927, the day of the official inauguration of the hospital, marked a distinct moment in the symbolic coherence of both the
endeavour to have a modern hospital built in the unlikely locale of St
Anthony, and the hospital itself as a symbolic marker of the mission's
accomplishment and future aims. It was prior to its official inauguration
that the hospital could be perceived as a distinctly built object, taking
on such temporary symbolic valences as that of the purpose and importance of American industrial education for the mission's largely male
labour force, evinced through the figureheads of McNeill and Mesher,
as well as the crucial role of the constructive agencies of architecture,
as the July 1927 issue of *Among the Deep Sea Fishers* shows. From architects to engineers to foremen, the parade of actors involved in the
materialization of the hospital prior to its inauguration differs from its

gaining officialdom through the presence of colonial governors, governmental representatives, IGA executives, and members of the clergy. Overlying these actors, of course, was the hospital's divine consecration, those "hearts and hands" of Grenfell's practical philanthropy that could act on and advocate for an action-based approach to missionary pursuits. Immediately after the dedication of the hospital, the collected audience sang the "Hospital hymn":

Spirit of Truth, we call
On Thee, this house to bless,
Give Wisdom, strength and grace to all
Who here Thy name confess.
Spirit of Mercy, bring
Thy balm the sick to heal;
And make the weary ones to sing,
Who shall Thy presence feel.
Spirit of Peace, descend,
Thyself the Heavenly Dove.
Let care for souls and bodies blend
In ministries of love.[32]

This Anglican hymn, sung to dedicate to God "houses, places, and things" was usually grouped in hymnbooks with such institutions and objects as a home for the aged, a burial ground, a church bell, and an organ.[33] Here it marks the reinsertion of the hospital into the mission's apparatus of Christocentric works. While Grenfell, in his speech to the audience after the singing of the hymn, would conclude by paying "special tribute to the two native Labrador men, Mr Edgar McNeil [sic], foreman of the construction, and to Wilfred Mesher, superintendent of electrical and plumbing equipment, through whose untiring efforts the difficult work of building and completing this structure was accomplished,"[34] it would mark the passing of the hospital from a "structure," with all its attendant processes of construction, to a concrete reality. That is, the hospital's symbolic valence as an architectural process would become a necessary if unintentional erasure, an overcoming and recasting of the work behind its very materialization – once one of its concrete blocks became a cornerstone, the hospital started to move towards ceasing to be an instructive "structure" and site of materialization of otherwise anonymous labour.

In the context of the mission, the St Anthony hospital did indeed mark a departure from the "make do," wood-frame ethos of the previous hospital, one that had certainly echoed the prevailing vernacular in the region that largely came out of necessity and expediency – those two guiding forces of the vernacular tradition – with the local knowledge and materials at hand working their way into its final form and function. The opportunity to build an entirely new and, more importantly, contemporaneous medical institution, entirely "modern in its spatial attitudes" and, in this instance, its construction practices, befitted the mission's goal of instituting standards of comparison by which to measure the health and general well-being of their regional population.[35] As such, soon after its completion, the new St Anthony hospital received an A-1 certification from the American College of Surgeons (an accomplishment that J.T.H. Connor discusses more fully in chapter 10 in this volume). It would seem difficult to think of the St Anthony hospital on a continuum with similar building types of the period – most notably, Delano's ornate and spa-like hospitals for his wealthy clients on Long Island.[36] Yet, in gaining the ACS certification, the mission, already with a longstanding practice of bringing in highly qualified specialists from the United States, Canada, and the United Kingdom, could claim to have thoroughly modernized northern Newfoundland, and by extension, Labrador's medical infrastructure. "In 1927 this hospital was rated A-1 by the American College of Surgeons," as Curtis writes, "and so put an on equal standing with the leading hospitals in the United States and Canada."[37] This infrastructure, however, was no longer predicated on an "at-handness" in the mission's construction practices supervised and coordinated by the likes of McNeill, but rather was seeking to place the new St Anthony hospital on precisely that continuum of medical-architectural and practical modernity that such publications as *The Modern Hospital* would feature in its pages. The particularities of its missionary purpose, colonial context, and cost-conscious design and construction make the hospital an embodiment of just such a medical modernity that was neither rooted in the past nor looking to the future:

"The overall image of the modern factory for healing was simply too sterile or too scary for post–World War I society. Good health was still related in a real way to traditional values, through the symbols of home and the values associated with traditional architecture. Hospitals, in fact, relied on the likeness of the big, safe house to convince middle-class city dwellers that their chances were as good there as at home, especially to those who might pay much-needed extra fees for semiprivate or private accommodation."[38]

In a place such as St Anthony, with its missionary class system of, on the one hand, fisherfolk, and, on the other, mission workers and volunteers, the hospital was both a charitable institution and an anchor of a modern architecture – that is, one built of steel frame and reinforced concrete. In this context, architectural design reflected not merely the exigencies of medical technical evolution, but also the evolution of materials and engineering techniques that could be imported to northern Newfoundland; hence, again, the importance of McNeill and Mesher in the execution of the project. As Emma Demarest would point out in the earliest issue of *Among the Deep Sea Fishers* looking to shore up support for the hospital,

> To us in the States, accustomed as we are to the vagaries, delays and annoyances accompanying the employment of expert union labor, it is remarkable that unskilled Newfoundland labor can undertake the erection of this large building, keep the cost well within the estimate and in all profitability have the hospital ready for opening ahead of schedule. This certainly shows the adaptability of the Newfoundland fishermen, who build their own homes, their boats and schooners, also the remarkable work of the Grenfell Mission in developing this adaptability. The Mission has not only cared for sick bodies, but it has provided opportunity for industrial education, which has resulted in turning out two such fine men as Edgar McNeil and Wilfred Mesher, capable of managing so important an undertaking.[39]

Adaptation was indeed one consequence of the new hospital. While it certainly did not institute a shift from a labour practice such as fishing to that of carpentry (as the mission's small-scale mill projects had already gone down this road), it did provide evidence to the fisherfolk themselves, the mission's local workers and volunteers, and the IGA's network of donors, that "architecture," in its modernizing sense, had been built. In the context of the St Anthony hospital, however, the agency and authorial coherence of "the architect" has to be put under question. The mission's expansive program of "industrial education," though limited in number to such figureheads as McNeill and Mesher who would make the long trip to Pratt, could also encompass a host of modernizing construction practices that could make this predominantly medical intervention into a thoroughly spatial and architectonic one as well. In this sense, to understand the mission's making of northern Newfoundland and Labrador, simply "'knowing space' is not enough – trigonometric formulae, engineering structures, shaping the land and dwelling on it." Rather, as Rob Shields writes, "we need to know about 'spacing' and the spatializations that are accomplished through everyday activities, representations, and rituals."[40] The shift in spatial practice, instigated by the new St Anthony hospital project, could be an architectural cause in its double sense – both a philanthropic goal to be achieved and a precipitating event in the fisherfolk's understanding of spatial transformation. "The hospital of today is not a thing within four walls; it is not a house that shelters the sick; it is a state of mind. It permeates the whole community; out from its walls radiate all its influences. Like educational institutions everywhere, it teaches and trains those who are to minister, and these in their turn go out into the community and carry its blessings."[41]

Thinking about the mission's particular understanding of architectural authorship may also be relevant in past and present colonial and postcolonial contexts wherein a politics of space is sedimented and contested, built over and reshaped through a wider spectrum of missionary or metropolitan practices. The Grenfell mission played a prominent role in literally re-forming the spatial practices and materialities of the colony's settler population that had, in their own right, supplanted a pre-existing indigeneity. As a colonial actor, their means of "making" new spatial practices in northern Newfoundland and Labrador can be placed alongside other colonial practices and environments wherein "the ontological and material cannot be extricated from the epistemo-

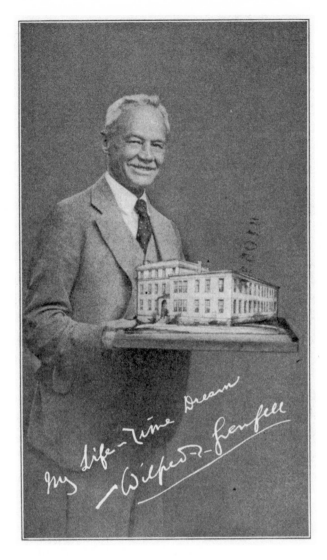

Figure 9.7 Wilfred Grenfell and new St Anthony
hospital, "My life-time dream." "Frontispiece,"
ADSF 23 (October 1925): 98

logical and discursive."[42] Alongside medical change came environmental
change. The fisherfolk, as a settler population, were playing out multiple
stages of colonial influence – both through inheritance and missionary
instruction. By participating in the building of a "modern" hospital in
northern Newfoundland, they could thus make a newfound claim for
their own "indigeneity."

This is an important nuance in the "material" life of Edgar McNeill that I have assembled here. It signals to what extent a figure such as McNeill and his life are bound up across these registers of ontology and materiality, of having lived and made things; of epistemology and discourse, of having learned and believed in his world and thus, in turn, been recorded through speech, writing, photography, and film. While I certainly do not want to conflate or limit McNeill's lifetime to the building of the mission's 1927 hospital, I trust this episode shows how "material agency," particularly as it is made manifest through the "counter-biography" I performed here, can reconfigure how we read the sedimentary layers of meaning present in such a material artifact as a building. If the 1927 hospital was ultimately claimed for the mission as a whole, and if its origin story belies its importance as Grenfell's own "life-time dream" (figure 9.7), then it could follow that its ongoing semantic instability, much like John Hornsby's understanding of the immaterial longevity of the then-"modern hospital," can live on, equally along with and in, the varied materialities and agencies of the always recent past.

American Aid, the International Grenfell Association, and Health Care in Newfoundland, 1920s-1930s

J.T.H. Connor

With the exception of an astounding number of physician autobi-
ographies that occasionally connect with Wilfred Grenfell and his mission, studies of cottage hospitals and other institutional histories, for
the period before Newfoundland joined Canada, medical historical
studies generally ignore the private medical mission.[1] Conventional wisdom has instead maintained a state-based perspective of health-care delivery that, without organizational support or intervention (religious or
state), medicine and health care throughout the island was substandard
to non-existent in this pre-Confederation era. To shed light on the full
scope of medicine and surgery practised in the island, a research team
is therefore examining the internal clinical records of the main mission
hospital in St Anthony up to 1940.[2] As a complementary step to this
ongoing investigation, this chapter examines published hospital reports
for both this hospital and the Notre Dame Bay Memorial Hospital
(NDBMH) in Twillingate, which had a close affinity with the International Grenfell Association. Through narrative and statistical profiles
of hospital in- and outpatient activities, admissions/discharges, surgical
procedures, and death rates in the 1920s and 1930s, this study shows
that these two hospitals were the most professionally connected and advanced in Newfoundland. The United States played a significant role in
this regard, in funding and material donations; in providing medical
staff, supplies, collegial clinical consultations, and ancillary services;
and in building and accrediting hospitals. In essence, it was primarily

American aid that laid the foundation for an independent health-care system in northern Newfoundland that thrived and survived long enough to become absorbed by the public government scheme. This discussion thus illustrates the transition of Grenfell's vision from that of a Victorian British imperial Christian charity to a twentieth-century American philanthropic enterprise geared toward social progress; as well, it suggests that historiographical concepts such as periphery/metropole, urban/rural, or core/margin may not be useful when assessing the clinical significance of institutions, especially in Newfoundland, where there were strong connections to the United States.

THE ECOSYSTEM OF HEALTH-CARE DELIVERY IN PRE-CONFEDERATION NEWFOUNDLAND

There was no centralized system of health-care delivery in Newfoundland before Confederation; instead, several different modes and models of formal and informal patient care and financing functioned independently of each other, yet frequently were interlinked. In 1935, for example, ninety-three doctors practised in Newfoundland, which had a population of approximately 300,000: thirty in the capital city of St John's, with its population of around 40,000; fifty distributed thinly along the east coast; seventeen along the south and west coasts; and about ten others in five small towns. This distribution meant one physician for about 1,300 people in the only real urban area, compared with one physician for 4,700 for all outports that might rise as high as one for 7,000 people in more remote regions. Hospitals were few for the whole island. St John's had five institutions: two dating from the nineteenth century, including an asylum. The other St John's Victorian-era hospital, the General, was adequately equipped for the period with six wards, an aseptic operating room, a modest diagnostic laboratory, and radiological apparatus. The building was centrally heated and electrified, and sections were connected by telephones. Around 1917, it admitted approximately 1,500 patients annually, who stayed, on average, for about twenty-three days; a death rate of about 4 per cent was reported, which was not atypical.[3] Two smaller denominational hospitals were established in 1922 and 1923; and a tuberculosis sanatorium in 1917. The combination of charity aid, municipal and government funds, fee for service, and religious duty supporting these hospitals, along with their organization, was similar to many small city situations elsewhere. Indeed, a contemporary evaluation by a British administrator who was a member of the appointed Commission of Government that from 1934 oversaw the affairs for Newfoundland concluded that St John's had a "medical organization which in its human as in its material resources need fear no comparison with that of any other city of its size in the Empire."[4] Three small hospitals were established elsewhere in Newfoundland in company towns for workers (although, as with Grenfell mission hospitals, they served the wider geographical area): one in the mill town of Grand Falls, built in 1909; one in the mill town of Corner Brook, built in 1925; and one in the mining town of Buchans, by 1928.

In 1930, the Newfoundland government released the recommendations of a royal commission on health matters that drew attention to the "similarity of the Scotch settlers' condition" to that of Newfoundlanders: isolation, problematic land communication, poor economic conditions, and a dependency on the fishery. Because of this similarity, the model of the Highlands and Islands Medical Service in Scotland, which was implemented after the First World War and provided doctors, nurses, and hospital services to the scattered population of northern Scotland, was to act loosely as a model for Newfoundland.[5] Calls to build small, regional hospitals in locations around the island first dated to just after the First World War, especially following the great influenza epidemic. "Hospitals Needed at Extern Points" – to provide for the physical welfare of those who lived in outports – was the thrust of one newspaper story. The efforts of Grenfell, his staff, and their hospitals in the North notwithstanding, it continued, this matter was tantamount to "culpable neglect." Grenfell himself wrote about the need for "bay hospitals" to be established in key locales such as Twillingate, so that people would not have to travel great distances for timely health care. He further appealed to the populace to turn this issue into an electoral matter.[6] Such pleas, however, would not be heeded (with the exception of a hospital in Twillingate, as will be discussed) until the Commission of Government took over the administration of Newfoundland. Between

1936 and 1952, eighteen hospitals were built along the southwest and eastern coastlines, with a few others inland; eight of them were operational in the 1930s. Cottage hospital buildings often resembled a large suburban bungalow and originally were equipped on the main floor with two four-bed wards; isolation quarters; operating room; office and dispensary; nurses' workroom; and kitchen, dining, and laundry facilities. Residence rooms for doctors and nursing staff were on the upper floor. As they were readily accessible by water, or on land by foot, cart, and sled, cottage hospitals attended quickly to the myriad occupational injuries incurred in the dangerous outdoor jobs of fishing, hunting, and lumbering, along with other medical emergencies; these institutions also endeavoured to promote preventive medicine within the communities they served. Financially, cottage hospitals were generally effective, as all physicians were on a government salary, which helped contain expenses; augmenting government funding were annual subscriber fees (for example, ten dollars for family coverage) collected from patients. A subsequent government report drew several complimentary comparisons between Scotland and Newfoundland with respect to their cottage hospitals;[7] and an external consultant's report prepared for the Newfoundland government at mid-century concluded that while isolation was an issue for medical staff, their medical qualifications were "high," the system was of "tremendous *value to the people*," and that these institutions were "quite well-equipped and the *surgical results* have been excellent."[8]

Nurses were much more prevalent in the health-care ecosystem of pre-Confederation Newfoundland than their modern-day counterparts who typically work in institutional settings. Paradigmatic in this regard was Myra Bennett (1890–1990), a nurse-midwife who arrived from England in 1921 to settle in Daniel's Harbour, a coastal community situated roughly midway between the southern limit of that serviced by the IGA and the closest cottage hospital, Bonne Bay at Norris Point. In addition to her own medical work over the next half century, Bennett trained and/or upgraded the skills of local midwives, who were another ubiquitous feature of community life.[9]

Clergymen also performed some medical work: Grenfell may have been a doctor turned missionary, but the reverse could also be the case.

Rev. H.J.A. MacDermott, a British Christian missionary who served for the first third of the twentieth century in Fortune Bay on the Burin peninsula, related his dual role as "doctor"; indeed, the foreword to his 1938 autobiography by H.M. Mosdell, then chief government physician, described MacDermott as "Dr Mac" repeatedly and matter-of-factly.[10] After his formal retirement from the clergy in 1934, Mac-Dermott was retained as a consultant to the Department of Public Health and Welfare (through Mosdell, who was the secretary), with duties that included sailing on its maiden voyage with the *Lady Anderson* (a 100-foot personal luxury motor yacht of an American tycoon that was purchased by the Newfoundland government, renamed, and refitted as a floating medical clinic) to visit communities in his former "parish" to investigate welfare conditions and to refer tuberculous patients to St John's for treatment.[11]

The *Lady Anderson* would undertake numerous voyages to the eighty-seven small outports that comprised the settled areas of the southwestern shore with a scattered population of about 11,000. Surviving accounts of these trips are rich in detail.[12] Additionally, the coastal mail steamers acted as ambulances for sick patients being transferred among IGA institutions and other larger hospitals. The ss *Clyde* brought hundreds of people to Twillingate, who would flock to the outpatient department of the NDBMH; the *Clyde* might also undertake emergency missions to transport seriously sick patients. The ss *Kyle* had a government-paid medical officer to treat people ashore and onboard when the ship docked at its many stops along the coasts. Medical students served in this capacity in the early 1930s and mid-1940s, and the role of senior medical student as medical officer continued well into the late-1950s.[13] Although a patchwork of sorts, these boats connected physicians, nurses, patients, hospitals (urban and rural), families, and communities all around Newfoundland and Labrador – so much so that a mainland consultant concluded the "*boat service* has been very helpful" in transporting doctors and shuttling between nursing stations and nearby hospitals.[14]

Against this patchy background of regional health care in this period, the IGA, with its dozen hospitals and nursing stations, numerous hospital boats, and extensive staff of qualified medical personnel, constituted a standalone health-care system. With its locus of activity in northern New-foundland and coastal Labrador, the broad range of services of the main hospital in St Anthony, along with those of the NDBMH in Twillingate, attracted patients from areas outside their primary catchment areas.

TWILLINGATE AND ST ANTHONY HOSPITALS: EXCEPTIONS AND EXEMPLARS

Lack of centralization, as implied by the description of the health-care delivery ecosystem in Newfoundland, was probably advantageous for the scattered and isolated nature of outport settlements. Two historically unexamined "nodes" of this ecosystem – the hospitals at Twillingate and St Anthony – augmented the provision of health care. Analysis of their activities highlights the degree to which the IGA, unlike any other institution or government body, had an impact on the provision of health care for the whole island. Furthermore, this analysis considers the connection between external aid and health-care delivery, and how crucial it may have been; and uncovers the range of treatments available as well as the level of care offered and its apparent effectiveness.

International Aid: The Role of the United States

International aid embraced money and much more. In 1937 total rev-enue for the IGA was about $135,000. Of this amount, $10,000 was a grant from the government of Newfoundland, which was just marginally lower than patients' fees and donations received ($11,000); the remain-ing $113,500 was received from "friends and supporters" of Grenfell Associations of America, New England, Canada, Great Britain and Ireland, and Newfoundland (see figure o.1 in the introduction). These data illustrate the dependence of the IGA on contributions from the United States, which accounted for over 60 per cent of all funds. As well, that all government funds amounted to only 7 per cent illustrates how comparatively irrelevant was officialdom to the existence of Gren-fell's operation. Supplementing these funds were material donations of all kinds.[15] An unexpected representation of American aid was hospital chart forms: for years hospital admission records were prepared on standardized forms bearing the imprint of Boston's Massachusetts General Hospital. These printed forms included racial categories of "White" and "Colored" for patients, reminding users of their American origins; these categories were often modified to identify the more important local marker of patients' religious denomination. Other hospital stationery in use at St Anthony for laboratory reports derived from the New York Department of Public Health and also Boston's Peter Bent Brigham Hospital surgical service for anaesthesia charts.

Vitally important, too, was "aid-in-person" through the steady supply of temporary young workers and established practitioners. Many Americans served, including WOPs who would become rich, famous, and powerful. In 1926 about 83 per cent of the volunteer staff complement in IGA hospitals was American, compared with 2 per cent from Britain; by 1939 just before Grenfell died, 52 per cent were of American origin, but the British component had risen to 19 per cent. Yet numbers do not reveal the total impact on the mission, especially for the American involvement. Dr John Little (1875–1926) and Dr Charles Curtis (1887–1964), Grenfell's successive right-hand medical men in St Anthony, both graduated from Harvard Medical School. Curtis joined Grenfell in 1915 after being inspired by him during a speech given at Yale University; he would eventually succeed Grenfell as the IGA's leader in the mid-1930s until his retirement in 1959. A newly built hospital opened in 1968 in St Anthony was named the Charles S. Curtis Memorial Hospital, which still flies both the Union Jack and the Stars and Stripes outside the building.[16] In addition were those American specialists who routinely signed up for months of work and were advertised by Grenfell to residents around the island: Dr Joseph A. Andrews in particular stands out for his service to the mission over sixteen years of summer visits from early June until late fall, all not only voluntary but also supported by his own surgical equipment and payment for his own expenses. Originally from New York, where he had been president of the Academy of Medicine, Andrews was lauded for the innumerable eye operations he performed. Dr Frank D. Phinney of Cincinnati succeeded Andrews as the mission's volunteer ophthalmologist. Every summer from 1928 until his death a decade later, Phinney served in the St Anthony hospital and also in those in Battle Harbour and Indian Harbour, along with many floating clinics onboard the IGA's *Strathcona* as it sailed the Labrador coast. Along with performing countless eye operations to remove cataracts as well as other procedures that staved off blindness, he refracted many cases of defective vision. Not only was all of this clinical work free of charge, but Phinney's form of American aid extended to raising sizeable funds at home to purchase equipment for the hospital in St Anthony. The fact that a few women medical specialists also volunteered suggests an aspect of missionary activity that was often integral to their medical training; for instance, Dr Emma E. Musson, an ear, nose, and throat specialist from Philadelphia who was on faculty at the Woman's Medical College, travelled to St Anthony and Labrador with a recent medical graduate of the same school, Dr Elizabeth F. Clark. Graduates of the Woman's Medical College undertook missionary work in such places as China and India; however, Musson subsequently lectured and wrote about her experience to encourage other medical personnel to volunteer for the Grenfell mission.[17] American physicians stateside greatly aided the mission's medical work as well. Clinical specimens from St Anthony were often sent for analysis to institutions like Johns Hopkins University in Baltimore or the New York State Department of Health in Albany. Clinicians who were known for their specific areas of expertise, such as neurosurgeon Harvey Cushing and cancer specialist Joseph Bloodgood, were sent details of cases admitted to the St Anthony hospital for their opinions about diagnoses and treatment; notably such expert opinions were never sought from British colleagues or from doctors in St John's – only the American connection counted.[18]

The building and inauguration of the new IGA hospital in St Anthony was a major event that also involved substantial American support. The approximately forty-bed, fully equipped new hospital officially opened in July 1927. The hospital cost $120,000 to build, with all but about $2,000 donated from the United States; the building itself, made of steel girders and concrete blocks and equipped with electrical power, central heating, and extensive plumbing, was the most modern and most substantial structure in the community.[19] The costs of the architectural design were also a gift from the architect William Adams Delano, a staunch supporter of Grenfell and all that he did.[20] The actual design, construction, and opening of this hospital are more fully described in Rafico Ruiz's chapter in this volume.

An analogous yet slightly different situation obtained in Twillingate, a small but prosperous settlement situated roughly midway on the steamer route between St John's and St Anthony on the central eastern coast. When people in the region decided to erect a hospital in the memory of local men who died in the First World War, they approached Wilfred Grenfell for guidance. This hospital, the NDBMH, was never an IGA hospital, but Grenfell was instrumental in its establishment by recommending its architect and first medical director. The architectural firm of Delano and Aldrich of New York City catered primarily to the elite of America, and again Delano himself designed the NDBMH without fee. Even more significant was the fact that the Commonwealth Fund (CF), a philanthropic foundation located in New York and based on oil revenues, contributed tens of thousands of dollars to help build the hospital; later the hospital expanded with the help of another CF grant of $50,000. CF annual reports often drew attention to the dedication and devotion of the people who were served by the hospital, noting that they comprised a population of about 50,000 fishermen and their families scattered along 300 miles of coastline (more people to care for than in St John's, and over a vast area). This funding from America was unique: the CF did not support any other comparable institution outside of the United States.[21] The NDBMH opened in 1924 with a grand ceremony and was one of the best equipped hospitals in Newfoundland; it was also likely one of the best equipped rural hospitals anywhere. For example, around 1936 the NDBMH acquired an electrocardiograph machine (ECG) to undertake cardiac examinations. Apparently no hospital in the capital of St John's could match this; it was not until the late 1920s and early 1930s that this technology was becoming widely accepted, even in leading teaching and research hospitals in the United States and Britain.[22]

The NDBMH's first medical director, Dr Charles E. Parsons, led a long line of graduates from North America's leading medical school, Baltimore's Johns Hopkins University. While still an undergraduate Amherst College student, Parsons first became connected to Grenfell in 1913 as a teacher; in 1916 he returned as a medical student assistant. After graduation in medicine from Hopkins in 1919, he served at the IGA hospital in Battle Harbour, Labrador, before taking up the post at Twillingate in 1924. For the next decade, he oversaw the running of the hospital; his successor, Dr John Olds (1906–1985), who continued for the next forty years, was a Hopkins graduate (class of 1931). Johns Hopkins was also the source of many nurses in the hospital, along with visiting medical students or recently graduated doctors. For example, Robert Ecke (1909–2001) first spent the summer of 1934 as a senior medical student at NDBMH, then intermittently from 1937 to 1941 as a junior doctor, and returned in 1947–48 as acting medical director to relieve Olds temporarily. This pattern meant that, again, as with St Anthony, people of a remote settlement of bay and island communities had constant access to some of the best-trained doctors and staff in North America. Perhaps even more so than St Anthony, however, NDBMH was an American enclave (with very little British influence): the Stars and Stripes was flown outside the hospital, and the important American holiday of Thanksgiving was always celebrated. A major social difference between these institutions was that alcohol (and tobacco and parties) was never in short supply at the Twillingate site, while Grenfell's prohibitions for staff were imposed in St Anthony.[23]

Performance Indicators: The Role of American Standards

Both these hospitals relied on the full spectrum of international aid, which especially flowed north from the United States. Although they functioned independently (unlike, for example, cottage hospitals operated by the government), they were part of the health-care ecosystem in Newfoundland, serving tens of thousands of patients across massive areas and along extensive coastlines. At the same time, they were exemplars: the IGA's main hospital in St Anthony and the NDBMH were both accredited in 1927 by the standards committee of the American College of Surgeons (ACS).[24] This accomplishment is not to be underestimated. Hospital accreditation standards for 1927 were the most stringent since the ACS initiated its standards program in 1915; in 1926 the first official ACS standards manual was published. In brief, an approved hospital had to have a clearly identified cadre of medical staff who were all licensed MDs who had graduated from acceptable medical schools (i.e., those deemed worthy in the post-1910 Flexner Report world of North American medical education). The institution had to have clear rules, regulations, and policies governing its daily operations; medical staff members were to meet regularly to review their clinical performance; and medical records of patients were to be thorough, comprehensive, accurate, well maintained, and available. The preparation and availability of recorded hospital data were important aspects for accreditation, and there appears to have been an emphasis on this function by North American institutions (and for all intents and purposes St Anthony and Twillingate were very much American institutions). A report on the NDBMH conducted in 1933 on behalf of the Commonwealth Fund by an American doctor, Beeckman Delatour, specifically commented, "The histories and records of the patients in the hospital are of the highest standard. The histories are carefully and thoroughly carried out and could be used for the compilation of facts in any research work. Careful bedside notes are kept, with complete records of medication, laboratory reports, and operative procedure. The charting is splendidly done. Final and discharge notes are made. In short, all records are carried out in such a way as to be of value for future reference."[25]

It was also required for accreditation that there be medical supervision of diagnostic and therapeutic facilities such as clinical laboratories (that is, chemical, bacteriological, serological, and pathological) and the X-ray department. It is perhaps not surprising that hospitals led by Hopkins and Harvard graduates, model schools to Flexner's mind, would fare so well, even in Newfoundland. However, that the St Anthony and Twillingate hospitals met these conditions is testament to both their staff and their physical plants: of the approximately five hundred comparable small hospitals (those with from twenty-four to fifty-nine beds) the ACS surveyed across North America, at this time more than 80 per cent failed to pass muster.[26]

The fact that that these two hospitals were in the approved 20 per cent for North America and were the only ones in Newfoundland to be accredited by the ACS was met with the "greatest satisfaction" by Grenfell.[27] In his updated autobiography published in 1932 only a few years after accreditation, Grenfell glowingly recalled the achievement. The impetus for his inviting the ACS to review the two hospitals, he noted, was a snub by the St John's medical establishment, who maintained that no hospitals existed beyond the capital city. Grenfell could prove that many patients purposefully travelled from St John's to St Anthony for treatment. "There was enough of the old Adam left in us," he recounted, "to make us smile when we learned that we were the only hospitals in the Colony that had been granted the coveted honour."[28] Nevertheless some in St John's apparently remained unimpressed, leading to a unified defence mounted from the two normally competing newspapers in the capital. Commenting on the good work done by the "admirable institution" in St Anthony, the *Daily News* thought it "well to recall that the Hospitals in St Anthony and Twillingate were awarded standardization by the American College of Surgeons, which is equivalent to professional recognition of both institutions, as of the first class, in equipment and service." A leader in the *Evening Telegram* even addressed the question of standardizing hospitals as "to the adoption of which objection is made here in some quarters on the grounds that it is an American idea." To undermine this objection, the newspaper referred to the recent hospital standardization activities of the British Medical Association which "so closely resemble the principles laid down by the American College of Surgeons as to make them for all intents and purposes parallel." It then listed the British standards alternately with those of the ACS and invited comparison; the obvious conclusion was "there is little point in the objection that has been made."[29]

Medical and Surgical Profile

There is thus ample evidence that the two accredited hospitals were doing a solid job, but what exactly was being accomplished medically and surgically? What patient conditions were admitted? What were their outcomes? Where did the patients come from? What treatments were undertaken? Is it possible to reconstruct hospital performance from clinical accounts? The medical audit and site visit conducted in 1933 by Dr Beeckman Delatour (himself an American IGA alumnus and long-time supporter) for the CF provides answers to some of these questions for the NDBMH. The ninety-bed hospital admitted 926 patients from 1931 to 1933; another 3,000 people were treated in the outpatient department for these years. The general mortality rate for the hospital was 4.4 per cent, which was reduced to 2.2 per cent if "hopeless" tuberculosis and cancer cases were not included; the post-operative mortality rate was about 2 per cent. Deaths due to tuberculosis accounted for 26 per cent of all hospital deaths, while other infections accounted for about the same percentage of deaths, meaning that half of all deaths occurred from infection. The distribution of medical to surgical cases treated was 35–65 per cent, respectively. Chronic pulmonary tuberculosis, upper respiratory tract infections, and heart conditions were the most common medical illnesses; most prominent within the surgical category were ear, nose, and throat operations (tonsillectomies, adenoidectomies) and others involving the gastrointestinal system (such as appendectomies). Many blood transfusions, pneumothorax treatments (intentional collapsing of the lung for the treatment of pulmonary tuberculosis), and the preparation of plaster casts were performed. In all, 1,965 operations were conducted from 1931 to 1933. Although the NDBMH did not undertake many births (about 1 per cent of all operative cases), interestingly the visiting physician commented on what he considered to be a large number of gynecological cases, which he attributed to the "prevalent use of midwives and consequent poor obstetrical aftercare" aggravated by the habit of the new mothers who are "up and at hard work long before involution of the uterus has taken place." This observation appears to be less critical of the practice of midwives and more a social comment on the occupational lot of Newfoundland outport women. Nonetheless, the number of operations performed specifically for women's complaints for this two-year period only is remarkable: hysterectomies (sixteen); oophorectomies (removal of ovaries) (twenty-two); perineal repairs (twenty-four); and tubal ligations and sterilizations (thirty-two). In all likelihood, many of these procedures were required clinically, but one wonders if some were not also elective surgery as a form of birth control.

The medical and surgical schedule undertaken by the sole permanent medical director of the NDBMH and his two part-time assistant physicians (along with two occasional, visiting third-year medical students) was clearly a full one. But added to such clinical duties were other laboratory and related tasks: about 400 diagnostic X-rays were taken and processed each year, along with an annual average of 1,800 blood, urine, and bacteriological tests. Also, for the period 1931–33, eleven autopsies were performed. The overall report based on these extensive data and an inspection of the hospital's more than adequate facilities concluded that the NDBMH was doing admirable work with good esprit de corps, especially taking into consideration the widely scattered population it served.[30]

A more detailed statistical profile of the St Anthony hospital can be assembled for the decade after the new hospital building opened, from reports published annually by the IGA in its magazine, *Among the Deep Sea Fishers*.[31] From 1926 to 1937, 7,702 patients were admitted, of whom 201 (2.61 per cent) died, a rate about normal for the era.[32] There were also 36,560 outpatients treated (i.e., patients treated briefly in the hospital, but who were not formally admitted to it), bringing the total cases treated to 44,262. The average duration of in-patient stays for the period ranged from 22 to 34 days, with an overall average of 28.4 days, a number again about normal for the era. The cost per patient per day in 1929 was $2.84, but declined to $1.22 by 1937; these costs were comparatively lower than for other hospitals at the time. Reports from 1927 to 1931 and for 1933 helpfully identify the patients' place of origin; not surprisingly, as now confirmed from the clinical records themselves (see table 0.2 in the introduction), most inpatients (46 per cent) came from the St Anthony district (a region defined at the time by the hospital), along with most outpatients (65 per cent). The next largest groups of in-patients and outpatients came from districts on either side of the peninsula abutting St Anthony. With 86 per cent of all patients travelling from the larger St Anthony area (although it covered an area of over 4,000 square miles), it is clear that the hospital's primary function was as a regional facility. The hospital's physician in charge, Charles Curtis, described its role in this regard in his report for 1933: "Our hospital centre at St Anthony is unique in Newfoundland. We operate in a territory where there are no local doctors, from La Scie on the east coast to Ferrole on the Strait of Belle Isle. The people can look to this hospital only for help in time of sickness." He also observed that more patients were coming to the hospital "from distant parts of the country."[33]

The remaining 14 per cent of patients identified between 1927 and 1933 did in fact come from across the entire island, including the capital of St John's, and also from coastal Labrador. There are two explanations for this group of patients: on one hand, many itinerant fishermen and their families along with ships' crew lived in areas distinct from St Anthony but, en route, needed to stop at the hospital for acute illness or injury. On the other hand, patients were referred to St Anthony from other IGA hospitals, notably one in Battle Harbour, Labrador, because of the hospital's advanced medical and surgical services; they also travelled to St Anthony on their own volition, or sometimes by referral, for treatments that were unavailable elsewhere in Newfoundland, notably radium treatment for cancers. So popular was the hospital that local newspapers routinely identified patients who travelled for treatment there, published expressions of gratitude for their treatment there, or ran notices from Grenfell himself to alert residents of visiting specialists for particular kinds of treatment.[34]

As was the case with the NDBMH, the most likely reason for admission between 1927 and 1937 was for a surgical procedure – just under half of all inpatients: general surgery accounted for 39 per cent of admissions, while an additional 7 per cent were for orthopaedic reasons. Just over one-third of patients were medical cases; obstetrical and gynecological cases were roughly equal to those who received radium treatment (approximately one-tenth each). As noted, the death rate was about 3 per cent – but for what reasons might patients die? Again, as with NDBMH, half of known recorded deaths was due to infections, and about 40 per cent of the infections was attributable to tuberculosis. The next two largest identifiable causes of death were cancer and cardiovascular disease, at much lower rates than infections, of about 6 per cent each.

Both the preponderance of surgical cases treated and the prevalence of tuberculosis at St Anthony invite further analysis. The range and performance of operative surgery was comparable to, yet more comprehensive than, that of the NDBMH: ear, nose, and throat; gastrointestinal; general; neurological; ophthalmological; urological; gynecological and obstetrical; orthopaedic; and dental. Not uncommon were the removal of tonsils, adenoids, mastoids, cataracts, epitheliomas of the lip, abscesses, and appendixes, as well as corrective surgery for cleft palates and harelips. Amputations of fingers, hands, legs, and

breasts, along with circumcisions, were also undertaken. Within orthopaedics there were many bone grafts and joint surgeries performed,
but the most common procedure involved the preparation of plaster
casts for individual limbs and whole bodies, which numbered in the
hundreds. Obstetrical work included Caesarean section and forceps
deliveries, but mostly involved "normal deliveries," which averaged
about thirty-four annually; there are only rare references each to in-
duced abortion and sterilization, although cases of dilatation and curet-
tage were not uncommon.[35]

The extraction of teeth was commonplace (numbering in the tens of
thousands), but while extractions were the line of first resort in dental
surgery across Newfoundland and Labrador, at St Anthony restorative
and preventive dentistry was practised. Root canal procedures along
with fillings using amalgam, cement, and synthetic porcelain were done
frequently. This innovation was the influence of American-style dentistry
and its practitioners, whom Grenfell acknowledged in 1927 in a tribute
to their volunteer work over the past twenty years. For instance, during
the summer of 1926 Dr Roger J. Edwards of Harvard Dental School volunteered in St Anthony along with Mrs Elta LeBlanc, a dental hygienist
from Boston; likewise Drs Morton (Harvard), Rieger (Columbia), and
Merriam (Harvard) volunteered, along with dental assistant Miss Florence France (Columbia).[36] Between 1910 and 1930, seventy dentists –
all of whom trained at premier American dental schools – undertook
voluntary work with the IGA, according to a study by Peter Bellingham.
These practitioners worked in St Anthony and in Labrador (as far north
as Hopedale, even in winter), raised funds in America for equipment and
supplies, distributed toothbrushes and toothpaste, and undertook oral
hygiene preventive measures such as educational programs for children
along with their dental clinical sessions dedicated to extractions and
restorative work. The novelty of all this activity was underscored by
Grenfell in his characteristic manner: "The gospel of prosthetic and pro-
phylactic dentistry in a distant, foreign country on a scale of this kind is
entirely unique in the world's field of dentistry, as far as I can find."[37]

Surgery was inextricably linked to tuberculosis. Although the pulmonary form of this disease was the most common, infection could
have developed in almost any bone or organ. Accordingly, resections of

knees and elbows, spinal bone grafts, amputations of feet and hands, and removal of testicles were all performed to combat tuberculosis. Standard procedures for pulmonary tuberculosis are all recorded. Lung collapsing and "refills" (artificial pneumothorax) were first reported in 1935 (135 times), 440 times in the following year, and 353 times in 1937. While this procedure was later discredited for being ineffective, performing it in St Anthony (and at Twillingate) when it was first widely advocated in the early to mid-1930s ably demonstrates that IGA and NDBMH doctors kept abreast clinically. A full examination of the problem of tuberculosis is beyond the scope of this discussion other than to say that it was well recognized as a major concern that was addressed in keeping with prevailing modes of treatment; in brief, it is clear that the institution in St Anthony, even more than the one in Twillingate, in addition to being a general hospital, also functioned at a relatively high level as a sanatorium.

The documented use of radium in St Anthony is quite remarkable and again underscores the role of American aid in both materials and personnel and how well connected the hospital was to the mainstream of medical thinking, despite its remote location. According to Grenfell, the first radium arrived around 1918 and was the gift of the Ladies Club of Sewickley, Pennsylvania; he noted that the hospital had approximately fifty milligrams, which at the time may be estimated to be worth about $6,000. (The Women's Club of Sewickley Valley, founded in 1897, remains a well-to-do organization for the promotion of "education, moral and social measures." It is based just outside of Pittsburgh, home to the Radium Chemical Company, Inc., founded in 1914 as a subsidiary of Standard Chemical Company and the primary producer of radium in the United States at the time.) In several pleas, Grenfell made clear that the supply of radium was limited while demand was great; indeed, St Anthony was the only place it was available in Newfoundland and north of Halifax, Nova Scotia, on mainland Canada. Published IGA reports show that for 1929 and 1930 there were only, respectively, 11 and 13 people treated; by 1936 and 1937 these numbers had risen dramatically to 177 and 279, respectively. Cancers treated by radium included carcinomas, epitheliomas, lymphosarcomas, and sarcomas of the prostate, tongue, uterus, rectum, cervix, lip, face, jaw, neck, and breast. What the outcomes were in all these cases is unknown, but there were some who were "cured."[38]

Patients from all around, including St John's, travelled to seek treatment. One case study is especially instructive, as it underscores the main themes of this discussion. An entry in red ink in the St John's General Hospital General Register of Patients for August 1931 to September 1936 noted that a woman from nearby Bell Island diagnosed with carcinoma of the cervix was "transferred to St Anthony Hosp 13/11/35 for Radium treatment." From IGA records we know that one month later she was admitted to the hospital in St Anthony, where she stayed until discharged on 11 May 1936. During this six-month period, the patient was treated by Dr Harrison E. Kennard, who had graduated from Harvard Medical School in 1926. At the time Kennard was a senior medical trainee, the Massachusetts General Hospital was a leader in radiation therapy, and in 1925 it became the site of the first tumour clinic in the United States. Thus as St Anthony was equipped with radium and, as important, had personnel who knew how to deploy this highly radioactive material, this woman was able to receive care and treatment that matched that offered by the best and most modern hospitals in North America. On 20 December 1935, two small metal canisters each containing forty milligrams of radium were inserted into her cervical canal and left in place for 31½ hours; on 1 January this procedure was repeated, but for 30 hours. On 4 February and then again on 18 March, two more radiation doses were administered with forty milligrams of radium for 30 hours and 31 hours, respectively. In total, this patient received around 5,000 millicurie hours of radium, which was then the standard unit dose measurement for radiation therapy. Throughout this treatment, she suffered several reactions to the radium such as elevated temperature and vomiting; her hemoglobin level also dropped and her left leg was greatly swollen, which prompted her doctor to surmise that the carcinoma had invaded her femoral vein. Nonetheless, her condition when discharged, was noted as "improved." On the basis of other sources it appears that this woman died in 1940 in Bell Island; if so, perhaps her life was extended somewhat as the result of her treatment at St Anthony, which would not have been possible without aid from America in key ways.[39]

"Statistics, however, no matter how complete they may be, are but a feeble means by which to convey more than a general idea of the incalculable value of a hospital," noted an editorial in February 1928 in the St John's *Evening Telegram* referring to the IGA hospital in St Anthony (a comment that could equally be applied to the NDBMH in Twillingate). The editorial continued by highlighting the remoteness of the institution, yet noting that this was not an impediment, for it was

situated in a locality cut off from communication with the outside world for months at a time, and yet equipped with all the latest appliances known to medical science, and staffed by highly skilled doctors and nurses. The devotion of the staff to the work of their profession is best evidenced by their voluntarily foregoing everything that one associates with life in a city, in order to minister to the sick in a place remote from friends and their accustomed surroundings.
...
If such were not the case, few of those who make the sacrifices inseparable from work of this kind, and expose themselves to dangers and hardships in the pursuit of their calling, could long hope to survive the ordeal.[40]

The St Anthony hospital indeed was well equipped and staffed, its performance admirable by many standards. But the real point for this observer was that all that had been accomplished had to be understood against the background of the isolation and remoteness of the hospital's location: the place was "cut off from ... the outside world"; the staff were deprived of "life in a city" and removed "from friends"; to do one's job was an "ordeal" that demanded sacrifices. Clearly, for this writer the *city* was the centre or core of Newfoundland, and St Anthony (or, for that matter, Twillingate) was to be portrayed for readers in St John's as at the *margin*. Perhaps residents of London, Boston, or New York City might also have shared this perspective, but based as they were in a "metropole," they probably perceived St John's itself, if not all of Newfoundland and Labrador, as being at the periphery. In this respect, while the use of concepts such as centre/margin or metropole/

periphery and urban/rural is useful, the implicit assumptions embedded within these terms can be challenged, even within a post-colonial historiographical context: it may not be wise to assume that the "centre/core/metropole/urban" always leads, while the "margin/periphery/rural" is usually backward.[41] As shown in this discussion, St Anthony and Twillingate hospitals led those in St John's in many ways, including their medical technology, such as, for example, radium therapy and electrocardiography. A corollary is that these institutions on the "periphery" qua hospitals were modernizing and civilizing agents for their "rural/remote" locales. These buildings were the most substantial and dominant ones in their small communities, not just because of their architectural style and permanent construction materials and infrastructure (girders and concrete, compared with modest wooden frame structures typically with neither indoor plumbing nor electrical power), but also owing to the exotic technology housed in them. Moreover, their staff complement was primarily well educated and urbane; even if they did forego "everything one associates with life in the city," they brought a bit of the city with them in the form of ideas and culture. By the same token, many chose a life at these hospitals (even if only temporarily) for the very reason that they were on the periphery and remote. Dr Robert Ecke, who first served as a Johns Hopkins medical student in the NDBMH in Twillingate in 1934 and who returned there regularly until the early 1940s, mused in his diary that while he liked a hot bath and a comfortable bed, he also had a "strange yearning for the remote and idyllic remoteness" of the North. On his arrival there was not an operating radio to be found, but over the years the "frontier" kept retreating and "gradually refinement has crept up on us."[42] Similarly, a British physician with "escapist tendency" who signed on for service with the Grenfell mission from 1928 to 1929, at Harrington Harbour in Quebec, and then briefly at St Anthony, desired to get "away from the grime of London."[43]

The hospitals in St Anthony and Twillingate were also, in current terminology, economic drivers. They offered steady as well as seasonal employment; they attracted funds that were one way or another circulated in the local economy. Although not nearly as developed, the socioeconomic effects of Newfoundland's cottage hospitals and medical staff may be viewed similarly. In many ways hospitals in general were of "incalculable value." Indeed, taking all medico-socio-economic-cultural parameters into consideration for all the hospitals, hospital ships, and personnel (doctors, nurses, and male and female lay practitioners) in Newfoundland and Labrador – including those of the Grenfell mission – the metaphoric concept of an ecosystem seems to describe best the health-care situation for the 1920s and 1930s. Dr H.M. Mosdell suggested a program of centralized health-care delivery was not the model to follow for Newfoundland and maintained that more cottage hospitals and field services ought to be considered rather than expanding the main hospital in St John's. To his mind, "prejudiced and uninformed critics" did not appreciate "the wisdom, necessity or advantage of elaborating *local* public health policies" (my italics).[44] In reality during the two decades studied here, with important aid of the Grenfell mission, a majority of settled areas had access to care from a multidisciplinary range of primary health-care practitioners and institutions – much more than is generally held to have been the case; moreover, elements of these services were truly second to none. Independent corroboration came later from an unexpected American source. Preparation for the installation of American military bases in Newfoundland at the onset of the Second World War (eventually totalling 100,000 troops), which solidified an earlier trend of American aid, required a full review of conditions likely to affect American personnel; in this review US Assistant Surgeon General R.A. Vonderlehr reported that "the provision for medical care of the people in Newfoundland at public expense is more effectively developed administratively than in any part of the United States."[45]

Vonderlehr and others could have also noted how this provision of medical care was positively influenced by funding from the American public to Newfoundland and Labrador through philanthropic avenues like the Grenfell mission. The concept of philanthropy is not unique to the United States, but it was "reinvented" there at the turn of the twentieth century with creation of the legal entity known as the foundation, which helped shelter excess corporate profits. This astonishingly wealthy generation of businessmen who became philanthropists, in this case for medicine, were, as Stephen C. Wheatley notes, "bent on rationalizing social organization just as they had made their fortunes rationalizing economic organization."[46] In this regard, the role of the Commonwealth Fund in Newfoundland and its support for the NDBMH stands out. Concomitant with the rise of the foundation was the invention of professionally organized intensive fundraising by consultants in the early 1900s for philanthropic purposes such as "non-profit" religious, youth, educational, and medical groups. For example, the pioneering firm of Ward, Dreshman & Reinhardt of New York City raised almost two billion dollars during the first half of the twentieth century; among its clients of hospitals, churches, and colleges was the Grenfell organization, for which the sum of one million dollars was secured.[47] And of course augmenting that large sum was the stream of funds raised from the steady donations from many Americans, along with their seemingly endless gifts in kind and free time. Thus, despite the perceived drawback of being "situated in a locality cut off from communication with the outside world for months at a time," much-needed and appreciated international aid in many forms, especially from the United States, allowed many to pursue their calling in the Grenfell mission. Might the IGA have been able to achieve its myriad goals during the 1920s and 1930s without aid from Americans? Possibly. But it could never have been as prosperous as it was during this formative period and become a medical "centre," albeit on the periphery.

Editors' Conclusion
An American Operation

These essays about the Grenfell medical mission in Newfoundland and Labrador expose the variety and depth of the resources behind Dr Wilfred T. Grenfell's extensive organizational activities, which, in the vein of myth-making, have tended to be credited mainly to his vision and efforts. Instead, authors here reveal that during the period in which Grenfell was at the helm of his organization, the mission-turned-association was a complex enterprise, with a dense transnational network of supporters, primarily from the United States, including those drawn from among the close connections that Grenfell and his American wife Anne Grenfell built with Americans. The American focus has provided a unique avenue for us to explore what was a very large, distributed enterprise over a large region during the first half of the twentieth century. It has also allowed us to emphasize the broader (North) American and social influences of the time that essentially eclipse the progressive goals of either Grenfell the man or the mission that bore his name.

Although the IGA exists today in different form and purpose, the early strong American presence in the organization and the region did not necessarily continue after the Second World War, or particularly after Newfoundland joined Canada. After Grenfell's death, the American influence was still there but then operated within an entirely different international and cross-border Canadian-American perspective. The IGA itself noted the external change, with hope, right after the vote in Newfoundland to join Canada: "It is expected," the editor of *Among the Deep Sea Fishers* observed, "that the system of government for Newfoundland under confederation will not be greatly different from 'responsible government' in practice [one of the two vote choices], with certain limitations owing to the overall power of the federal government at Ottawa." After Confederation, anticipated in 1949, the editor concluded, "we look forward with good heart to a future of increased effectiveness and prosperity for the proud island of Newfoundland, Britain's oldest colony, in common with the great democracy of Canada."[1] Moreover, as a result of the war, the IGA had already ceased some of its longstanding operations such as the sale of IGA industrial department goods within the United States.[2] The cover of its magazine, too, adopted a graphic design in 1943 that signalled a new, more modern era. As well, in the same year that Newfoundland voted to join Canada – and in the same issue of the IGA magazine – an important change within the organization occurred with the death of its executive director, Cecil Ashdown, who had served the IGA for decades from chartered accountant auditing and stabilizing the mission's finances in 1912 through prime mover of the establishment of the IGA, finance committee chair, and executive director from 1936 until his death in 1948.[3] After 1949, everything changed in the world of both the colony and the mission.

To understand an enterprise that operated in a different political framework and in a completely different world before the Second World War, chapter 1 by James K. Hiller provided necessary background information about the political (mainly imperial) and social context of Newfoundland and Labrador from 1890 to 1940. He outlined the general condition of the colony, the migratory fishery from Newfoundland to Labrador – the initial reason for Wilfred Grenfell's first voyage to the region in 1892 – and the progressive expansion of the Grenfell mission's work into fields other than, but allied to, health care. As Hiller indicated, the more ambitious Grenfell became, the greater his reliance on external philanthropy. Grenfell looked increasingly in particular to the "deeper pockets" of supporters in the United States by 1914 before cutting ties with the UK-based Royal National Mission to Deep Sea Fishermen. In effect, Hiller observed, Grenfell's mission became an American operation. It was isolated geographically, but Grenfell also isolated it, to some degree, organizationally and socially from resources in Newfoundland. Hiller considered why the reaction of Newfoundlanders to the mission could be ambivalent, or in some instances, hostile. A central problem, he concluded, was that Grenfell and his supporters sought to impose unfamiliar and foreign programs on a conservative and traditional society. An outcome of this attempt was the creation of "a colony within a colony," rather than the development of an organizational structure that worked alongside, and engaged in mutual benefit with, existing institutions and structures.

In the next chapter, Jennifer J. Connor examined the social and organizational architecture of Grenfell's enterprise that was constructed from various fin-de-siècle "movements." She demonstrated how Grenfell capably tapped into the mission movement, settlement house movement, and student volunteer movement, as well as broad social reform movements, to embed his northern activities within transnational networks of mission activities. A heavy emphasis in Grenfell's work was the recruitment and deployment of many young upper-class Americans to work in Newfoundland and Labrador. As she delineated, Grenfell's appeal, carried throughout promotional activities by his followers, increasingly conveyed the message that the region's population shared Anglo-Saxon ancestry with these Americans, especially to highlight the racial and linguistic connections this poor population had with American donors and volunteers.

Chapter 3 by Ronald L. Numbers presented a key concept in Grenfell's multi-faceted approach to his mission: the gospel of right living. Grenfell's long association with Dr John Harvey Kellogg, the leading health reformer who was based in Battle Creek, Michigan, illustrates similarities and differences in pragmatic approaches to this concept, which encompassed moderation in all things (with an emphasis on diet) and abstinence in some things (notably alcohol, tobacco, spices), all towards a healthy body and a healthy mind. Both physicians projected an image of manliness, and both turned increasingly from evangelical religion to eugenics and the Social Gospel. Both also promoted each other in their own publications. As Numbers showed, Grenfell not only portrayed Kellogg as a "good angel to our work" through Kellogg's significant food donations to the mission, but he also praised Kellogg's food products for their easy assimilation and preparation, nutritive value, and low cost – all important considerations for people of Newfoundland and Labrador and for the mission's aim to improve public health in this northern region.

As Grenfell's enterprise expanded and drew on monetary gifts from wealthy donors, as Heidi Coombs-Thorne explained in the next chapter, this financial support depended on a carefully crafted public image that depicted Grenfell's mission as a deserving and responsible organization. However, as Coombs-Thorne demonstrated, the actions of one administrator, the superintendent of the King George V Seamen's Institute in St John's, threatened to discredit the entire mission and destroy the public favour that Grenfell had been building for twenty years. A scandal that called into question the accounting practices of the mission culminated in August 1912 with the superintendent, Charles Karnopp, being convicted of misappropriation of funds and sentenced to six months in jail. Karnopp's conviction laid bare the mission's administrative and accounting problems and consequently had a significant impact on the mission and its future. It signalled a large-scale restructuring of the mission; the eventual break from the parent mission, the RNMDSF; and the establishment of a systematized organization – all handled, to a great extent, by Cecil Ashdown, the auditor who had uncovered the fraud and who would ultimately manage the financial affairs of the IGA and work with Wilfred Grenfell for the next four decades. Indeed, as Coombs-Thorne argued, the events surrounding the arrest and conviction of Karnopp and the growing influence of American philanthropy on Grenfell and his activities led to the incorporation of the International Grenfell Association in 1914.

Together, these four chapters comprise Part I: Shaping the Grenfell Mission, making a valuable contribution to scholarly understanding of the IGA's organizational structure and its cultivation of supporters, allies, and donors, particularly throughout the United States. This latter emphasis is in contrast to connections that have been drawn commonly between the mission's British parent organization, the RNMDSF, and Grenfell's work in northern Newfoundland and coastal Labrador. Research by these four contributors shows how organizational connections to Great Britain were relatively short-lived in terms of the mission's organizational history, and how the mission strategically shifted its focus and attention towards American support and its attractive and financially lucrative model of middle-class philanthropy in order to ensure a steady supply of funds, volunteer workers, and donated goods, while enhancing the mission's reputation.

While these analyses alone cannot plumb the full extent of the mission's organizational structure, they do point to a number of areas for future research. One aspect could be the development of non-denominational non-governmental humanitarian aid in the twentieth century as reflected in the work of Grenfell in particular. This concept was emphasized by an article in a Battle Creek, Michigan, newspaper in a brief comparison of the careers of Kellogg and Grenfell when the two men celebrated their birthdays in 1940. In this meeting of Kellogg and "the Labrador doctor," it noted, "more than 116 years of medical experience and humanitarian service was represented." After outlining Grenfell's work, the article stressed again that his "half century of splendid achievement ... has been solely that of humanitarian service." When Grenfell died several months later, the newspaper again described him as a "humanitarian" who had been knighted for building hospitals and organizing humanitarian work.[4]

Significantly, this collection does not address the religious aspect of the mission's activities, albeit their unobtrusive, non-denominational, and voluntary nature. Workers, however, were required to sign up for service as teetotal Christians,[5] and physicians were expected to preach in communities, onboard ship, and in hospital wards, or to perform funeral services for different Protestant faiths as part of their mission service, sometimes out of necessity and upon request from residents as the only professional around.[6] The connections with belief systems in general, including those related to health, might perhaps be traced in their changing circumstances – and to the perception of Grenfell's values. For instance, Grenfell's memory was being used at the sanitarium in Battle Creek, Michigan, for Canadians, in a kind of tourist guide patter, long after his death and the time period for these chapters. A lifestyle article in 1961 in a national Canadian magazine, *Maclean's*, told readers that "Oscar Engen, your treatment supervisor, tells you casually as he tucks you into a hot-fomentation bed to simmer, that this very bed was particularly pleasing to Sir Wilfred Grenfell after the cold of Labrador."[7]

Of course, there is no evidence that Grenfell ever did this or would agree with this statement – and in fact, Grenfell along with most mission workers travelled by boat in the region during summer, when harbours became free of ice – but this account foregrounds the myth-making that had occurred about Grenfell the man and the assumption that a Canadian visitor to the sanitarium would recognize and value him as an icon to emulate. The myth of the man may no longer resonate with Canadians but is still invoked locally when those in the region seek to resurrect or reinvent the spirit behind Grenfell's resourcefulness. A meeting of government and community representatives late in 2017 to explore the "untapped potential" of the Northern Peninsula region around St Anthony included one researcher's suggestion to rebuild the gardens and greenhouses established by Grenfell's mission: because Wilfred Grenfell's intention was to bring food security to the people of the region, his important message was to teach them "to do things themselves, to sustain themselves, not just do it and leave."[8]

In general, the Grenfell mission's links to other missions and religious organizations, including its early connections to the Moravian mission in Labrador, could be explored, especially with respect to strong, organizationally supportive connections in the United States. The IGA's Fifth Avenue offices in New York, for example, were in the building constructed by the Presbyterian Church to house its missionary work, in a centrally located area known locally as "Paternoster Row" for its collection of churches and ancillary organizations. The domestic and foreign missions department, as with other church groups at the time, included the Women's Board of Home Missions of the Presbyterian Church. Other early tenants of the Presbyterian Building, as it was then known, were religious publishing houses and the Women's National Sabbath Alliance.[9] Not only did the IGA have its headquarters here, at 156 Fifth Avenue, but the entire building block of 154–8 Fifth Avenue also contained the offices of the publisher Fleming H. Revell at 158 Fifth Avenue. Revell was a major publisher of Grenfell's early books about Labrador and those by Norman Duncan that were based on Grenfell; furthermore, Revell provided space in the basement for donations to the mission prior to their shipment to Newfoundland and Labrador via the Red Cross Line, arrangements that Revell also made for the shipper's free transportation to St John's.[10] Study of these American and religious organizational connections, if possible, might uncover more information about the way in which the IGA operated as a corporate enterprise.

The methods of transportation were integral to the mission's operation and organizational structure in coastal areas: yachts, yawls, schooners, and other kinds of vessel – which were usually donated to the mission – ferried supplies (including clothing for exchanges and library materials for lending) and passengers (including patients, hospital staff, volunteer workers, and visiting mission supporters) to, from, and around the mission's widely dispersed premises. These vessels, too, have not been examined, including the important medical work conducted from and through these ships, especially the *Strathcona* with Dr Wilfred Grenfell as travelling physician.[11] Nor have the methods of ground transportation, especially during winter as physicians learned how to use a komatik and dog teams as they travelled for hundreds of miles around the mission's premises that were open year-round.

The collection's next six chapters form Part II: The Grenfell Enterprise in Motion to identify and examine key aspects of the mission's operations up to the 1940s. John R. Matchim's chapter 5 used sports history as an entry into the cosmopolitan character of the mission. With sprawling industrial cities in Great Britain and North America, and few spaces left for imperial expansion, concerns about emasculation and "race suicide" were common upper- and middle-class concerns. In keeping with such widely held contemporary views, Grenfell believed that physical activity cultivated a healthy mind and that sport and exercise were as essential to mission activities as they had been in Grenfell's own public school education in Britain. Grenfell's own prowess as an athlete, his adherence to muscular Christianity, his belief in physicality for both work and leisure, and his emphasis on men's physical activity, all demonstrated this belief in action. Importantly, Matchim argued that the combination of sport physical activity, drawn from the national games and attitudes of mission staff and volunteers, formed an integral part of the ethos of the mission, and furthermore, that such activity reflected the issues of class, gender, race, and imperialism. In this wide social context of beliefs about masculinity and a proper education, the prospect of working in the seemingly inhospitable regions of the Grenfell mission appealed to generations.

Emma Lang and Katherine Side studied another key aspect of Grenfell's belief, essentially a moral one that underpinned his mission: aiding people through dignity and work, not through their pauperization by charity. Grenfell specified that donated clothing and goods were to be obtained through the systematic exchange of labour and not through charitable distribution. As Lang and Side indicated in chapter 6, the mission's receipt and exchange of new and second-hand clothing was central in its goal of self-reliance for local populations, as a twofold means for helping them to escape potential exploitation by local merchants and to convey respectability on them – which included imparting middle-class values, expressed partly through dress. Assistance in this process was sought especially from across North America, and from the United States in particular. Supporters sent regular clothing donations to St Anthony, the mission's central collection point. Lang and Side argued that this process was the principal means through which the mission established its connections with, and tracked the support of, its many locally based branches and through which it communicated its primary messages about cultivating self-sufficiency among recipients. As well, for its part, the mission developed and marketed cloth for its windproof and weatherproof efficiencies; sales of this "Grenfell cloth"[12] highlighted Grenfell's connection to the North and aided the mission's work.

Research conducted by Lang and Side for this chapter led to the development of a bilingual travelling exhibit, *Tangled Threads / Fils Entremêlés*, which was displayed at museums, three of which were former Grenfell mission stations, on Newfoundland's west coast during summer 2017.[13] This kind of scholarly focus on material culture aspects of the mission invites similar studies related to other kinds of donation to the mission, which included not just bedding and equipment for hospital wards but also communications equipment (radio, typewriter), domestic equipment (sewing machine, spinning wheel), and many other items such as theatrical costumes.[14]

A little-known strand in the institutional history of the IGA is the semi-autonomous and short-lived White Bay Unit, located south of St

Anthony. By exploring the origins and activities of this unit in chapter 7, Mark Graesser drew attention to another under-reported feature of the mission: the placement of summer "teachers" in coastal communities. More accurately characterized as community development workers, these volunteers played roles and often had experiences that were quite different from those of health-care workers, institutional staffers, and male WOPs based at the various Grenfell hospitals and nursing stations. Elizabeth Page, a university graduate from New York, was the driving force behind the White Bay Unit, and her work, along with that of her supporters, challenges perceptions about the singular assertion of authority and control over Grenfell's enterprises and its workers. Graesser demonstrated that Page undertook her own recruitment, managed personnel, and personally secured much-needed resources; he argued that her activities identify her as an IGA "builder" in the mould of other well-educated, self-reliant, progressive American women who led the evolution from medical mission to fully institutionalized social reform organization. Page's interplay with the IGA in New York and St Anthony, and her vision of self-reliance, contrasted with institutionalized dependency that was exercised under the auspices of the IGA.

While these chapters identified American support within and to Newfoundland and Labrador, many contributions in the collection also alluded to the valuable work done stateside on behalf of Grenfell's enterprise throughout this period. As with the religious connections in New York, more could be explored from this perspective, particularly in the market for, and sales of, products of the cottage industry. Mission stores were established in New York and Philadelphia as outlets for home industries in support of the mission, along with Dog Team taverns and tea houses in Vermont and Connecticut. In 1938, the dozen summer volunteers who worked in these latter establishments were acknowledged as a separate part of the Staff Selection Committee report.[15] Similarly, study of the American societies and associations that routinely worked in tandem with the IGA, such as the Needlework Guild of America (which, despite its name, was dedicated to both sewing and purchasing new clothing for the mission),[16] might augment our understanding of the broad-based networks that Grenfell tapped for his work.

The mission's distinctive hooked mats have received some scholarly attention,[17] but other aspects of its material culture remain unconsidered. For instance, the IGA's Victoria Street offices in London played a central role in the production of some of the IGA's print materials, including postcards. Produced for distinct markets in Great Britain, the United States, and Canada, Christmas cards and calendars were sold annually to support the mission's activities. Such materials constitute what contributor Rafico Ruiz has referred to elsewhere as the IGA's "media infrastructure" that accompanied and complemented its organizational and physical structures and that enhanced the transnational transmission of the IGA's central purposes.[18] Additionally, although the mission's emphasis in its promotional material rested squarely on what it perceived to be the culturally related Anglo-Saxon people actually served by the mission, in order to sell its unique brand and consequently, its products, its crafts depicted Inuit people in characteristic attire and activities. The tension between these two public-outreach activities and their outcomes by the later twentieth century could be explored more fully in studies of Grenfell's mission.

The dissemination of printed material was an essential part of the mission's public relations operation and was an area in which Grenfell himself made a substantial contribution as a writer, artist, and photographer. Grenfell's impromptu sketches often accompany his signature on fly-leaves of his books, and his signed card designs are still sold. His designs were also used for hooked mats, and his whimsical sketches adorn and illustrate at least three books; they also appear as illustrations in early clinical records of the mission.[19] Indeed, because Grenfell was an inveterate scribbler, always sketching and doodling in addition to writing, it is perhaps not far-fetched to see a link between his visual imagination at play in these creative forms and in shaping a medical mission and association. As the chapters in this collection illustrated, Grenfell saw the Newfoundland and Labrador region as a white canvas on which he had free rein to sketch his own structure for large-scale social reform: health care, food and nutrition, education for the body and mind, warmth and protection, and home-based commercial enterprises.

Future examinations of the mission's cultural engagement and output might study the industrial department's gendered enterprises in wooden toy making, weaving, and drawing and painting. The former two activities appear to have been earmarked for those who were considered in need of lessons in industriousness, whereas the latter activities, drawing and painting, were often considered the purview of the mission's volunteer workers. Some of the visiting artists to the mission became well known. They include British-born, watercolour artist and mission volunteer Rhoda Dawson, whose work is included in the collection of the Victoria and Albert Museum, London. Educated at the Hammersmith School of Art and Royal Academy Schools, London, Dawson began working with the IGA's industrial department in 1930; between 1930 and 1935, she completed ninety-one watercolour paintings of Newfoundland and Labrador.[20] Also known for his watercolours was British-born corporate executive Cecil S. Ashdown, who had guided the financial affairs of the IGA for almost forty years. Ashdown's watercolours specifically of Newfoundland and Labrador appeared on mission Christmas cards and were included in large exhibitions.[21] Later representations of the mission include the graphic design of New York–based book illustrator LeRoy Appleton, which from 1943 graced the cover of *Among the Deep Sea Fishers*.[22] (See p. 100 in this volume.)

Drama also awaits study in the context of the mission on which it was based. For example, volunteer Florence Clothier's *She Canna Perish: A Play of the Labrador Coast* debuted at Vassar College in 1926 and was published by the Vassar Experimental Theatre in 1933. Clothier also wrote *Right Machinery: A Drama in Three Acts*, a play set in Tilt Cove, Newfoundland, that appears to have been based on her mission experiences.[23] Dawson also wrote plays about mission life, at least three of which are known.[24] Similarly, the mission had a well-established tradition of staging two musicals per year, at Christmas and Easter, that might provide insights into the cultural life of the organization. Indeed, scholars might study the broad introduction of cultural traditions by mission workers, not just play and games, but also holiday customs. For instance, Arthur Wakefield, a British physician who frequently served with the mission in Labrador, humorously described in 1910 his unrecognized role as Santa Claus. After a gruelling fifteen and a half-hour's walk back to Cartwright from a medical journey, arriving on Christmas Eve, Wakefield wrote, Santa Claus duly arrived the next day:

"Children and adults were alike charmed, for there was scarcely a person present who had ever seen Santa Claus or a Christmas tree before." The children told Wakefield for days afterward they were sorry he had not been there to see him.[25] Toys to place under the Christmas tree had been sent to Cartwright by "New England friends and marked, 'For Dr Wakefield's Christmas trees.'"[26]

Cultural and social reform included the mission's training and educating people of Newfoundland and Labrador, both within the region and at American institutions. As Helen Woodrow explored in chapter 8, examination of this activity extends Graesser's discussion of community-based teachers in White Bay while linking to the next chapter by Rafico Ruiz. Unusual for Newfoundland (Labrador had a more limited and poorly developed system of education), Grenfell insisted on a non-denominational approach to education that was funded almost entirely by the mission. Significantly, Woodrow showed how the mission schools differed dramatically from those run from the 1920s by the government's Department of Education, with oversight by church denominations: the mission attracted qualified teachers, had more teaching rooms and resources, and employed a curriculum that offered practical training. She also analyzed the mission's involvement with the Carnegie Corporation of New York, which twice gave an annual grant that financed a portion of the mission's practice of providing select individuals with educational opportunities outside of Newfoundland and Labrador. This support was administered through the mission's United States Educational Committee, by Anne Grenfell. Most beneficiaries attended schools and colleges in the New England states, and many received education in trades. The cooperation of American institutions also made it easier for residents of Newfoundland and Labrador to study in the United States. Woodrow outlined Grenfell's close association, in particular, with Berea College in Berea, Kentucky. Founded in the mid-nineteenth century as the first interracial and coeducational college in the American South with goals similar to Grenfell's (including temperance and the dignity of labour),[27] Berea College provided educational and vocational training for disadvantaged Appalachian populations.

Finally, to illustrate the impact of the mission's education on local residents, Woodrow included four condensed life stories of individuals who lived in northern Newfoundland or Labrador and who benefited from training, education, and employment with Grenfell's enterprise. Their recollections revealed their own perspectives on play, clothing donations, hospital appointments, agricultural endeavours, and certification (which was important for the hospital and also for education). With the foundation provided here by Woodrow, together with discussions by Graesser and Ruiz, a fuller picture of the mission's educational priorities and practices could be developed that captures the entire scope of mission initiatives in informal education, including apprenticeship (among hospital ward maids, for instance) and libraries (which again were aided by donations from the United States and are examined elsewhere by co-editor Jennifer J. Connor[28]).

The construction of a new modern hospital in 1927 to replace its predecessor at St Anthony afforded Rafico Ruiz insight into another of the residents whom the mission trained and employed – in this instance, alongside a lasting physical structure. As Ruiz indicated in chapter 9, perceptions of the Grenfell mission as an institution were defined by its metropolitan philanthropic networks and by its prime representatives of New York's Fifth Avenue elite, who included the architect in charge of the hospital project, William Adams Delano (who decades later served as vice-president of the Grenfell Association of America). Yet, Ruiz noted, underlying this metropolitan narrative of fundraising and philanthropic concern was the actual labour involved in building what was, according to Grenfell, the most modern hospital in the British Empire: coordinating the collection of materials and their arrival in St Anthony, and contending with local building technologies and practices.

Edgar ("Ted") McNeill, a Labrador-born ward of the mission, would prove to be one of the mission's most adept builders and the foreman in charge of the project. McNeill had acquired his education, with assistance from the mission, at the School of Science and Technology of the Pratt Institute in New York. Ruiz assembled a counter-biographical sketch that suggests how McNeill was part of a broader network of local manual labourers involved in erecting the St Anthony hospital that could provide a "made in Newfoundland" authenticity to the northerly modernity of the institution. In the process, McNeill would prove how this seemingly alien building type was co-produced by both off-island and on-island institutional, material, and human components, capital, and equipment from New York, as well as a local labouring population with newly acquired skills, construction mettle, and a longstanding work ethic. Ruiz also included some of his interview with Dorothy McNeill, Ted McNeill's daughter, and his chapter uniquely combined two narrative registers, the analytical-historical and the oral, in order to reassess the role of a foreman such as McNeill in the institutional identity of the mission and indicate how McNeill could stand in for anonymous and difficult-to-trace fisherfolk labourers who were involved in the construction of the mission's medical and philanthropic infrastructure.

The mission's operations occupied prominent spaces in Newfoundland and Labrador, and the layout of towns such as St Anthony are still shaped by the mission's historical presence and activities. It is ironic that some of the purpose-built buildings that were the mainstay of the IGA stand today as part of Newfoundland and Labrador's heritage tourism industry and still draw substantial numbers of visitors from outside the province. While analyses have relied heavily on the mission's textually and visually based archival traces, future consideration might encompass this aspect of its material culture and its effects on the province's built environments. These examinations could also extend to the mission's forays into agriculture (including experimental farm and related seed experiments), animal husbandry, and Grenfell's short-lived livestock project that began with the importation of a reindeer herd and Sami herders from Norway.[29] Grenfell's agricultural and animal husbandry projects are abundantly documented in photographic collections, which themselves remain understudied artifacts.

Finally, through analysis of the published clinical and surgical reports of the mission hospital in St Anthony and the Notre Dame Bay Memorial Hospital in Twillingate in the 1920s and 1930s, in chapter 10 J.T.H. Connor uncovered the scope of the mission's health-care activities. After outlining the modes of health-care delivery in the region, Connor demonstrated how the mission hospital activities spotlight the significant role played by the United States in sending funds and material donations; in providing medical staff, supplies, collegial clinical consultations, and ancillary services; and in building and accrediting hospitals. More importantly, Connor showed how these two hospitals had an impact on health care on the island of Newfoundland and how they illustrate the transition of Grenfell's vision to a twentieth-century American philanthropic enterprise geared toward social progress. His study counters views about St John's as the region's only modernized location for medical care and confirms that, with this American support, the St Anthony hospital, with exception only of the Notre Dame Bay Memorial Hospital, was the most professionally connected and advanced hospital in Newfoundland. Connor argued that it was therefore American aid that laid the foundation in Newfoundland and Labrador for an independent health-care system that thrived and survived long enough to become absorbed by the prevailing public government scheme.

Regionally specific relations between the mission and the United States for health care could be examined further, including the involvement of medical staff at particular locales, such as the presence of New York's Columbia University students and staff at Spotted Islands, Labrador, and Baltimore's Johns Hopkins University's students and staff at Battle Harbour, Labrador. These long-term relationships may have shaped medical and social relationships and may have established long-lasting place-based associations and/or geographic connections. As well, comparative studies of the clinical work based on the records of government-funded or religiously affiliated hospitals in St John's with those especially of the IGA hospital in St Anthony would further augment understanding of the respective roles of both kinds of institution within the health-care ecosystem for the island of Newfoundland.

This volume's focus on the IGA's organizational and operational visibility can be regarded as a first step in uncovering and understanding the mission's organizational structure, its operations and its networks. As indicated briefly in this conclusion, there is still much to offer future researchers. The complexities of the IGA's activities are well apparent in this collection: its activities were ambitious, its geographic reach was wide, and its support base was broad. Its networks and beneficiaries extended across geography, borders, and continents in complex ways. Far from being in a remote and distant locale, these philanthropic activities brought Newfoundland and Labrador closer to similar projects undertaken by social missions and moral reformers elsewhere, particularly in the United States. Because Grenfell's unique amalgam of social reform and philanthropy went largely unchallenged by Newfoundland's successive governments, the IGA was able to develop and provide its own models of health care, education, and, on occasion, justice.[30] Indeed, although some government and church leaders in St John's were publicly unhappy with the image that Grenfell broadcast about poverty among Newfoundlanders and Labradorians, they evidently were more than comfortable to relinquish to his mission's operations both the task and the cost of providing health care in particular. For at least fifty years, from the 1890s until the 1940s, as these chapters have shown, the Grenfell mission filled a vacuum in the much needed provision of medical and social services, and it addressed gaps created by the Newfoundland government's limited finances and administrative capacities and by the region's challenging geography.

Local residents, however, may hold different perspectives on Grenfell the man and on the work of his mission in their communities, especially those outside St John's, and residents' views likely change over time. As James Hiller explained, Grenfell received a mixed reaction at the time, and mission workers were not always received enthusiastically. Much work on this aspect of the mission needs to be undertaken for the period under study, although traces of residents' voices are difficult to locate. Newspapers afford one avenue. For example, the fact that writers in St John's criticized the kinds of "gentlemen" associated with Grenfell and his work (in this case, Dr A.W. Wakefield), who "strike the town with a sympathetic tone and splash advice around in wholesale quantities,"[31] contrasts with Newfoundland residents who wrote letters to the editor thanking the hospitals for their care, as indicated briefly in the chapter by J.T.H. Connor.[32] The voices of local, rural residents appear throughout this volume, although sometimes refracted through other published sources that derive extensively from the large literature of the mission, literature that may portray their voices in positive – or quaint – ways. As the chapters by Jennifer Connor, Emma Lang and Katherine Side in particular indicated, these published sources show how the IGA had imperialistic impulses to "uplift" the impoverished "Anglo-Saxon" people of the region at a time when missions were widely criticized for adopting this approach with other races.

Through similar "media traces," Rafico Ruiz focused his chapter on the work of local labour on the new hospital building in St Anthony – the "men behind the scenes" – but was able to extend the discussion by interviewing the daughter of the local builder. Perhaps from the vantage point of a generation removed from direct work with Wilfred Grenfell, she took special care to emphasize the degree to which residents of both Newfoundland and Labrador were not isolated, geographically or mentally, before and after Grenfell arrived. A potential inference that this need to explain to an outsider reflected reaction to the paternalism associated with Grenfell and his mission is made manifest in the publications of residents themselves. As revealed in the life stories that Helen Woodrow excerpted from residents employed or aided by the mission, their experiences were not unreservedly or consistently positive, and they might even depend on their geographic location within the mission enterprise. In one case, a paid farmer in Labrador was dismissed by one of Grenfell's longstanding supporters, Dr Paddon; in another, a young girl was abused in Ontario by a Grenfell teacher before returning to friends and family in St Anthony and embarking on IGA-sponsored training in the United States; and in another, a schoolgirl did not appreciate being told at a Labrador school she was lucky to have "nice clothes" when she missed her home and family, but had a much better experience later in St Anthony. Although recent oral histories have been undertaken about work for the Grenfell mission in later years of the twentieth century,[33] a full historical "bottom up" approach from local communities could form the basis of subsequent, more nuanced study of the Grenfell enterprise in its first fifty years in order to build on the one developed here as an initial foray into the topic.

Volunteer workers in the mission came from many countries other than the United States and Canada. The formal organizational structures, personal networks, or underlying religious or social motivations for these volunteers remain under-examined, as do organizational features of the IGA that followed a transatlantic route rather than the ties to continental North America explored in this collection. A notable gap, for instance, is the place of Ireland (which would presumably have been, after partition, Northern Ireland) in the London-based Grenfell Association of Great Britain and Ireland.

Nevertheless, as this collection demonstrated, it was American volunteer workers, and support provided by US-based societies, foundations, educational institutions and networks – mainly from the eastern seaboard – that above all afforded the modernity with which the IGA came to be associated and that was distinct from the reputation of Newfoundland and Labrador. Not all of the American influence at the mission was, in modern terms, entirely positive, however, as suggested by J.T.H. Connor elsewhere with respect to the sterilization in St Anthony of women deemed mentally unfit.[34] (Indeed, today the province itself struggles to clean up sites vacated by the US military in the 1960s.[35]) Some – especially in modern Canada – might wonder about American imperialism in the examples presented here of the attempts by mission volunteers to educate Newfoundland and Labrador children about American geography and culture. Indeed, the full extent of the mission's reliance on donated American reading materials, while identified elsewhere by Jennifer Connor,[36] has yet to be examined as one way in which American values may have been inculcated in local residents.

Yet the reliance of Grenfell's organization on both Americans and other nationalities of its personnel essentially continued the activities of a geographic region that for centuries had acted as a "crossroads of the world," as the result of the large fishing trade shared by many nations in the Atlantic waters around Newfoundland. Indeed, the region could be perceived as almost tailor-made in current terms for historical studies of transnationalism, the core interest of which rests on concepts of circulation, movement, and exchange – a global experience of interconnections and processes that are not contained within nations.[37] The fact that these concepts are inherent to missions in general is clearly indicated by their historians, who note that Anglo-American connections had long supported missionary work to convert the whole world to their shared view of Protestant Christianity,[38] and that missions developed international networks of colleagues through "recruitment, intermarriage, personal friendships, revival movements and scholarly exchanges."[39] At an early period, Grenfell's mission thus perhaps anticipated global secular trends in aid and development that would become more pronounced in the latter part of the twentieth century with the establishment of federal and non-government organizations for student volunteer work overseas.[40] These activities on the Yale University campus alone by then embraced a range of charities, notably the World Student Service Fund,[41] and the memoir of a later Yale summer volunteer therefore likened the Grenfell work to that of a federal organization, the US Peace Corps founded in 1961.[42] Ironically, the non-government Canadian University Students Overseas (CUSO) program had initially – and misleadingly – been popularly dubbed "Canada's Peace Corps."[43] Fuller study of Grenfell's mission within the context of the larger secular movements in the twentieth century that supported international aid would greatly advance our knowledge of the approaches taken globally.

As models of governance and philanthropy changed over time, so too did the area's fortunes. Philanthropy shifted in the IGA from Wilfred Grenfell himself towards custodianship by other, prominent mission workers, and eventually the role of the IGA was absorbed into the existing political, medical, and social landscape of Newfoundland and Labrador. Its legacy, however, remains embedded in the region's psyche. In light of the scholarly contributions made here and the abundance of archival materials and areas of consideration available, the Grenfell mission and its place in Newfoundland and Labrador through the twentieth century deserve continued scholarly consideration to expand knowledge of its complex organization, operations, and connections.

Notes

1 For the initial part of our discussion and table 0.2 from clinical records, we are indebted to J.T.H. Connor and to research assistant John R. Matchim, who was initially supported by a Canadian Institutes of Health Research grant (HOM-98740), to Jennifer J. Connor, J.T.H. Connor, Monica Kidd, and Maria Mathews. Statistics also derive from Grenfell Association of Great Britain and Ireland, *Medical Work in Labrador and Northern Newfoundland: Eleventh Annual Report*; and [International Grenfell Association], *A Few Facts about the Grenfell Missions*. See also Connor, Connor et al., "Conceptualizing Health Care"; and J.T.H. Connor, "'Medicine Is Here to Stay.'"

2 This estimate is based on travel times reported by Nigel Rusted to fifty ports of call for the 1930s: McKinnon, "Health and Medical Services Perspective of the Labrador Fishery," 16, 45, 50, MU-FLA. In later years this time was shortened to about nine days, presumably because of fewer stops at smaller outports: see Brian Rusted, "Diary of a Medical Student on the SS *Kyle.*"

3 See International Grenfell Association, "Our History"; Battle Harbour, "Historic Trust." For a review of later IGA activities, see Thomas, "The International Grenfell Association"; Thomas, "The International Grenfell Association. Part II"; and Thomas, *From Sled to Satellite.*

4 Simms and Ward, *Regional Population Projections for Labrador and the Northern Peninsula 2016–2036.* This report initiated media accounts of the region, which suggested that, among other things affected by this decline, the "local hospital, once the administrative home

for health care in the region, has also lost some of its influence": Terry Roberts, "'Just a Ghost Town, That's All': The Northern Peninsula and Its Population Predicament," CBC News Newfoundland and Labrador, 6 November 2016. https://www.cbc.ca/news/canada/newfoundland-labrador/northern-peninsula-population-plunge-1.3824345.

5   The Labrador-Grenfell Regional Health Authority delivers care to the people once served by Wilfred Grenfell through three hospitals, three community health centres, fourteen community clinics, and two long-term care facilities, north of Bartlett's Harbour on Newfoundland's Northern Peninsula and all of Labrador on the mainland of Canada (an area of approximately 193,000 square kilometres, with a population of around 37,000): see Labrador-Grenfell Regional Health Authority, "About Us."

6   Labrador-Grenfell Regional Health Authority, "Grenfell Foundation." Grenfell's image and quotation also appear on the website banner of the Faculty of Medicine, Memorial University of Newfoundland. From its establishment in 1967, the medical school has aimed to provide physician graduates to rural practices around the province.

7   Grenfell Historic Properties.

8   Battle Harbour, "History"; Grenfell Louie A. Hall Bed and Breakfast, "Our History."

9   Crimi, Ney, and Cobb, *Jewels of Light*, 96–7.

10 Coombs-Thorne, "Nursing with the Grenfell Mission"; Coombs-Thorne, "Conflict and Resistance to Paternalism"; Coombs-Thorne, "'Mrs Tilley'"; Coombs-Thorne, "'Such a Many-Purpose Job'"; Ruiz, "Sites of Communication"; Ruiz, "Media Infrastructure"; Ruiz, "Moving Image on the North Atlantic."

11 Ronald Rompkey, "Heroic Biography and the Life of Sir Wilfred Grenfell"; J.T.H. Connor, "Rural Medical Lives and Times"; J.T.H. Connor, "Putting the 'Grenfell Effect' in Its Place."

12 *Congregationalist*, "Patron Saint of Labrador," 14.

13 Grenfell, *Adrift on an Icepan*. To survive, Grenfell killed some of his sled dogs, huddled under their flayed bodies, and wore their skins along with his school rugby outfit.

14 For example, Johnston, *Grenfell of Labrador*.

15 Duncan, *Doctor Luke of the Labrador*; Duncan, *Dr Grenfell's Parish*; Duncan, *Adventures of Billy Topsail*; Duncan, *Billy Topsail, MD*. Duncan protested in his book *Dr Grenfell's Parish* that his fictional *Doctor Luke* was not based on Grenfell ("To the Reader," [8]).

16 For example, Grenfell, *A Labrador Doctor*; Grenfell, *Forty Years for Labrador*.

17 Porter, "Religion, Missionary Enthusiasm, and Empire," 240; Buckner, "Creation of the Dominion of Canada," 77. This literature has been widely acknowledged but studied in piecemeal fashion, often with respect to the role of women in its production; see, for example, Sarah Robbins, "Woman's Work for Woman"; Schoepflin, "Mythic Mission Lands"; Gerson, *Canadian Women in Print*, 140.

18 For an example of Pomiuk's writing from Battle Harbour, see "Pomiuk's Letter to Mr Martin, 1897," in Petrone, ed., *Northern Voices*, 77.

19 "Kirkina"; "Jottings from the Grenfell Association of America"; Charles Curtis, "It Should Be Told," 5.

20 For print copies of these instructions, see Grenfell Historic Properties Collection, Florence F. Fuller photograph album (1926–7); and PAD, IGA Fonds, MG 63.2138, c 1940, box 63, "Instructions for Staff Members."

21 Grenfell, "Missions," 226–36. See also the journal entries and reports of the 1893 Grenfell voyage, which included time spent with the Moravian mission, in Curwen, *Labrador Odyssey*, 99–103, 126–8. Hans Rollmann has studied this mission extensively: see, for example, "Hopedale."

22 See the letter by Jas. Dove in St John's about the summer circuit to harbours of Methodist people around the Red Bay region, "The Home Work." For more discussion of this history, see Edgar Jones, "Early Work of the Church of England in Labrador."

23 Ronald Rompkey, *Grenfell*, ix. Of note, the 2017 apologies for treatment of Indigenous people in both IGA and Moravian institutions were directed primarily at the post-Confederation period 1949 to 1979 when thousands of Indigenous children were taken from their homes to attend residential schools. See "'A Painful Chapter of Canada's History': Read the PM's Apology for N.L. Residential Schools," CBC News Newfoundland and Labrador, 24 November 2017, https://www.cbc.ca/news/canada/newfoundland-labrador/trudeau-speech-nl-residential-schools-1.4417905; and Geoff Bartlett, "Tearful Justin Trudeau Apologizes to N.L. Residential School Survivors," CBC News Newfoundland and Labrador, 24 November 2017, https://www.cbc.ca/news/canada/newfoundland-labrador/justin-trudeau-labrador-residential-schools-apology-1.4417443.

24 Ronald Rompkey, *Grenfell*, xvi–xvii.

25 O'Brien, *Grenfell Obsession*; Hiller, "Social Issues in Early 20th-Century Newfoundland"; Curwen, *Labrador Odyssey*; Luther, *Jessie Luther*; Paddon, *Labrador Memoir of Dr Harry Paddon*; Ronald

Rompkey, "Sir Wilfred Thomason Grenfell"; Anne Budgell, *Dear Everybody*; Lombard, *Adventures of a Grenfell Nurse*; Frankel, *I Want to Know if I Got to Get Married*; Clothier, *It's a Glorious Country*; Side, "E. Mary Schwall."

26 Perry, "Nursing for the Grenfell Mission"; Bulgin, "Mapping the Self in the 'Utmost Purple Rim'"; Lush, "Nutrition, Health Education, and Dietary Reform"; Woodrow, "'Serve the World'"; Coombs-Thorne, "Nursing with the Grenfell Mission"; Coombs-Thorne, "Conflict and Resistance to Paternalism"; Coombs-Thorne, "'Mrs Tilley'"; J.T.H. Connor, "'Medicine Is Here to Stay'"; Coombs-Thorne, "'Such a Many-Purpose Job'"; Jennifer Connor and Coombs-Thorne, "To the Rescue."

27 Work on Wakefield's contribution to the Grenfell mission, and to Newfoundland and Labrador, is in progress. See Jennifer Connor, "'Flits' of Medical Personnel on the Grenfell Labrador Mission" (presented at the Health, Medicine and Mobility conference).

28 [International Grenfell Association], "Summer Staff"; [International Grenfell Association], "Staff and Volunteer Workers" (1915–1928), *ADSF* 13; *ADSF* 14; *ADSF* 15; *ADSF* 16; *ADSF* 17; *ADSF* 18; *ADSF* 20; *ADSF* 21; *ADSF* 22; *ADSF* 23; *ADSF* 24; *ADSF* 25; *ADSF* 26; [International Grenfell Association], "Report of the Staff Selection Committee" (1929–1939), *ADSF* 27; *ADSF* 28; *ADSF* 29; *ADSF* 30; *ADSF* 31; *ADSF* 32; *ADSF* 33; *ADSF* 34; *ADSF* 35; *ADSF* 36; *ADSF* 37.

29 While these American hospitals represented numbers of volunteers over these years, several Canadian hospitals represented individuals. Notable among them was the General Hospital in St John's, NL. Others were the Royal Victoria Hospital, and Montreal General Hospital in Montreal; Toronto General Hospital and Davenport (probably Hillcrest) Hospital in Toronto; Hamilton General Hospital; Victoria Hospital in London, ON; Homewood Sanitarium in Guelph, ON; Winnipeg General Hospital and Selkirk Mental Hospital in Manitoba.

30 Governor Sir Ralph Williams, quoted in Hiller, "Status without Stature," 134.

31 Governor Sir W.E. Davidson, quoted in Sheard, "Seamen's Institute," 146.

32 Jennifer Connor, "'Dispensing Good Books and Literature.'"

33 Greene, "Items from St Barbe Islands."

34 Bourne, "School at Englee," 27.

35 Ronald Rompkey, *Grenfell*, 195–6.

36 Jenny Higgins, "Truck System"; Cadigan, *Newfoundland and Labrador*, 108–9, 119–20.

37 Curwen, *Labrador Odyssey*, 170. See also Ronald Rompkey, *Grenfell*, 68–9, 89–90.
38 Chambers II, *Tyranny of Change*, 132–52; Ronald Rompkey, *Grenfell*, 108.
39 Smith, *Canada: An American Nation?*; Smith, *Doing the Continental*. For fuller discussion in the medical context, see Jennifer Connor, "Stalwart Giants."
40 For example, see Buxton and Acland, *American Philanthropy and Canadian Libraries*; Rochester, "Bringing Librarianship to Rural Canada"; Fedunkiw, *Rockefeller Foundation Funding and Medical Education*.
41 Wright, *Professionalization of History in English Canada*, 127–30.
42 Reeves, "Alexander's Conundrum Reconsidered"; Earle, "Cousins of a Kind."
43 Travellers included the philanthropist George Eastman, whose camera film innovation and popularization through his Eastman Kodak Company would be important in helping others to document mission premises, activities, and people: see Cuerrier, "Newfoundland and Labrador Photographs."
44 Byrne, "Selling Simplicity"; High, "Working for Uncle Sam"; High, "From Outport to Outport Base"; Pocius, "Tourists, Health Seekers and Sportsmen"; Neary, "'Mortgaged Property'"; Neary, *Newfoundland in the North Atlantic World*.
45 Earle, "Cousins of a Kind"; Reeves, "Alexander's Conundrum Reconsidered," 28; Reeves, "Newfoundlanders in the 'Boston States.'"
46 Reeves, "Newfoundlanders in the 'Boston States,'" 40–1.
47 Reeves, "Alexander's Conundrum Reconsidered," 27.
48 This occupational activity of Newfoundlanders has yet to receive scholarly attention. For popular discussions, see Jim Rasenberger, "Cowboys of the Sky," *New York Times*, 28 January 2001, http://www.nytimes.com/2001/01/28/nyregion/cowboys-of-the-sky.html; Rasenberger, *High Steel*; Jenish, "Raising Steel"; Betty Ryan, "Reaching for the Sky"; Thurston, "Fish Gang."
49 Earle, "Cousins of a Kind," 406.
50 Richard Gwyn, quoted in Earle, "Cousins of a Kind," 405.

CHAPTER ONE

1 The words *Royal* and *National* were added to the name in 1896.
2 Now the Royal London Hospital.
3 Treves (1853–1923) became a well-known surgeon, knighted in 1902.

He was associated with Joseph Merrick, "the Elephant Man," introduced the operation to remove the appendix, and operated on King
Edward VII in 1902. See Keith, "Treves, Sir Frederick."

4 Grenfell, *Labrador Doctor* (London, 1929), 31–2. The "Cambridge
Seven" included one person from the Royal Military Academy. In 1885
the decision of the seven to go to China as missionaries became sensational news.

5 McDevitt, *May the Best Man Win*, 11–13; Newsome, *Godliness and
Good Learning*, 216–39; Putney, *Muscular Christianity*, 1–19, 37–44.

6 A "public school" in Britain is an independent institution, usually secondary, that charges fees. It is "public" to those who can afford it.

7 Hopwood (1860–1947) was a civil servant on his way to the top. He
was knighted in 1906, became permanent undersecretary at the Colonial Office 1907–11, and was ennobled as Baron Southborough in
1917. See H.M. Palmer, "Hopwood, Francis John Stephens." His report can be found in Hopwood, "Newfoundland Fisheries and Fishermen." Though he had never been there, he called the Labrador fishery
"a remarkable and really scandalous state of things."

8 Armour, "Castles in the Air"; *ENL* (1984), 2:849–50, *s.v.* "Harvey,
Moses."

9 Gosling, *Labrador*, 454; Hiller, "O'Brien, Sir John Terence Nicholls."

10 I am grateful throughout for Ronald Rompkey's *Grenfell*, and Ronald
Rompkey, "Grenfell, Sir Wilfred Thomason."

11 Richards, *Snapshots of Grenfell*, 3.

12 The history of Newfoundland in the Grenfell period can be found in
Noel, *Politics in Newfoundland*; O'Flaherty, *Lost Country*; and Cadigan, *Newfoundland and Labrador*.

13 *Evening Mercury* (St John's), 21 October 1885.

14 Candow, *History of the Labrador Fishery*, 30–1.

15 *Census of Newfoundland and Labrador, 1891*, 388.

16 WGP, box 291, notebook. I consulted the Wilfred Grenfell Papers over
forty years ago, and the collection has since been reorganized. At that
time, the lists were in this location. Subsequent references to the Grenfell Papers will cite the fonds: see the finding aid by Tony Myrans and
Jane Elaine Gertz, "Guide to the Wilfred Thomason Grenfell Papers,"
MS 254, rev. 2012, Yale University Library, 2015, http://hdl.handle.
net/10079/fa/mssa.ms.0254.

17 The 1891 census listed 228 vessels from Conception Bay and 619 from
the northeast coast.

18 For example, *JHA*, "Report of Dr Skelton on Medical Visit"; *JHA*,
"Medical Report of Dr Forbes."

19 *JHA*, Act to Provide for the Better Accommodation of Female Passengers, 176–7.

20 *JHA*, Report of the Select Committee to Consider the Operation and Effectiveness of the Present Law, 173–9.

21 The question was settled by the Judicial Committee of the Privy Council in 1927.

22 *Census of Newfoundland and Labrador, 1891*, 453: Anglican, 1,749; RC, 354; Methodist, 604; "Other," 1,399.

23 This includes both St Anthony proper and its "bight." *Census of Newfoundland and Labrador, 1901*, 206.

24 The calculation is based on the population of the electoral districts of St John's East and West as given in the 1891 *Census*. The number living within the town's municipal boundaries was substantially lower.

25 During the Napoleonic Wars, Newfoundland fishermen had used parts of the eastern Northern Peninsula. After 1815 this was not possible.

26 Trade with the United Kingdom was slowly declining, while that with Canada and the United States was increasing.

27 See Curwen, *Labrador Odyssey*, 15–16, 21. O'Brien "expressed his disgust of both" political parties and sounded off about sectarianism and pervasive corruption.

28 Fitzpatrick, "Render unto Caesar?"

29 Gosling, *Labrador*, 462. On Grenfell's religious outlook, see Robinson, "Wilfred Thomason Grenfell." She calls him an "evangelical liberal," 26.

30 WGP, Bishop Jones to Grenfell, 24 January 1895.

31 WGP, Wilfred Grenfell to Jane Grenfell, 30 November 1892; 7 November 1893.

32 For a list of those attending the meeting convened by O'Brien on 27 October 1892, see Grenfell, *Vikings of To-day*, 222. There was one Roman Catholic present, probably in his capacity as president of the Legislative Council. *Toilers of the Deep* 8 (1893): 36–8. Eliot Curwen noted that there were no Roman Catholics at the christening of the steam launch *Princess May* in 1893: Curwen, *Labrador Odyssey*, 26.

33 It was suggested that this unusual degree of support was related to the approaching general election in 1893. See Curwen, *Labrador Odyssey*, xx, 16–17.

34 Writing to his mother from Hopedale in 1892, Grenfell stated, "Certainly these people are very affectionate and have the same feelings as we have, though not I believe quite so acute – that is death and loss of friends some appear not to feel – while others are like us." He bought a kayak and Inuit clothing. See WGP, Wilfred Grenfell to Jane Grenfell,

19 September 1892. In 1895 he referred to Inuit as "the quaintest little figures ... chattering, laughing, and pleased as children": Grenfell, *Vikings of To-day*, 175.

35 Officially the "Unitas Fratrum," and possibly the oldest Protestant sect – certainly pre-Reformation. Robert Gathorne-Hardy remarked, "I would not depreciate the excellent and well publicised doctor. But for one who has seen the work ... [of the Moravians] there must always be a regret ... for the consequent obscurity which has covered their two-centuries' labour": *Traveller's Trio*, 55.

36 Schumacher, "Anglo-Saxonism." See also Horsman, *Race and Manifest Destiny*, especially 62–77.

37 But Robert Bond, prime minister in 1906, told Governor Sir William MacGregor that he did not "consider it either necessary or justifiable that approaches be made to Missionary societies and private sub-scribers outside this Colony": National Archives, UK, Colonial Office 194/262, 207, Bond to MacGregor, 21 March 1906, encl. MacGregor to Elgin, 23 March 1906.

38 Governor MacGregor, a fellow doctor, told Grenfell in 1908 that he should "not touch politics in any form whatever." WGP, MacGregor to Grenfell, 30 November 1908.

39 Hiller, "Newfoundland Credit System."

40 Gosling, himself a prominent merchant, thought that the value of the co-ops was unproven and that they were undercapitalized. Gosling, *Labrador*, 469–70.

41 WGP, Wilfred Grenfell to Paul Hettasch, 15 October 1900. Hettasch had returned a shipment of clothes. Grenfell was also unhappy about the Moravian decision in 1896 to establish a mission station at Makkovik. He apparently thought that since Makkovik mainly served "settlers" rather than Inuit, the settlement should fall within "his" terri-tory. WGP, Letters 1910–40, Wilfred Grenfell to the Council of the Moravian Mission, 15 September 1910; Wilfred Grenfell to C.A. Mar-tin, 5 September 1910; C.A. Martin to Wilfred Grenfell, 24 October 1910. He told the MDSF council in 1926 that the Moravians were "dying out or getting out." RNMDSF, London, Papers Relating to the Grenfell Association Transfers, Report of a Council Meeting, 9 Decem-ber 1926, 18.

42 Grenfell was explicitly warned off from direct political involvement in the colony's affairs, and he accepted that advice. However, he was al-ways willing to supply his opinions to influential friends and acquain-tances in London, Ottawa, and elsewhere. He was for many years a welcome guest at Government House, a privilege that ended in 1921.

43 WGP, scrapbook 33, W.A. Munn to Wilfred Grenfell, 9 June 1896.
44 Ronald Rompkey, *Grenfell*, 89. Cash was more prevalent on the island
    of Newfoundland. In 1939 Grenfell wrote that the stores and other en-
    terprises had "cost me all I owned almost, because the people did *not*
    cooperate. They listened to others." WGP, Letters 1910–40, Wilfred
    Grenfell to Ethel Graham, 8 March 1939.
45 WGP, Letters 1910–1940, Wilfred Grenfell to W.L. Mackenzie King,
    17 September 1910.
46 The institute has recently been converted into expensive condominiums.
47 On the last point, see Perry, "Nursing for the Grenfell Mission," chap-
    ter 5; Fitzhugh, *Labradorians*, 49.
48 Richards, *Snapshots of Grenfell*, 83.
49 The phrases are taken from Rudyard Kipling's 1897 poem "Reces-
    sional."
50 Ronald Rompkey, in Paddon, *Labrador Memoir*, xxvi–xxvii. Paddon
    called Grenfell "a born autocrat." See also Ronald Rompkey, "Paddon,
    Henry Locke."
51 PAD, GN 2/5, file 225.C (3), H.R. Brookes for the Grenfell Association
    of Newfoundland to the Newfoundland government, [1919]. The
    percentages are approximations. For about the period 1914–16, the
    United States contributed 57.4 per cent.
52 RNMDSF, Report of a Council Meeting, 9 December 1926, 7.
53 Quoted by Ronald Rompkey, in Paddon, *Labrador Memoir*, xxx.
54 Mackay with Saunders, "Economy of Newfoundland," 131–3.
55 Reeves, "Newfoundlanders in the 'Boston States,'" 35.
56 Mackay with Saunders, "Economy of Newfoundland," 132. The num-
    ber in Canada peaked at 26,410 in 1931, and 23,971 in the United
    States in 1930.
57 Two further articles by W.G. Reeves are relevant here: "Alexander's
    Conundrum Reconsidered" and "Aping the 'American Type.'"
58 Mackay with Saunders, "Economy of Newfoundland," 146.
59 Mackay with Saunders, "Economy of Newfoundland," 139, 145, and
    appendices 6 and 13; Hiller, "Politics of Newsprint," 25–6.
60 Information derived from New Hampshire Genealogy & History at
    Searchroots, www.nh.searchroots.com; and Belvin, *Forgotten
    Labrador*, 96–7. See also Hollett, *Beating against the Wind*, 273. The
    winter station was at St Paul's River, the summer station on Caribou
    Island. I am also grateful to John Kennedy.
61 Ronald Rompkey, *Grenfell*, 72–4.
62 Ronald Rompkey, *Grenfell*, 91.
63 Ronald Rompkey, *Grenfell*, 110.

64 For a sympathetic analysis of Duncan's work, see O'Flaherty, *Rock Observed*, 95–102. Grenfell is discussed briefly, 85–6.

65 "Prince Pomiuk's Friend." See also Whiteley, "Story of Pomiuk."

66 See Hulan, "'Brave Boy's Story for Brave Boys.'"

67 Reissued in different editions; for example, with an introduction by Ronald Rompkey in 1992 by Creative Publishers (St John's); and most recently in 2016 by Flanker (St John's) with a foreword by Edward Roberts.

68 There is a full account of this incident in Ronald Rompkey, *Grenfell*, 141–9.

69 I have drawn on Porterfield, "Protestant Missionaries"; Sealander, "Curing Evils at Their Source"; and Emily S. Rosenberg, "Missions to the World."

70 The phrase is from Robinson, "Wilfred Thomason Grenfell," 3.

71 Letter from J. Moore in *Daily News* (St John's), 24 March 1894. A nasty attack followed from Rev. Selby Jefferson (a Methodist): Grenfell did more good in a summer than Moore "could have done in a century." *Daily News* (St John's), 6 June 1894. The newspaper thought the comment "uncharitable and unjust."

72 Ronald Rompkey, *Grenfell*, 102–3, 121–4.

73 WGP, cutting.

74 PAD GN 2/5, file 225-H, Petition to the House of Assembly, 12 June 1917.

75 PAD GN 2/5, file 225-H, statement in "Evidence Taken in the Grenfell Inquiry," 9 June 1917, 23.

76 WGP, box 291, A. Sheard to W.R. Stirling, 27 January 1913.

77 For a more extended discussion, see Hiller, "Social Issues in Early 20th-Century Newfoundland."

78 Grenfell, *Labrador Doctor* (1919), 282.

79 In addition, eight Labradorians and possibly fifty men from the Northern Peninsula served in the Naval Reserve. Six Labradorians served with the Canadian forces. This information is derived from "Labrador War Memorial"; and Patey, *Veterans of the North*, 36–142. See Ronald Rompkey, *Grenfell*, 185–8.

80 WGP, statement by Wilfred Grenfell, 5 June 1916, typescript.

81 PAD GN 2/5, file 225, "Evidence Taken on the Grenfell Inquiry," 133–77. Harry Paddon thought that Labrador was "not ready for co-operative methods": Paddon, *Labrador Memoir*, 126.

82 PAD GN 2/5, file 225-H, "The Report of the Commissioner of the Grenfell Inquiry," 1 November 1917; Ronald Rompkey, *Grenfell*, 195–6.

83 WGP, Wilfred Grenfell to Jane Grenfell (his mother), 10 June 1918.

84 The same question had been raised earlier in the century concerning the Reid Newfoundland Company.

85 The figures are rounded approximations.

86 Alexander, "Newfoundland's Traditional Economy," 20 (table 1).

87 Candow, *History of the Labrador Fishery*, 31.

88 Alexander's estimate is 1,500 to 2,500 per year between 1901 and 1945, "Newfoundland's Traditional Economy," 25. Candow thinks 1,000 to 1,500, *History of the Labrador Fishery*, 64. A memorandum in the Grenfell Papers (WGP) shows that 131,044 Newfoundlanders emigrated to the United States between 1925 and 1930, and 2,167 returned. From 1931 the United States tightened a 1917 act denying entry to anyone who might be a "public charge."

89 Accounts of this period can be found in Noel, *Politics in Newfoundland*, chapters 11–12; O'Flaherty, *Lost Country*, chapters 6–7; and Overton, "Economic Crisis and the End of Democracy."

90 WGP, cutting, *Western Star*, 5 October 1921.

91 Ronald Rompkey, *Grenfell*, 209–14.

92 WGP, cutting, *Evening Telegram* (St John's), 21 October 1922.

93 Ronald Rompkey, *Grenfell*, 264–5.

94 Junek, *Isolated Communities*, 113. See also 106.

95 John Kennedy, *People of the Bays and Headlands*, 153. More generally, see 147–58.

96 John Kennedy, *People of the Bays and Headlands*, 152.

97 Simms and Ward, *Regional Population Projections for Labrador and the Northern Peninsula, 2016–2036*.

CHAPTER TWO

1 Ronald Rompkey, *Grenfell*, 31–7, 107–10, 128–9.

2 Porter, "Religion and Empire at Home and Abroad"; Porter, *Religion versus Empire?*, 4.

3 Porter, "Religion and Empire at Home and Abroad"; Porter, "Religion, Missionary Enthusiasm, and Empire," 222.

4 Buckner, "Creation of the Dominion of Canada," 77; Porter, "Religion, Missionary Enthusiasm, and Empire," 229.

5 Porter, "Church History, History of Christianity, Religious History," 575.

6 Porter, "Religion, Missionary Enthusiasm, and Empire," 243.

7 Grenfell, *Forty Years for Labrador*, 93.

8   Hardiman, "Introduction," 16; *Christian Missions*, cited in Schoepflin, "Mythic Mission Lands," 72. It is not known whether this survey included Newfoundland and Labrador.

9   Porter, *Religion versus Empire?*; Walls, "British Missions."

10 Porter, *Religion versus Empire?*, 311–13.

11 Hardiman, "Introduction," 16–18; Edgar Jones, "Early Work of the Church of England in Labrador," 93.

12 Wong, "Local Voluntarism," 99; Ronald Rompkey, *Grenfell*, 106; Baehre, "Whose Pine Clad Hills"; Rompkey, "Introduction," in Luther, *Jessie Luther*, xxii.

13 Grenfell, *Down to the Sea*; Grenfell and others, *Labrador*; Grenfell, *Tales of the Labrador*. See also the following books that include some "Eskimo" content, including the story of Pomiuk, along with the focus on deep-sea fishers: Grenfell, *Off the Rocks*; Grenfell, *Harvest of the Sea*; Grenfell, *Vikings of To-day*. After 1914, references to "Eskimo" (including his much earlier lecture lantern slide images) seem to retreat from his publications; see, for example, Grenfell, *Labrador Days*.

14 Grenfell, *Forty Years for Labrador*, 93.

15 Grenfell, quoted in Curwen, *Labrador Odyssey*, 74; Edgar Jones, "Early Work of the Church of England in Labrador," 93.

16 Ronald Rompkey, *Grenfell*, 95.

17 "Missionary Business Men Are Need of the World," *Daily Star* (St John's), 19 October 1920, 1, 3.

18 Grenfell, "New Hospital for St Anthony," ADSF 23 (October 1925): 102.

19 Chambers II, *Tyranny of Change*, 293–4; Avery, "*Dangerous Foreigners*," 96.

20 Maxton, United Kingdom Parliament, Commons Sitting, 14 December 1933, 648. Quoted in Cullen, "What to Do about Newfoundland?," 110. For recent discussion of the British identity of Newfoundland as a white-settler colony within the British Empire, and its reconstruction politically as racial degeneration to facilitate imperial suspension of the colony's self-rule in 1933, see Cullen, "Race, Debt and Empire."

21 Grenfell, *Forty Years for Labrador*, 94; Greenleaf, "Introduction," xxv. At the risk of appearing immodest to compare myself with the recognized folklorist Elisabeth Greenleaf, I can attest that the same experience holds true for the modern visitor to Newfoundland. My first travels on land, around the Bonavista Peninsula in the early 1990s, elicited the same "shock" with the sudden feeling that I had been transported to Devon, so close in dialect and cadence was the speech around me to that of my own family in Torquay. Indeed, speech in Bonavista itself is so close today to that of Somerset as to be uncanny.

22 Carleton, "Notes on the Labrador Dialect," *P&S on the Labrador ...
Summer of 1922*, 12–15; reprinted in Carleton, "Notes," ADSF (1924).

23 The particular form of English, which included "words which are characteristically Newfoundland by having continued in use here after they died out or declined elsewhere," and that were "shared by Newfoundland speakers with those of their principal points of origin, especially the south-west counties of England and southern Ireland," was the focus of the much later publication, Story, Kirwin, and Widdowson, *Dictionary of Newfoundland English*: see "Introduction." Indeed, later scholars were to study such aspects of Newfoundland intensively: see Webb, *Observing the Outports*, 26–83.

24 Johnson, *Doctor Regrets*, 138, 146.

25 Armstrong, "Summer Resort Industrial Sales," 135. On his way to Harrington Harbour, Johnson similarly encountered laughter when he asked about the people: "No, the Coast People were definitely not Eskimo. ... The Eskimos were further north somewhere – certainly not on the Canadian Labrador": *Doctor Regrets*, 137.

26 Logan, "In the Land of the 'Chanty Punts,'" 132; Grenfell Association of Great Britain and Ireland, *Medical Work in Labrador and Northern Newfoundland: Sixth Annual Report*, 3; Eleanor Cushman, quoted in "Miss Cushman Gives Movies and Speech on Grenfell Work," *Vassar Miscellany News* 21, no. 29 (20 February 1937): 1.

27 Cutter, "Pioneer Library Work in Labrador."

28 Kverndal, *Seamen's Missions*, 273, 303, 397–8.

29 Gosden, *Friendly Societies in England*, 7.

30 On the Fishermen's Mission and its predecessor, the Royal National Mission to Deep Sea Fishermen, see their web page "Our History."

31 Hiller, "Nineteenth Century, 1815–1914," 85–6; Ronald Rompkey, *Grenfell*, 40, 77; Grenfell, *Forty Years for Labrador*, 139 (see also 68, 85–6, 140–1). See also Curwen, *Labrador Odyssey*, 170.

32 Grenfell, *Forty Years for Labrador*, 139–47; see 139.

33 James, "Reforming Reform"; Valverde, *Age of Light, Soap, and Water*, 140–2.

34 Ronald Rompkey, *Grenfell*, 108–10.

35 Ronald Rompkey, *Grenfell*, 108; Rompkey, in Luther, *Jessie Luther*, xxiv–xxxii.

36 On the notion of manliness, muscular Christianity, and its role in missions, see Ronald Rompkey, *Grenfell*, 10–11; Semple, "Missionary Manhood"; Imhoff, "Manly Missions." See also Daniel Coleman, *White Civility*, 128–67, for discussion of these notions in literature popularizing and inculcating "normative ideas of British civility": the muscular

Christian's physical strength balanced by a sensitive heart, Coleman argues, represented the ideal Canadian for the hard physical work of settlement and for the social work of building a new civil society.

37 Ramsay Cook, *Regenerators*, 175–6.
38 Edgar Jones, "Early Work of the Church of England in Labrador," 93.
39 Porter, "Religion, Missionary Enthusiasm, and Empire," 242; Porter, *Religion versus Empire?*, 248–9, 301–5; Phillips, "Changing Attitudes in the Student Volunteer Movement."
40 Porter, *Religion versus Empire?*, 305.
41 Grenfell, *Forty Years for Labrador*, 314–15; Grenfell, *Labrador Doctor*, 298.
42 Phillips, "Changing Attitudes in the Student Volunteer Movement," 132; Porter, *Religion versus Empire?*, 302.
43 *Evening Star* (Toronto), "Gathering in Aid of Missions," 10 February 1894, 1; *Evening Star*, "The Interest in Missions Grows," 15 February 1894, 1; "Missionary Convention," *Canada Presbyterian* 23 (21 February 1894): 1; "Foreign Mission Conference," *Presbyterian Review* 10 (22 February 1894): 607.
44 Phillips, "Changing Attitudes in the Student Volunteer Movement," 132.
45 Cushman, quoted in "Miss Cushman," 5. The mission's magazine *Among the Deep Sea Fishers* routinely provided details of the volunteers from American universities and colleges; for example, in 1911, students came from Harvard, Yale, Amherst, Williams, Dartmouth, Occidental, Princeton, Pennsylvania, Clark, St Marks, and Johns Hopkins: see [White], "Items from the New England Grenfell Association," *ADSF* 10 (July 1912): 29. For brief discussion, see Side, "E. Mary Schwall," 78.
46 Neil Rosenberg and Guigné, "Foreword to the 2004 Reprint," xvii.
47 "Grenfell Mission Seeks Aid in Labrador Work: Brooks House Sponsors Work with Men, Money," *Harvard Crimson*, 26 February 1932.
48 "The Missionary Movement," *Harvard Crimson*, 16 October 1919.
49 Grenfell, "Mission as Practical Religion," 60; Grenfell, "Sir Wilfred's Log," 174.
50 Musson, "Labrador," 199.
51 Both student papers have online versions, and the citations to them in the following discussion are drawn from Yale Daily News Historical Archive (of fully digitized copies), available at http://web.library.yale.edu/digital-collections/yale-daily-news-historical-archive; and *Harvard Crimson*, available in individual article transcripts at http://www.thecrimson.com. I am indebted to Monica Kidd for raising the initial question about how Grenfell recruited medical students, which steered me towards investigating this important aspect of his mission.

52 "Labrador Pictures Shown," *Yale Daily News* 150, 24 April 1934, 1.

53 D.B. Macausland, "Work of Grenfeil [*sic*] Mission Described: Trip Starts Late in June," *Harvard Crimson*, 16 February 1921.

54 "Grenfell Mission Aided by 'WAPS' [*sic*] from Harvard: Started in 1892 with a Single Hospital on a Schooner," *Harvard Crimson*, 12 March 1925.

55 "'Where There's a Will There's a Way" Motto of Grenfell Mission,' Says Yale Senior," *Yale Daily News* 138, 25 March 1931, 3.

56 "Dr Grenfell Wants Yale Men in Labrador This Summer," *Yale Daily News* 163, 28 April 1917, 6.

57 "Need University Men for Grenfell Mission: P.B.H. Committee Appoints Special Member to Take Charge of Enrollments Here – Volunteers Work in Labrador during Summer," *Harvard Crimson*, 18 February 1922. The Phillips Brooks House Association of Harvard University continues its mission of social service and social action. As its web page indicates, until the 1940s, it placed students at settlement houses, organized clothing and book drives, and financed missionaries to serve in Asia: see Phillips Brooks House Association, "Our History."

58 "What It's All About," *P&S on the Labrador … Summer of 1921*, [3]; "How It Started," *P&S on the Labrador … Summer of 1922*, 3. See also "History of the Station," *P&S on the Labrador … Summer of 1923*, 3–4; "History of the Station," *P&S on the Labrador … Summer of 1924*, 5–6.

59 The club has been active since 1894 as "the most comprehensive student activities organization in American medical education": see its web page, "About P&S Club."

60 McLaren, *Our Own Master Race*.

61 See "Yale-in-Labrador: Work with Grenfell," *Yale Daily News* 7, 2 October 1939, 2; "Dr Grenfell to Lecture on Work as Missionary," *Yale Daily News* 147, 14 April 1923, 3; "Dr Grenfell Will Lecture on Activities in Labrador," *Yale Daily News* 146, 13 April 1923, 1; "Lecture Will Be Given in Sprague by Dr Grenfell," *Yale Daily News* 60, 7 December 1927, 1, 7; Wilfred Grenfell, quoted in "Dr Grenfell Finds True Life in Arctic Wilds, Deploring Present Crowded Conditions in Cities," *Yale Daily News* 82, 20 January 1927, 5; "Opportunity Offered for Yale Men in Labrador," *Yale Daily News* 146, 3 April 1925, 2; [E.P. White], "'Carrying Thirty-Foot Logs or Burying the Dead, It's All in the Day's Work at Grenfell Mission in Labrador,' Says Undergraduate," *Yale Daily News* 139, 26 March 1931, 1; "Grenfell to Have Help of Many College Men," *Yale Daily News* 149, 7 April 1925, 3.

62 "Dr Grenfell to Speak on Work in Labrador," *Yale Daily News* 54,

1 December 1920, 4. On Paddon's views of Labrador, see Ronald Rompkey, *Grenfell*, 172–3; Rompkey, "Introduction," in Paddon, *Labrador Memoir*, xxvi–xxvii.

63 Harry Paddon, quoted in "Grenfell Mission Wants Four Yale Students to Work in Labrador This Summer," *Yale Daily News* 125, 11 March 1924, 1.

64 "Sir Wilfred Grenfell's Story Linked with Yale," *Yale Daily News* 21, 18 October 1933, 1.

65 "Grenfell Reviews Work on Coast of Labrador," *Yale Daily News* 58, 6 December 1920, 6.

66 "The White Peril," *Yale Daily News* 37, 11 November 1925, 1.

67 Grenfell, quoted in "Opportunity for Work with Labrador Mission," *Yale Daily News* 60, 8 December 1920, 1; "Grenfell to Have Help of Many College Men." See also *Yale Daily News* 95, 2 February 1923, 1; *Yale Daily News* 101, 12 February 1929, 1; *Yale Daily News* 132, 20 March 1929, 1.

68 Grenfell, quoted in "Opportunity for Work with Labrador Mission"; "Grenfell Association on University Budget," *Yale Daily News* 21, 19 October 1928, 2.

69 *Yale Daily News* 52, 29 November 1920, 2; *Yale Daily News* 53, 30 November 1920, 4.

70 "Speaking of Labrador," *Yale Daily News* 165, 2 May 1925, 2.

71 "The Press: Doctor, Lawyer, Indian Chief," *Harvard Crimson*, 11 January 1928. This concept of students' vacation volunteerism in developing countries of non-white populations to augment a career CV has become popular in the twenty-first century – known as "voluntourism" – and widely criticized, particularly as it often does more harm than good to the local community and appears to resurrect concepts of white colonialism. See, for example, the account of one American student volunteer from a girls' boarding school: Biddle, "Problem with Little White Girls, Boys and Voluntourism."

72 "Grenfell Wants Volunteers," *Yale Daily News* 139, 29 March 1913, 3.

73 "A New Land," *Yale Daily News* 44, 19 November 1925, 4.

74 "Speaking of Labrador."

75 "Another Outpost," *Yale Daily News* 26, 29 October 1925, 2; "New Grenfell School to Bear Name 'Yale,'" *Yale Daily News* 26, 29 October 1925, 1, 3.

76 See "Grenfell Association on University Budget"; *Yale Daily News* 43, 18 November 1925, 5; *Yale Daily News* 21, 23 October 1925, 1; *Yale Daily News* 29, 27 October 1939, 2.

77 "Sir Wilfred Grenfell's Story Linked with Yale."
78 Phillips, "Changing Attitudes in the Student Volunteer Movement," 132.

CHAPTER THREE

I am grateful to my friends Jim and Jennifer Connor for inviting me
back to Newfoundland and for providing me with copies of *Among the
Deep Sea Fishers.*

1 There is still no comprehensive biography of Kellogg, but see Schwarz,
   John Harvey Kellogg; Numbers, "Sex, Science, and Salvation," 218–20;
   Brian Wilson, *Dr John Harvey Kellogg and the Religion of Biologic
   Living*; and Markel, *Kelloggs.*
2 Numbers, *Prophetess of Health*, 177–83, 253–63. Regarding White,
   see also Aamodt, Land, and Numbers, *Ellen Harmon White.*
3 Ronald Rompkey, *Grenfell*, 22–3, 33, 83, 109–12; Grenfell, *What
   Life Means to Me*, 17–18. See also "How Dr Greenfell [*sic*] Became
   a Missionary," *Medical Missionary* 16 (20 February 1907): 82–3.
4 Grenfell, *What Life Means to Me*, 29; Ronald Rompkey, *Grenfell*, 167,
   192.
5 "The Visit of Dr Grenfell," *Medical Missionary* 16 (6 March 1907):
   75–6.
6 "How Dr Greenfell [*sic*] Became a Missionary," 64.
7 "Dr Grenfell at the Sanitarium," *Medical Missionary* 16 (20 March
   1907): 94, describing his visit on 25 February. See also "How Dr
   Greenfell [*sic*] Became a Missionary," 82–3; and "Address by Dr Wilfred T. Grenfell," *Medical Missionary* 16 (3 April 1907): 107–9.
8 Advertising section, *Good Health* 42 (November 1907): n.p.
9 Advertising section, *Good Health* 49 (August 1914): n.p.
10 "Note," *Medical Missionary* 17 [18] (7 April 1909): 257–8; editorial,
   Medical Missionary 18 (5 May 1909): 337; Grenfell, "Medical Missions in Labrador"; editorial, *Medical Missionary* 18 (5 May 1909):
   344–59; Reports from the Interdenominational Medical Missionary
   Conference, *Medical Missionary* 18 (June 1909): 460; Schwarz, *John
   Harvey Kellogg*, 207.
11 "Note," *Medical Missionary* 18 (September 1909): 529; editorial notes,
   Medical Missionary 18 (November 1909): 593; "Note," *Medical Missionary* 19 (May 1910): 130; Note, *Medical Missionary* 21 (January 1912):
   1–2; "Honored by His King," *Medical Missionary* 18 (5 May 1909): 339–
   40. Kellogg also from time to time dropped Grenfell's name in his own
   books; see, e.g., *Natural Diet of Man*, 68; and *Crippled Colon*, 280.

12 Grenfell, "Soul of Battle Creek." The Brook Farm Association was a transcendentalist experiment in communal living, founded in the early 1840s just outside of Boston.

13 Grenfell, "Dr Grenfell's Log on Land." On his dietary habits, see Grenfell, "Soul of Battle Creek," 279. On various contributions from Battle Creek, see [White], "Items from the New England Grenfell Association," *ADSF* 10 (October 1912): 27.

14 Mitchell, "Food Problems on the Labrador," 102; Poppleton, "Letter concerning Flower's Cove."

15 "Consumption from Fish"; Valen, "Citizens, Protect Your Property," 47. I am grateful to Katherine Side for bringing the latter article to my attention.

16 Grenfell, "Soul of Battle Creek," 277–8; Ronald Rompkey, *Grenfell*, 178.

17 Ronald Rompkey, *Grenfell*, 235.

18 Bentley Historical Library, University of Michigan, John Harvey Kellogg Papers, Anne Grenfell to John Harvey Kellogg, 21 June 1937; see also Ronald Rompkey, *Grenfell*, 280–1.

19 Ronald Rompkey, *Grenfell*, 290.

20 Vaughn, "Labrador Days in Florida."

CHAPTER FOUR

This research was supported by funding from the J.R. Smallwood Foundation, Memorial University. Special thanks to Greg Walsh, Melanie Tucker, and Kylea Thoms at PAD, The Rooms; Genevieve Coyle and staff at Manuscripts & Archives, Yale University; and David Harvey, retired correctional officer from Her Majesty's Penitentiary in St John's.

1 For more on the role of the King George V Seamen's Institute during the sealing disaster, the First World War, and the influenza epidemic, see Coombs-Thorne, "'Radiating Center of Helpfulness.'"

2 "Grenfell Missions' Plans: Reorganizing with Central Board – Karnepp [*sic*] Theft a Lone Incident," *New York Times*, 4 September 1912.

3 Ronald Rompkey, *Grenfell*, 176.

4 Sir Edward Morris, who was also then prime minister of Newfoundland.

5 Ronald Rompkey, *Grenfell*, 171.

6 Sealander, "Curing Evils at Their Source."

7 Zunz, *Philanthropy in America*, 2.

8 Zunz, *Philanthropy in America*, 2.

9 Crocker, "From Gift to Foundation," 215.

10 Ronald Rompkey, *Grenfell*, 134. Karnopp met Sage in 1910 while fundraising for the institute and asked for $20,000 towards the cause; Sage agreed to $5,000. See MU-FMA, Coll-002: Dr Cluny MacPherson fonds, series 3: IGA file, folder 1, Charles Karnopp to Cluny MacPherson, 20 April 1910.

11 Ronald Rompkey, *Grenfell*, 130.

12 Ronald Rompkey, *Grenfell*, 130.

13 WGP, 254-1-320, John D. Rockefeller (New York) to Grenfell (New York), 17 March 1911.

14 LAC, William Lyon Mackenzie King Collection MG 26, Primary Series Correspondence (J1), vol. 29, Mackenzie King (Denver, CO) to John D. Rockefeller (Hot Springs, VA), 21 November 1915. King had his own connections to Rockefeller, having served as director of the Department of Industrial Relations of the Rockefeller Foundation during the First World War. See Mackenzie King Collection, MG 26 J1, vol. 32, Jerome D. Greene, secretary of the Rockefeller Foundation (New York) to W.L. Mackenzie King, 8 June 1916.

15 WGP, 254-1-28, Grenfell to Miss White, 30 July 1910.

16 Indeed, funding universities and libraries were among Carnegie's top priorities. See Sealander, "Curing Evils at Their Source," 224.

17 Grenfell, *Forty Years for Labrador*, 228–9.

18 Grenfell, *Labrador Doctor*, 13th ed., 268.

19 WGP, 254-9-49, R.S. Cassels (Toronto) to Abram Sheard (St John's), 3 October 1912.

20 Merchant Walter Baine Grieve donated a property at Battle Harbour, which became the first "Grenfell" hospital on the coast: Ronald Rompkey, *Grenfell*, 52–6.

21 "Donations and Contributions," ADSF 1 (July 1903): 20.

22 For more on the life of Julia Greenshields, see Jennifer Connor and Coombs-Thorne, "To the Rescue." Since the Canadian branches were more established and active than the American branches at this time, Canadian activities dominated the ADSF in its early years, and in 1907 Greenshields begged American readers to keep her apprised of their activities: "Our Magazine is intended to record American doings as well as Canadian; but unless news of them is sent to us, we cannot carry out the intention of the little paper!," ADSF 4 (January 1907): 3.

23 Grenfell, "American Jottings," *Toilers of the Deep* (1903): 150–1; and ADSF 1 (July 1903): 1.

24 See, for example, "Labrador Medical Mission: Work among the Fishermen and Settlers along 600 Miles of Bleak Coast Line Described by a

Physician Who Has Devoted Ten Years to It," *New York Times*, 26
April 1903; and Grenfell, "American Jottings."

25 Ronald Rompkey, *Grenfell*, 111.

26 For more about Lyman Abbott's influence on Grenfell and contribution
to Grenfell's success in the United States, see Ronald Rompkey, *Grenfell*, 109–16.

27 Grenfell, "Dr Grenfell's American Tour," ADSF 3 *(*April 1905): 7.

28 Ronald Rompkey, *Grenfell*, 117.

29 Ronald Rompkey, *Grenfell*, 89.

30 WGP, 254-1-24, Grenfell (*Strathcona*, St John's) to unknown, 16 June
1910.

31 For example, in order to help out the St Anthony store, Grenfell loaned
them $1,000 in shares and also paid off $1,500 of their debts. See WGP,
254-1-37, Grenfell (St Anthony) to Munn, 10 October 1910. See also
WGP, 254-1-24, Grenfell (*Strathcona*, St John's) to unknown, 16 June
1910.

32 WGP, 254-1-254, Edgar Jones to Grenfell, 6 April 1897.

33 WGP, 254-1-254, Edgar Jones to Grenfell, 12 April 1897.

34 WGP, 254-1-37, Grenfell (St Anthony) to Delano (New York), 10
October 1910.

35 WGP, 254-1-228, Jennie Gray to Grenfell, 13 June 1910.

36 For example, in August 1910, he randomly asked Jennie Gray, office
secretary for the GAA, to purchase sixty barrels of fuel oil to be forwarded to St Anthony. See WGP, 254-1-24, Grenfell to Gray, 7 June
1910. See also, WGP, 254-1-227, John Grieve (Battle Harbour) to
Grenfell, 24 September 1910.

37 WGP, 254-1-24, Grenfell to Mr Halsey, 4 June [1910].

38 WGP, 254-1-33, Grenfell to Arthur Estabrook, 15 September 1910.

39 WGP, 254-1-24, Grenfell to Jennie Gray, 7 June 1910; and 254-1-28,
Grenfell to William [Stirling], 26 July 1910.

40 WGP, 254-1-24, Grenfell to unknown/creditors, 16 June 1910.

41 WGP, 254-1-24, Grenfell to Gray (New York), 1 June 1910.

42 WGP, 254-1-30, Grenfell to H.G. Matthews, 22 August 1910.

43 WGP, 254-1-30, Grenfell to H.G. Matthews, 22 August 1910.

44 WGP, 254-1-39, Grenfell (Parkgate) to Wood, 1 March 1911.

45 WGP, 254-1-26, Grenfell to the chairman of the Finance Committee,
MDSF, 20 June 1910.

46 WGP, 254-1-25, Grenfell to W.C. Job, John Harvey, John Ayre, S.
Milley, Royal Stores, E.J. Horwood, Rothwell and Bowring, and
John Munn, 18 June 1910.

47 WGP, 254-1-26, Grenfell to Julia Greenshields, 21 June 1910.

48 WGP, 254-1-35, Grenfell (*Strathcona*) to Delano (New York), 21 September 1910.

49 WGP, 254-1-36, Grenfell (St Anthony) to Franklin, 27 September 1910.

50 WGP, 254-1-183, John Munn (St John's) to Grenfell, 3 October 1910.

51 WGP, 254-1-37, Grenfell (St Anthony) to Munn, 10 October 1910.

52 WGP, 254-ACC-88-M22, Grenfell to Stirling, 11 October 1911.

53 WGP, 254-1-39, Grenfell (Parkgate) to Wood, 1 March 1911.

54 WGP, 254-ACC-88-M22, Grenfell to Stirling, 22 November 1911.

55 John Mason Little to Mrs John Mason Little Sr, 5 March 1911, quoted in Ronald Rompkey, *Grenfell*, 165.

56 Ronald Rompkey, *Grenfell*, 166.

57 Lougee, "Items from the Grenfell Association of America," 41.

58 WGP, 254-1-266, Lougee (New York) to Grenfell (St Anthony), 31 August 1910.

59 WGP, 254-1-228, Gray (New York) to Grenfell, 20 September 1910.

60 WGP, ACC-88-M22, Grenfell (Groton, MA) to Stirling, 1 December 1911.

61 WGP, 254-9-67, Charles F. Karnopp, pamphlet on the Seamen's Institute, "Some Vital Facts concerning the Proposition for a Fishermen's and Seamen's Institute at St John's, Newfoundland."

62 The institute did not open for occupancy until 19 December 1912. See PAD, MG 63-2215, scrapbook, invitation to formal opening and "Opening the Doors for Use & Occupation" agenda.

63 WGP, 254-1-25, Grenfell (SS *Strathcona*, St Johns) to Judge Prowse, 18 June 1910. For more on the Rowton Houses, see Higginbotham, "Workhouse."

64 Grenfell, "Urgent Call for Help," ADSF 3 (July 1905): 6.

65 WGP, series 9, folder 67, "Some Vital Facts concerning the Proposition for a Fishermen's and Seamen's Institute at St John's, Newfoundland."

66 WGP, series 9, folder 67, "Some Vital Facts."

67 Pennoyer and Walker, *Architecture of Delano & Aldrich*.

68 MU-FMA, Cluny Macpherson collection, Coll-002, "King George the Fifth Seamen's Institute, St John's, Newfoundland: The Girls' Department – A Home for the Daughters of Fishermen and Seamen."

69 WGP, series 9, folder 67, "Some Vital Facts."

70 PAD, MG 63.1921, IGA fonds, Finance Committee, St John's: 1914, King George the Fifth Seamen's Institute, Comparative Statistics Relating to the Loss during 1916.

71 Seton, *College Y*, 7, 146.

72 "Institute," ADSF 6 (January 1909): 10.

73 "Institute," ADSF 6 (January 1909): 11.

74 In fact, other meetings of the institute committee were also held at Government House. WGP, series 1, folder 33, Grenfell to Charles Karnopp, 15 September 1910. See also "Institute," ADSF 6 (January 1909): 10.

75 MU-FMA, Cluny Macpherson collection, Coll-002, file 3.02 King George V Seamen's Institute, 1911-59, Sir Edward Morris (London) to P.T. McGrath (St John's), 10 June 1911.

76 PAD, MG 63.1913, Karnopp (St John's) to Jose Machado (Ottawa), 24 May 1912.

77 PAD, MG 63.2214, Grenfell Association of Newfoundland, Diaries, Scrapbooks, and Publications; News Clippings, 1909–13; Buckingham Palace to Wood (London), 13 May 1912.

78 For example, see WGP, 254-9-1, Karnopp (St John's) to Philip Newel (Seldom-Come-By), 22 September 1909.

79 For example, see "Institute," ADSF 5 (July 1907): 1–2.

80 In September 1910, Grenfell wrote to Karnopp, "I have written to Miss Greenshields to place $1,000 to you [sic] account, the Institute account, so you will be able to pay the bill you referred to." WGP, 254-1-31, Grenfell (Strathcona) to Karnopp, 2 September 1910; and 254-1-33, Grenfell (St Anthony) to Karnopp, 15 September 1910.

81 PAD, Grenfell to Lougee (New York), [September 1910].

82 WGP, 254-1-43, Grenfell to Mum, 20 August 1912.

83 PAD, Grenfell (Boston) to Jose Machado (Ottawa), 25 November 1911.

84 "Dr Grenfell's Work Is All to Be Merged," Sun (New York), 1 September 1912.

85 "Careless Methods Blamed," Allentown Leader, 3 September 1912.

86 "Manager Karnopp of Grenfell Institute Arrested Tuesday Night: Charged with Embezzling $1,000 from Its Funds," Evening Chronicle (St John's), 8 August 1912.

87 "Grenfell Mission Business Corporation after Official's Dishonesty," New York Herald, 8 September 1912.

88 WGP, 254-1-255, Karnopp to Grenfell, 5 September 1910.

89 WGP, 254-1-255, Karnopp to Grenfell, 5 September 1910.

90 PAD, GN 1-3A, Wilson S. Naylor (Wisconsin) to Grenfell (St John's), 30 November 1912.

91 PAD, GN 1-3A, Naylor to Grenfell, 30 November 1912.

92 PAD, MG 63, microfilm, Van Dyke to Grenfell, [20] August 1912.

93 PAD, GN 1-3A, Naylor to Grenfell, 30 November 1912.

94 "Karnopp Pleads Guilty and Gets Six Months," Evening Telegram (St John's), 10 August 1912.

95 PAD, GN 1-3A, Naylor to Grenfell, 30 November 1912.

96 "Karnopp Pleads Guilty."

97 For example, see "Grenfell Mission Robbed: Superintendent of Institute Is Charged with Theft," *Montreal Gazette*, 10 August 1912; "Dr Grenfell Causes C.H. Karnopp's Arrest: Superintendent of Institute Charged with Misusing $1,000 Mission Funds," *Globe* (Toronto), 12 August 1912; "Stole Mission's Funds? C.H. Karnopp, Superintendent, Arrested, Charged with Theft," *Toronto Star*, 12 August 1912.

98 "Misuse of Funds of Grenfell Missions in Labrador Charged," *New York Herald*, 2 September 1912.

99 "Grenfell Mission Business Corporation after Official's Dishonesty," *New York Herald*, 8 September 1912.

100 "Nations Will Join in Move to Right Grenfell Mission: Administration of Labrador and Newfoundland Work to Be Reorganized," *New York Herald*, 8 September 1912.

101 "Grenfell Missions' Plans: Reorganizing with Central Board – Karnepp [*sic*] Theft a Lone Incident," 4 September 1912.

102 PAD, MG 63.2214, Grenfell Association of Newfoundland, Diaries, Scrapbooks, and Publications; News Clippings, 1909–13, "Tales of Graft in Grenfell Mission Only Partly True: Investigation Shows That One Agent Now in Prison in Newfoundland Was Guilty of Theft," *World*, 4 September 1912.

103 WGP, 254-9-24, Sheard (St John's) to Stirling (Chicago), 30 January 1913. R.S. Cassels was a prominent Toronto lawyer who was married to a cousin of Julia Greenshields.

104 WGP, 254-9-24, Sheard (St John's) to Stirling (Chicago), 30 January 1913.

105 By May 1913, Cassels confirmed that Greenshields would never return to work for the mission. See PAD, MG 63-37, "Montreal Branch, Correspondence (Transcriptions), 1912–19," R.S. Cassels to Miss Fleet, 25 January 1913; PAD, MG 63-1981 "Cots – Endowed: 1913–37 (NY Permanent File), R.S. Cassels (Toronto) to Francis H. Wood (London), 5 May 1913.

106 PAD, GN 1-3A, Naylor to Grenfell, 30 November 1912.

107 WGP, 254-1-255, Karnopp (Penitentiary, St John's) to Grenfell, 16 December 1912. Karnopp and his wife, Martha, had many loyal friends in the city, including St Andrew's Presbyterian Church, which stood by him and voted to keep his name on the church roll as a member in good standing.

108 MU-ASC, Florence Miller Fonds, COLL-016, 6.01.001, Martha Karnopp

(Winnetka, IL) to Florence Miller (Topsail, NL), 11 November 1949. For more on the life of Phoebe Florence Miller, see Hallett, "Class unto Itself."

109 The RNMDSF would later be replaced by the Grenfell Association of Great Britain and Ireland, created in 1926.

110 Cecil Ashdown to RNMDSF, reprinted in *Toilers of the Deep* 1912 (12): 294.

111 The first Board of Directors included W.F. Archibald and Edgar Bogue, RNMDSF; Cecil S. Ashdown and William R. Stirling, GAA; Clarence J. Blake and Reginald A. Daly, NEGA; Herbert B. Ames and Jose A. Machado (Labrador Medical Mission, precursor to the GLMM); and W.C. Job and Robert Watson, GAN. See *First Annual Report of the International Grenfell Association*.

112 Ronald Rompkey, *Grenfell*, 176.

113 Patients were expected to pay as much as they could afford towards this cost but would not be refused treatment if they were unable to pay. PAD, MG 63-1921, "Finance Committee: St John's," Minutes of the First Meeting Held at St Anthony, 3 October 1914; and Minutes of the Third Meeting Held at St Anthony, Newfoundland, 3–8 October 1916.

114 WGP, 254-ACC-88-M22, Grenfell to Stirling, 8 October 1916.

115 Ronald Rompkey, *Grenfell*, 175.

CHAPTER FIVE

1 Terry Roberts, "The Decline of the Northern Peninsula: More Than a Story for This Journalist," CBC News Newfoundland and Labrador, 10 November 2016, https://www.cbc.ca/news/canada/newfoundland-labrador/northern-peninsula-my-ther-home-1.3841720.

2 Colin Howell, *Blood, Sweat, Cheers*, 7.

3 Colin Howell, *Blood, Sweat, Cheers*, 7.

4 Robidoux, *Stickhandling through the Margins*, 4.

5 Burstyn, *Rites of Men*, 4.

6 In Newfoundland and Labrador, an "outport" community refers to a small fishing settlement that supplied cod to the primary port and capital of St John's.

7 Korneski, *Conflicted Colony*, 7.

8 Korneski, *Conflicted Colony*, 7.

9 Howell and Leeworthy, "Borderlands."

10 Judy McGrath, "Labrador Pastimes," 4.

11 Colin Howell, *Blood, Sweat and Cheers*, 5–6.

12 Halverson, *Entirely Synthetic Fish*, 5.

13 Erdozain, *Problem of Pleasure*, 85.

14 Mangan, *Games Ethic and Imperialism*, 169.

15 Gorn and Goldstein, *Brief History of American Sports*, 82.

16 Heggie, "Sport (and Exercise) Medicine in Britain," 252.

17 Zirin, *People's History of Sports in the United States*, 34.

18 Zirin, *People's History of Sports in the United States*, 34.

19 Putney, *Muscular Christianity*, 129.

20 Putney, *Muscular Christianity*, 129–30.

21 Hobsbawm, *Invention of Tradition*, 290. Hobsbawm commits a minor error here (or major, depending on one's affiliation with the club) in referring to Huddersfield AFC as Huddersfield United.

22 Heggie, "Sport (and Exercise) Medicine in Britain," 252.

23 Although soccer was becoming a universal obsession and badge of British working-class identification, its popularity was in no way deemed healthful or nationally beneficial by the country's elites. Drinking in the terraces, gambling on match outcomes, and fighting over club and sectarian allegiances ensured that soccer would be viewed with suspicion and contempt by the British Establishment until well into the twentieth century. But criticism of terrace behaviour was just one expression of a deeper concern, for the professionalization of sport had "redefined athletics as work, and connected sport to the struggle between labour and capital" (Colin Howell, *Blood, Sweat, Cheers*, 6). While sport was deemed desirable and beneficial by elites, the co-option of sport by unruly working-class spectators and athletes – and its transformation into something suited to their particular needs – amounted to an unwelcomed act of subversion.

24 Goldblatt, *Ball Is Round*, 88–9.

25 Zirin, *People's History of Sport in the United States*, 5.

26 Colin Howell, *Blood, Sweat, Cheers*, 5.

27 Shackle, "Rebirth of Women's Football."

28 Zirin, *People's History of Sport in the United States*, 13.

29 Zirin, *People's History of Sport in the United States*, 13.

30 Croci, "(Association) Football."

31 Croci, "(Association) Football," 11.

32 Croci, "(Association) Football," 6–7.

33 Croci, "(Association) Football," 10.

34 W.J. Higgins, "Football in Newfoundland," 4.

35 Stirling, "Ice Hockey in Newfoundland," 151.

36 While Grenfell and his peers first attempted to remove the snow themselves, they quickly "tired of this plebeian chore" and a labourer was hired. For a full discussion of the origins of hockey in Newfoundland,

see Ben Jesseau's excellent unpublished essay "A Most Interesting Game." Jesseau demonstrates the importance of hockey as cultural bond between Newfoundlanders and Canadians long before Confederation in 1949.

37 Graham, *Ready ... Set ... Go!*, 64.

38 Graham, *Ready ... Set ... Go!*, 121.

39 Graham, *Ready ... Set ... Go!*, 121.

40 "Bell Island," *NQ* 1, no. 1 (July 1901): 3.

41 Colin Howell, *Blood, Sweat and Cheers*, 5.

42 Colin Howell, *Blood, Sweat and Cheers*, 5.

43 One of Grenfell's rescuers recalled that the doctor "had learned everything else but to stay off bad ice." Taylor and Horwood, *Beyond the Road*, 47.

44 "Battle Harbour Jottings," 23.

45 Grenfell, *Labrador Doctor*, 21.

46 Ronald Rompkey, *Grenfell*, 10.

47 Quoted in Robert MacDonald, *Sons of Empire*, 33.

48 "Battle Harbour Jottings," 23.

49 "Battle Harbour Jottings," 23.

50 Agnes E. Hamilton, "Football in Labrador," 95.

51 Robert MacDonald, *Sons of Empire*, 54.

52 Robert MacDonald, *Sons of Empire*, 55.

53 Nicholson, *Fighting Newfoundlander*, 97.

54 Wakefield, "St Anthony Items," 11.

55 Wakefield, "St Anthony Items," 11.

56 Ronald Rompkey, *Grenfell*, 105.

57 Zecher, "Annual Sports on the Ice at St Anthony," 121.

58 Zecher, "Annual Sports on the Ice at St Anthony," 122.

59 Warren, "Winter Sports, St Anthony, 1920," 47.

60 Warren, "Winter Sports, St Anthony, 1920," 47.

61 Wakefield, "St Anthony Items," 5.

62 Zecher, "Annual Sports on the Ice at St Anthony," 122.

63 Warren, "Winter Sports, St Anthony, 1920," 48.

64 Zecher, "Annual Sports on the Ice at St Anthony," 123.

65 Heidger-Osborne, "Sports Day at Harrington," 46.

66 Heidger-Osborne, "Sports Day at Harrington," 46.

67 Warren, "Winter Sports, St Anthony, 1920," 48.

68 Hospital admission record #1640, St Anthony Hospital, International Grenfell Association. Access to these anonymized clinical records for this research on sports was provided by Jennifer J. Connor, Faculty of Medicine, Memorial University of Newfoundland.

69 Grenfell, "Dr Grenfell's American and Canadian Tour," 24.
70 Grenfell, "Donation from the Philadelphia Nationals," 95.
71 "North Wind: From New England," 118.
72 George Reynolds, "Mission Stations," 14.
73 The Inuit also had a distinct version of "football": "The football is a small round ball made of sealskin and stuffed with reindeer hair. In Labrador, as in Greenland, it is whipped over the ice with a thong loop attached to a wooden handle. It can be caught in the air and returned with terrific force with this instrument": "Balls," 44.
74 Ronald Rompkey, *Grenfell*, 105.
75 "Balls," 45.
76 George Reynolds, "Mission Stations," 14.
77 "Balls," 46.
78 Hospital Admission Record # 0039; 0220; 1321; 1961; 3081; 5209; 5446; 6419; 7139; 7725; 8330; 8397, St Anthony Hospital, International Grenfell Association. Access to these records provided by Jennifer J. Connor.
79 Shannon Ryan, *Ice Hunters*, 269–70.
80 Scott, "Play at the Newfoundland Seal Fishery," 64.
81 Scott, "Play at the Newfoundland Seal Fishery," 65.
82 "Skating," 43.
83 Coates, "Item from Mud Lake Hospital," 27.
84 Leonard Tucker, "Hockey."
85 Wall, "R.C.A.F. Station, Goose, Labrador," 9.
86 Bledsoe, "Christmas-Tide at North West River," 11.
87 Withers, *Rock Harbour*, 127.
88 Robin McGrath, "Traditional Games of Newfoundland and Labrador," 7.
89 Robin McGrath, "Traditional Games of Newfoundland and Labrador," 7.
90 Robin McGrath, "Traditional Games of Newfoundland and Labrador," 7.
91 Forsyth, "Sport on Labrador," 97.
92 *Among the Deep Sea Fishers* is largely silent on Indigenous sport. While one tribute for Grenfell's birthday noted that he had participated in a "white man–Indian shoot" and "kayak race against Eskimos" ("Birthday Broadcasts," 7), and a photograph shows a group of Inuit children and adults posing with a soccer ball, such references are exceptional and brief.
93 Robin McGrath, "Traditional Games of Newfoundland and Labrador," 13.

94 Hutchings, "Labrador-Inuit Games Report," 18–19.
95 Hutchings, "Labrador-Inuit Games Report," 20.
96 Hutchings, "Labrador-Inuit Games Report," 10.
97 Hutchings, "Labrador-Inuit Games Report," 11.
98 Hutchings, "Labrador-Inuit Games Report," 11.
99 Byrne, "Introduction of Moose," 9. See also Byrne, "Selling Simplicity."
100 Grenfell, "Labrador," 92.
101 Grenfell, "Labrador," 107.
102 Grenfell, "Labrador," 99.
103 Kinsey, "Seeding the Water as the Earth," 531.
104 Byrne, "Introduction of Moose," 9.
105 Pocius, "Tourists, Health Seekers and Sportsmen," 49.
106 Pocius, "Tourists, Health Seekers and Sportsmen," 69.
107 Overton, *Making a World of Difference*, 196.
108 Overton, *Making a World of Difference*, 197.
109 Overton, *Making a World of Difference*, 198.
110 Hustins, *Rivers of Dreams*, 70.
111 Hustins, *Rivers of Dreams*, 73.
112 Hustins, *Rivers of Dreams*, 81.
113 Byrne, "Introduction of Moose," 9.
114 "Northern Pastimes: I – Fishing," 50.
115 "Northern Pastimes: I – Fishing," 50.
116 Overton, *Making a World of Difference*, 203.

CHAPTER SIX

1 Sweeny, *Why Did We Choose to Industrialize?*, 122.
2 The Depression era presents specific economic and political circumstances. For the effects of the Depression on Newfoundland and Labrador, see Alexander, "Newfoundland's Traditional Economy and Developments to 1934"; Cadigan, "Battle Harbour in Transition"; and Overton, "Self-Help, Charity, and Individual Responsibility." Some of the economic and political challenges of this period are addressed directly in Cullen, "What to Do about Newfoundland?"
3 Personal communication, Beverly Bennett, The Rooms.
4 John Kennedy, *Encounters*.
5 John Kennedy, *Encounters*, 226.
6 PAD, IGA fonds, file MG 63.2101, box 63, Board of Management of the International Grenfell Association, Minutes 1924; Luther, *Jessie Luther*, 280.

7 The ss *Strathcona* was acquired by Grenfell in 1899; it was a donation from Donald Alexander Smith (Lord Strathcona). The ss *Strathcona* was outfitted to include X-ray equipment, a dispensary and "emergency cots," and clothing. See O. and M., "Strathcona's Secretary's Report"; and Jenny Higgins, "Grenfell Mission."

8 Clothing and its connections to pauperism through charity are noted in the inaugural issue of ADSF. The magazine's first column notes, "It must be borne in mind that the clothing and other articles sent to Labrador are not as a rule given to recipients. Whenever possible, work is asked in exchange; fuel for the hospitals and boats being obtained in this way and the pauperizing element eliminated" (April 1903, 2).

9 The quality of mats was controlled by the mission's Industrial Department. Each mat was assigned a dollar value based on its quality. See "St Anthony Mat Industry." For a history of hooked mats in Newfoundland, see Laverty, *Silk Stocking Mats*. Some clothing was used in the manufacture of mats in the Industrial Department; these items were recorded, and payment for their value was invoiced to the Industrial Department.

10 Anne Budgell, *Dear Everybody*.

11 King, "Reclothing the English Poor"; Peter Jones, "Clothing the Poor"; Richmond, *Clothing the Poor*; and Richmond, "'Indiscriminate Liberality Subverts the Morals," 52.

12 Richmond, "'Indiscriminate Liberality Subverts the Morals,'" 53.

13 Richmond, *Clothing the Poor*, 199.

14 Richmond, *Clothing the Poor*.

15 Richmond, "'Indiscriminate Liberality Subverts the Morals,'" 59.

16 Richmond, "'Indiscriminate Liberality Subverts the Morals,'" 56.

17 After working with the Mission to Deep Sea Fishermen in the North Sea since 1889, Grenfell travelled to the Labrador coast in 1892. See Ronald Rompkey, "Grenfell, Sir Wilfred Thomason"; Ronald Rompkey, *Grenfell*.

18 Ronald Rompkey, *Grenfell*, 193.

19 Worth, "Developing a Method for the Study of the Clothing of the 'Poor,'" 70.

20 The first clothing store director at St Anthony was Dorothy Stirling, from Chicago. PAD, IGA fonds, M 63.2138, box 68, Circular of Information, 1940.

21 See ADSF 22 (July 1924): 54; ADSF 23 (January 1926): 176; and ADSF 24 (October 1926): 128.

22 Women, men, and children may have participated unequally in

exchanges. As men's capacity for labour exchange was limited by the seasonal nature of the fishery, women and children likely compensated for men's unavailability through their labour.

23 In addition to illustrating Grenfell's public lectures, his 1,371 magic lantern slides could also be borrowed by church groups, Sunday schools, philanthropic organizations, and later, by IGA branches. A set about Grenfell's work accompanied a prepared script by Frank Killam of Brockton, MA, and provided for $5 per lecture to raise funds. See *ADSF* 6 (July 1908): 4.

24 Sweeny, *Why Did We Choose to Industrialize?*, 123.

25 See Cadigan, "Battle Harbour in Transition"; and Sweeny, *Why Did We Choose to Industrialize?*

26 Sweeny, *Why Did We Choose to Industrialize?*, 215.

27 Cadigan excludes those individuals employed by merchants, by the church, in policing roles, and as justice of the peace in Battle Harbour, "Battle Harbour in Transition," 130.

28 Baine Johnston donated the building that Grenfell used as a hospital in Battle Harbour and had a vested interested in the well-being of fishers and their families.

29 Cadigan identifies merchants with whom fishers in Battle Harbour likely conducted business: Slades, Baine Johnston, the Hudson Bay Company and Moores: "Battle Harbour in Transition." On the basis of an assessment from Judge Prowse in 1895, Kennedy identifies fifteen merchants and their agents who operated in locations throughout Labrador, including Battle Harbour: *Encounters*, 79.

30 Grenfell, "Doctor Grenfell's Log," 12.

31 What was contested was the special privilege extended, from the colonial government to the mission, permitting the receipt of goods, including clothing donations, without a duty applied to them: see PAD, Colonial Secretary's Office, 1917, box 33, files 22.5.H, folder 1, special files, IGA: Report and Evidence of Enquiry into the Affairs of the IGA, 1917.

32 See Overton, "Economic Crisis and the End of Democracy"; PAD, MG 884.17, box 1, *History of the Dorcas Society*; and Sexty, "Dorcas Society," 34.

33 Overton, "Self-Help, Charity, and Individual Responsibility," 80.

34 *ADSF* 1 (April 1903): 2.

35 [White], "Items from the New England Grenfell Association," *ADSF* 10 (October 1912): 24.

36 [White], "Items from the New England Grenfell Association," *ADSF* (October 1912): 24.

37 [White], "Items from the New England Grenfell Association," *ADSF* (October 1912): 24.

38 Julia Greenshields played a key role in organizing clothing drives from her Toronto home: Jennifer Connor and Coombs-Thorne, "To the Rescue." The Labrador Needlework Guild of Canada was based in Toronto, and the Grenfell Labrador Medical Mission was based in Ottawa; the Grenfell Association of America was based in New York; the New England Grenfell Association was based on Boston; and the Grenfell Association of Great Britain and Ireland was headquartered in London. See Macklem, "Report of the Labrador Needlework Guild of Canada," 12; and Ronald Rompkey, *Grenfell.*

39 Anne Budgell, *Dear Everybody*; Ronald Rompkey, *Grenfell.*

40 Richmond, *Clothing the Poor*, 226.

41 Richmond, *Clothing the Poor*, 221.

42 Richmond, *Clothing the Poor*, 212, 221.

43 The first Annual Meeting of the American-Labrador Branch of the Needlework Guild of America was held in Pilgrim Hall, Boston, on 23 May 1908. (The Coast-to-Coast branch of the Needlework Guild of America, which supplied clothing from elsewhere in America, was administered from New York.) See Tatnall, "Report of the American-Labrador Guild of America," 11; and Tatnall, "Seventh Annual Report of the Needlework Guild," 60–1. For a history of the American-Labrador branch, see Tatnall, "Effort for the Grenfell Mission," 111. Individual membership in needlework guilds was open to men, women, and children. It required a monetary donation, or the donation of two new, purpose-made articles of clothing or linen. Directors in individual branches organized clothing and collected cash donations. See Concord Free Public Library, Concord, MA, Concord New England Branch of the Grenfell Association, Minutes 27 January 1926; and Alice Fernald See, West Concord Union Church, Concord, MA, Minutes, 6th Annual Meeting, Concord New England Branch of the New England Grenfell Association, 1931.

44 Despite the central role played by IGA chapters in New York and Boston, there are relatively few traces of their activities in local newspapers. This may be because charitable work by the middle classes, particularly women, was expected. See Tatnall, "Effort for the Grenfell Mission."

45 Tatnall, "Report of the American-Labrador Guild of America," 11.

46 Knitting patterns were provided for "beanie caps": "Needlework Guild Notes," *ADSF* 40 (January 1943): 123; and mittens, "Needlework Guild News," *ADSF* 41 (October 1943): 91.

47 Beatrice Farnsworth Powers Collection, MS 125, Sophia Smith Archive.
    For a discussion of the popularity of the tam-o'-shanter, see Picken,
    Language of Fashion, 21.

48 Anne Budgell, *Dear Everybody*; and PAD, IGA fonds, MG 63.2101, box
    63, file Board of Management of the International Grenfell Association,
    Minutes 1924.

49 Later, denim would also prove to be a durable, versatile, and valued
    fabric. It would be used to make dresses, pinafores, overalls, dickies
    (pullover parkas), curtains, chair covers, tablecloths, and canoe seats:
    see Berthelsen, "Blue Denim."

50 Hopkins, "Adventures in the Clothing Department," 125.

51 Cadigan, *Newfoundland and Labrador*.

52 PAD, IGA fonds, "Clothing Department Annual Report, 1924–1925."

53 This wardrobe includes one of each of the following: undervest, "un-
    derdrawers," a "combination" (an American term for one-piece "un-
    derdrawers," also called a "union suit" in Atlantic Canada), pair of
    wool trousers, wool shirt, cotton shirt, pair of wool socks and pair of
    cotton socks, heavy sweater, nightshirt, shoes, coat and hat. PAD, IGA
    fonds, "Clothing Department Annual Report, 1924–1925."

54 PAD, IGA fonds, "Clothing Department Annual Report, 1924–1925."

55 PAD, IGA fonds, "Clothing Department Annual Report, 1924–1925."

56 PAD, IGA fonds, "Clothing Department Annual Report, 1924–1925."

57 Mayou, "Sketches of Dr Grenfell's Work," 14.

58 Claudio, "Waste Couture," A449.

59 See "Directions for Making Mittens." On knitwear, also see "Notes
    and Comments," ADSF 16 (January 1919): 179. Also see Duley, "Un-
    quiet Knitters of Newfoundland," 60; and Scott, "Cuffs, Vamps, Trig-
    ger Mitts and Drawers," presentation at Newfoundland Historical
    Society, February 2016.

60 Trigger mittens have separate sheaths for the thumb and index finger,
    making it possible to shoot a gun with one's hand covered. See Storey,
    Kirwan, and Widdowson, *Dictionary of Newfoundland English*, 582.
    For 1924–5 clothing inventory, see PAD, IGA fonds, box 98, file
    63.2084, Clothing Department Annual Report, 1924–5.

61 According to the *Dictionary of Newfoundland English*, a vamp is a
    thick woollen oversock that covers the foot. *Vamp* is also used as a verb,
    meaning "to darn a sock": see Storey, Kirwan and Widdowson, *Dictio-
    nary*, 128, 593. Vamps were valued because they prevented chafing in
    rubber boots (Scott, "Cuffs, Vamps, Trigger Mitts and Drawers").

62 ADSF 1 (April 1903): 2.

63 Hopkins, "Adventures in the Clothing Department," 125.

64 Anne Budgell, *Dear Everybody*, 55.
65 Anne Budgell, *Dear Everybody*, 56.
66 Harriet Cook, "'Down' North," 26.
67 PAD, Colonial Secretary's Office, 1917, box 33, files 22.5.H, folder 1, Special Files, IGA: "Report and Evidence of Enquiry into the Affairs of the IGA."
68 Anne Budgell, *Dear Everybody*, 56. The stores also were sites for distribution of reading material, and in 1926 the mission's library work itself was overseen by the clothing department: see Jennifer Connor, "'Dispensing Good Books and Literature,'" 378, 382.
69 Ruiz, "Media Environments," presentation at Memorial University of Newfoundland, January 2016.
70 Ruiz, "Media Environments."
71 PAD, IGA fond, Circular of Information.
72 Emphasis in original letter. CGC, loc. 13I, box 1, folder 6, Carolyn Galbraith to Frances Stilwell, 3 October 1926.
73 CGC, loc. 13I, box 1, folder 6, Carolyn Galbraith to Frances Stilwell, 29 October 1926.
74 In this collection, individual photographs are separated from correspondence; it is not possible to determine the photograph to which Galbraith refers.
75 CGC, Galbraith to Stilwell, 29 October 1926.
76 Waste wool may refer to an inferior quality of wool that included short and/or unclean fibres. PAD, IGA fonds, "Clothing Department Annual Report, 1924–5."
77 PAD, IGA fonds, "Clothing Department Annual Report, 1924–5."
78 Italics ours. A print copy of these instructions is included in the Florence F. Fuller photograph album (1926–7), Grenfell Historic Properties collection, St Anthony, NL; Fuller, from Waterville, Maine, was a summer volunteer. Also see PAD, IGA fonds, box 68, file 63.2138, 1940, *Instructions and Information for Staff and Volunteers*, ca 1940.
79 PAD, IGA fonds, *Board of Management of the IGA*, Minutes.
80 In the 1917 Squarey Enquiry, a further contravention of the mission's clothing policy is discussed: a volunteer at the Spotted Islands hospital sold clothing to raise money for the dispensary. Brought to Grenfell's attention, the situation was rectified by payment of the applicable duty. See PAD, Colonial Secretary's Office, 1917, "Report and Evidence of Enquiry into the Affairs of the IGA," 141.
81 PAD, Colonial Secretary's Office, 1917, "Report and Evidence of Enquiry into the Affairs of the IGA," 141.
82 PAD, Colonial Secretary's Office, 1917, "Report and Evidence of

Enquiry into the Affairs of the IGA," 141. Knickerbockers are pants, sometimes banded, that fall just below the knee without covering the lower legs and ankles. Fashionable among women in the 1920s, they were also worn by men for sports: Picken, *Language of Fashion*, 85.

83 Jessie Luther's summer packing list for women volunteers included "oil-skin coat (long), sou'wester hat, rubber boots, moccasins, two or three sweaters, two woollen skirts (of stout material that will not tear easily), canvas or khaki skirt and waist, bloomers, three or four pairs woollen stockings (thin), two pairs woollen stockings (heavy), "plenty of cotton stockings," lightweight underwear, medium [weight] underwear, cotton underclothing, two or three flannel nightdresses, warm bathrobe, one good house gown, one good street skirt, one or two linen or cotton gowns, a linen skirt, several thin shirtwaists, two or three woollen shirt-waists, a pair of "high heavy tan tramping boots," one pair of sealskin boots, ordinary boots, pumps and "tan and black, plenty of them," a woollen cap, a good (travelling) hat for church, two pairs woollen gloves, kid gloves for church, "a heavy ulster" (a daytime overcoat, usually with an attached cape), vamps for skin boots, a leather coat (short), and a canvas hat. See Luther, "Labrador Clothing and Routes." Her winter list, also published in the same issue, included heavier clothes, as well as additional items that were to be purchased by staff and volunteer workers at the mission's St Anthony location. Grenfell cloth, which was manufactured by Haythornthwaite Sons, in Lodge Mill, Burnley, England, was available after 1923 (likely only to staff and volunteers because of its cost); sealskin boots were made in the mission's Industrial Department: PAD, MG 63.2075, box 94, 10th Annual Meeting, Minutes 1923.

84 Galbraith to Stilwell, 29 October [1926].

85 CGC, loc. 13I, box 1, folder 6, 1926, Carolyn Galbraith to Evelyn Haviland, 17 September [1926?].

86 Perry, "Nursing for the Grenfell Mission"; see also Loder, *Daughter of Labrador*.

87 Punctuation in original, CGC, loc. 13I, box 1, folder 6, 1926, Carolyn Galbraith to Mrs Lucy Clapp, 13 February 1926. Greta Ferris, Hart-ford, CT, was also a volunteer worker at L'Anse aux Loup, Labrador.

88 Cadigan, "Battle Harbour in Transition."

89 Punctuation in original. Grenfell, "Battle Harbour," 112.

90 Grenfell, "Log of the ss *Strathcona*," ADSF 12 (January 1905): 15.

91 In this context, "inside" clothing likely refers to what was unlikely to be worn publicly. Maud Alexander was also a volunteer nurse at the

mission; she married volunteer staff doctor James C. Janney. See Luther, *Jessie Luther*, 321. After 1926, Dorothy Stirling, who was also a friend of Anne Grenfell, is recorded as the director, Clothing Store: PAD, MG 63.2077, box 94, Minutes, Board of Directors: 1917–1922, 11th Annual Report 1926.

92 Hopkins, "Adventures in the Clothing Department," 124.
93 Ronald Rompkey, *Grenfell*, 274.
94 Anne Budgell, *Dear Everybody*, 56.
95 PAD, IGA fonds, box 33, file 22.5, 1917, Report and Evidence of Enquiry into the Affairs of the IGA (including Petition).
96 Cadigan, *Newfoundland and Labrador*, 168.
97 PAD, MG 63.2075, box 94, IGA, 10th Annual Meeting, Minutes 1923.
98 The letter included assertions about the excessive use of liquor, and acts of public immorality, including allegations of adultery, by local officials. PAD, box 33, file 22. 5, Correspondence to [Magistrate] Mr R. Squarey, 23 August 1917.
99 PAD, Colonial Secretary's Office, 1917, "Report and Evidence of Enquiry."
100 In 1929, the director's position was salaried as permanent staff and approved by the IGA Board of Directors: see PAD, IGA fonds, MG 63.1944, box 85, Minutes of the Executive Committee IGA, 1928–61.
101 PAD, Colonial Secretary's Office, 1917, "Report and Evidence of Enquiry," 293.

CHAPTER SEVEN

I am grateful to George Wislocki for providing me with the Florence Clothier letters.

1 The biographical information on Muir has been assembled from fragmentary online sources, primarily census records, college catalogues, and yearbooks. A Muir Family Reunion website compiled by Douglas J. Graham in 2012 contains a brief biography, which cites early family letters written by Muir. I have made some inferences to reconcile conflicting information and to fill gaps.
2 Muir, *Ethical System of Adam Smith*.
3 Fingard, "College, Career, and Community," 31.
4 Muir, "People on the Labrador and Their Needs," 38.
5 Muir, "People on the Labrador and Their Needs," 35–41; and Muir, "Summer School at Red Bay," 31–4.
6 Muir, "Summer Work at Eddies Cove," 21.

7 Only six of the seventy-one were recorded in 1908–13. Others may
   have gone unrecorded, as systematic annual staff reports appeared only
   from 1914 onward. The number of individuals was somewhat fewer
   than seventy-one, as some made repeated visits.

8 PAD, IGA fonds, MG63.1943, vol. 1, IGA Board of Directors Minutes,
   November 1916, 148.

9 Ewing, "Education Department," 53–5.

10 Most of the biographical information on Page is taken from EPHP,
   "Guide to the Elizabeth Page Harris Papers."

11 Harper, "Missionary Work of the Reformed (Dutch) Church."

12 Elizabeth Hazelton Haight, "The Vassar Units for Service Abroad,"
   Vassar Miscellany News 3, no. 1 (28 September 1918): 4.

13 EPHP, box 57, folder 1233, Muir to Page, 7 February 1921. Grenfell
   mission correspondence in EPHP is stored in boxes 57–60, folders
   1233–1339, grouped sequentially by date; subsequent references will be
   only to the correspondence and its date in this collection.

14 EPHP, box 57, folder 1233.

15 Katharine Blayney suggests that the first medical trip to White Bay by
   the *Strathcona* occurred in 1920 or 1921: Blayney, "Nutrition Work in
   White Bay," 123.

16 For a more extensive outline of White Bay history and socio-economic
   conditions in the 1920s, see Clothier, *It's a Glorious Country*, 16–19.

17 EPHP, Page to Muir, 21 November 1921. An expanded version of this
   report was published as Page, "Educational Department: White Bay,
   Newfoundland."

18 Blayney, "Nutrition Work in White Bay," 123–5.

19 Although most of her time in St Anthony had focused on the industrial
   work, Page had also met with Marion Moseley, a volunteer whose arrival in St Anthony in the summer of 1920 resulted in a more concerted
   "nutrition and child welfare" effort by the Grenfell organization. Moseley had received some training by Dr William Emerson in Boston, who
   pioneered in developing protocols for identifying and responding to
   childhood nutritional deficiencies. He particularly advocated health
   education aimed at schoolchildren and mothers. In 1921 Moseley recruited and coordinated several volunteer "nutrition workers" in St
   Anthony and communities along the traditional IGA coastal areas. She
   welcomed the opportunity proposed by Page to emulate her work in
   White Bay. See Moseley, "Third Year of Health Work"; and Lush, "Nutrition, Health Education, and Dietary Reform," 124–45 and 149–50.

20 EPHP, Page to Mary [Card], 3 January 1925. I can find no record of

approval in the Minutes of the Board of Directors, so Page may have been referring to approval by the Staff Selection Committee.

21 EPHP, Page to Grenfell, 7 April 1922.

22 EPHP, Grenfell to Page, 31 March 1922.

23 EPHP, box 57, folders 1234–7.

24 Page, "Educational Department: White Bay, Newfoundland"; Page, "Growth of the White Bay Work." Page encouraged her accomplices to submit articles on their work to the mission quarterly. Articles concerning the White Bay Unit may be found in the following issues of ADSF: January 1922 (two articles), January 1924, April 1924 (three articles), July 1924, January 1925 (two articles), July 1925, and October 1930.

25 EPHP, Watson to Page, 2 November 1922; and Page to Watson, 22 November 1922.

26 PAD, IGA fonds, folder MG63.2138.

27 This section is based primarily on Page, "Growth of the White Bay Work," correspondence in EPHP, and the letters of Florence Clothier (cited below). Lush, "Nutrition, Health Education, and Dietary Reform" (chapters 4 and 5) offers an extended description and interpretation of the White Bay work, and Page's role, using many of the same sources. However, she views the White Bay Unit more narrowly, essentially as a "nutrition" enterprise like the "travelling nutrition units" operated elsewhere under the direction of Marion Moseley and Elizabeth Criswell. She refers to Page as a "nutrition worker," whereas Page had a greater personal interest in the industrial work and in promoting community development through her summer teachers. She consistently referred to herself as "Secretary of the White Bay Unit."

28 EPHP, Page to Houghteling, 6 May 1924.

29 See Clothier, *It's a Glorious Country.*

30 In "Nutrition, Health Education, and Dietary Reform," Lush provides an account of the evolution of interest in dietary reform within the Grenfell mission from 1893 to 1920, in relation to the emerging American scientific and vocational interest in nutrition and health education (see chapters 2 and 3).

31 PAD, folder MG63.2084, IGA Board of Directors Minutes, 9 December 1922. Report of the Executive Officer (Arthur Cosby) for 1923.

32 In 1925 these teams were supplanted by the appointment of two fully qualified district nurses under the auspices of NONIA, whose duties would encompass the public health dimension of the IGA workers. However, a travelling dentist continued to be assigned to the White Bay Unit until 1926.

33 For a more detailed account of Page's industrial work, see Laverty, *Silk Stocking Mats*, 19–22.

34 As an example, among her papers there are carbon copies of lengthy letters typed on her "trusty Corona" while aboard the *Loon*.

35 PAD, MG63.1928, "Report of the White Bay Unit for 1925," typescript (November 1925).

36 PAD, MG63.1928, "Report of the White Bay Unit for 1925," typescript (November 1925).

37 The acquisition and funding of the *Loon* is documented in dozens of letters from October 1924 to April 1925, EPHP folders 1273–86. In late 1926, as she was severing her ties with the IGA, Page wrote about the "Status of Loon." She had apparently heard that it had been taken to the West Coast without permission. She declared that $3,500 of "White Bay money," plus $500 of "personal money," had gone into the boat and equipment, and that the boat remained the property of "White Bay." If it was not needed there, the mission could rent it for $300 a season, but was not permitted to have the furnishings, tools, etc. EPHP, undated note [November 1926, folder 1314]. It is not known whether this note was sent to IGA authorities. A boat named the *Loon* was reportedly operated by the mission in Lake Melville, Labrador, in 1944: Anne Budgell, *Dear Everybody*, 121–2.

38 The schoolteachers were left entirely for Page to manage; although Ethel Gordon Muir continued to come to Labrador along with many other teachers every summer until 1930, she had no involvement with Page or White Bay after 1921.

39 EPHP, Page to Crowe, 23 January 1924; Crowe to Page, 5 March 1924; Page to Crowe, 26 March 1924; Page to Elliot, 26 March 1924; Crowe to Page, 4 June 1924; Card to Page, 9 July 1924.

40 EPHP, Blackall to Marks, 30 May 1924.

41 EPHP, Page to Blackall, 13 May 1924; Blackall to Page, 21 May 1924; Page to Walter, 22 May 1925.

42 EPHP, Page to Allardyce, 24 April 1925.

43 EPHP, Clothier to Page, undated [early 1926].

44 EPHP, Muir to Page, 9 May 1922, and 13 May 1922.

45 PAD MG63.1928, Correspondence 1928. "Report of the White Bay Unit for 1925," [November 1925].

46 EPHP, Page to Card, 3 January 1925. Mary Card was an old Vassar / White Bay Unit hand who had been the nutrition worker for two summers and spent winters in St Anthony.

47 Page to Criswell, 9 May 1925.

48 See House, *Way Out*.

49 EPHP, Allardyce to Page, 18 August 1924.
50 EPHP, Page to Cleveland, 15 November 1924.
51 EPHP, Allardyce to Page, 9 April 1925.
52 EPHP, Houghteling to Page, 19 April 1925.
53 EPHP, Page to Allardyce, 3 July 1925. Florence Clothier provides a wry eye-witness account of Page's efforts to organize the NONIA committee in Jackson's Arm: *It's a Glorious Country*, 179–80.
54 EPHP, "Work in White Bay," [15 December 1926], 4.
55 MU-ASC, COLL-151, Newfoundland Outport Nursing and Industrial Association, NONIA Annual Reports; House, *Way Out*.
56 [International Grenfell Association], "Report of the Staff Selection Committee," *ADSF* 27 (July 1929): 91.
57 In 1958 Charles Curtis wrote a reminiscence of the IGA educational efforts over fifty years: see his "Willingly to School." His essay included reference to Ethel Gordon Muir's early placement of young women in summer teaching posts, and a brief account of the "unit" operated in White Bay "in the 1930s" by Page, Tallant, Card, Clothier, and Criswell.
58 EPHP, Mrs Bennet F. Schauffler to unnamed "Friends," 3 April 1969.

CHAPTER EIGHT

Archival research was supported by a grant from the J.R. Smallwood Foundation, Memorial University.
1 References to this training in the mission's magazine, *Among the Deep Sea Fishers*, were often meagre; for example, "Bessie [of Labrador, sister of Fred] graduated in the Mechanics Institute of Social Science of Rochester, New York." See Grenfell, "Educational Fund," 46.
2 Bourdieu, *Distinction*; Lane, *Pierre Bourdieu*; Michael Grenfell, *Pierre Bourdieu*; Seidman, *Contested Knowledge*.
3 Antikainen and Komonen, "Biography, Life Course, and the Sociology of Education," 149.
4 Newfoundland was granted status as a self-governing colony in 1854 and became a dominion of the British Empire in 1907.
5 Rury, *Education and Social Change*.
6 Graves, *Girls' Schooling during the Progressive Era*, xvii.
7 Fischer and Hout, *Century of Difference*, 10–12.
8 *JHA*, "Resolutions to Be submitted by Mr Murray to a Committee of the Whole House, May 8, 1890."
9 *Report of the Public Schools of Newfoundland under Roman Catholic School Boards for the Year Ended 31st December 1917*, xxiii.
10 Cremin, *Popular Education and Its Discontents*, 13.

11 "Report of the Public Schools of Newfoundland under Methodist Boards for Year 1922–23," 108.

12 McCann, *Schooling in a Fishing Society*, 82.

13 John Kennedy, *People of the Bays and Headlands*.

14 *JHA*, "Report of an Official Visit to the Coast of Newfoundland by the Governor of Newfoundland during the Month of August 1905," 351.

15 *JHA*, "Report of an Official Visit to the Coast of Newfoundland by the Governor of Newfoundland during the Month of August 1905," 356.

16 CCNYR, International Grenfell Association, 1921–46, box 186, folio 8, Vincent Burke to Frederick Keppel, 14 May 1928.

17 Davis, "Itinerant Teacher 1923–5."

18 Maud Chaulk, "We Liked the Outdoor Life."

19 "Education Act 1903," 99. Amalgamated schools were sometimes called common schools. The name *amalgamated* was discontinued in favour of the word *integrated* in May 1969.

20 Cliff Robbins, "Amalgamated Schools of Newfoundland," 31. In 1920 the government enacted legislation creating a Department of Education. Seven years later new legislation replaced the department with a Bureau of Education. This new arrangement meant all power lay in the hands of the superintendents of the major churches. In essence, the government had no effective control over the education system.

21 It was known as the Muddy Bay School, but outsiders called it the Gordon School. It was the first non-denominational school in Labrador. See Clara Gordon, *Labrador Teacher*, 46n5.

22 Henry Gordon, *Labrador Parson*, 52.

23 Best, "School Days," 42.

24 Powell, "Charlottetown," 57–8. The author writes that a school was the first priority when people moved to Charlottetown in 1951 from New York, Nick's Cove, and other small settlements in St Michael's Bay. Powell was born in Carbonear, Newfoundland, in 1921 and moved to the forgotten coast in 1936.

25 Barnes, "History of Education in Newfoundland."

26 William Hamilton, "Society and Schools in Newfoundland," 141.

27 Hiller, "Social Issues in Early 20th-Century Newfoundland," 31.

28 Abe, "Muscular Christianity in Japan," 14.

29 Grenfell, *Labrador Doctor* (1948), 175. The first edition of this book was published in 1919.

30 Hickman, "History of Education in Newfoundland," 47.

31 PAD, Wilfred Thomason Grenfell Collection, MG 327, reel 114, W.W. Blackall to Edward Morris, 20 September 1910.

32 Squarey, "Newfoundland Government Inquiry," 160.

33 For examples of the contribution of women in the American south, see Katherine Reynolds and Schram, *Separate Sisterhood.*

34 The Gordon School at Muddy Bay was taken over by the Grenfell mission at the request of Henry Gordon. A fire destroyed the building in 1928, and the school was rebuilt at Cartwright. It was then called Lockwood School, in recognition of Mrs Joseph Lockwood of Concord, Massachusetts, who financed the new school and dormitory.

35 Criswell, "School Health Work in Labrador," 1089.

36 Whisnant, "Second Level Appalachian History," 118.

37 Katherine Reynolds and Schram, *Separate Sisterhood,* 57.

38 John Kennedy, *People of the Bays and Headlands,* 152.

39 MU-ASC, collection MF-117, Wilfred Grenfell to Nathaniel Stuart Noel, 18 September 1926.

40 Rowe, *Education and Culture in Newfoundland,* 127. Eskimo or Inuit children attended Moravian schools on the north coast of Labrador in the 1920s unless they were living at the St Anthony Orphanage. Other children attending the St Anthony School at that time stayed at the orphanage.

41 Paddon, *Labrador Memoir,* ix.

42 John Kennedy, "Impact of the Grenfell Mission," 202.

43 Grenfell, *Challenge of Labrador,* 12.

44 Charles Curtis, "It Should Be Told ... Part II." See also PAD, Grenfell Collection, MG 327, reel 113, Moret to Wilfred Grenfell, 2 December 1931.

45 On 24 November 2017 Prime Minister Justin Trudeau apologized on behalf of all Canadians for the treatment of Innu, Inuit, and NunatuKavut children who attended the Yale School at North West River, the Lockwood School in Cartwright, and the St Anthony Orphanage and Boarding School, three schools operated by the IGA and the Moravian Boarding Schools at Nain and Makkovik. These schools also served settler populations.

46 Paddon, *Labrador Memoir,* 82.

47 Stewart, "Letter from Lockwood School," 167.

48 Devens, "'If We Get the Girls,'" 228.

49 Crane, "Across the River," 15.

50 Lemare, "I Liked to Tease."

51 Loder, "Early School Days," 38. More discussion of Millicent Blake Loder and her IGA experience is provided below.

52 Bertha Chaulk, "Coombs Family History."

53 *Report of the Public Schools of Newfoundland under Methodist Boards, 1920,* 65.

54 The current mandate of the Pratt Institute is to provide education in the liberal arts and sciences, and train architects, creative artists, and information professionals: "About Pratt."

55 "Men behind the Scenes," 67.

56 Badger, "Wilfred Bertram Mesher"; Mesher, letter to the editor; Pratt Institute, "Machine Construction Class of 1916," 41.

57 Sergeant Archibald Ash of Red Bay, a member of the Royal Newfoundland Regiment, was killed in action at Sailly-Saillisel, France, on 23 February 1917.

58 "May Pardy," 37.

59 "Notes and Comments," ADSF 15 (April 1917): 23.

60 Grenfell, *Labrador and North Newfoundland,* 10.

61 PAD, IGA Collection, MG 63, box 86, file 63.1943, vol. 1, 28–9 March 1914 to 22 November 1932, meeting minutes, 6 May 1920.

62 Lagemann, *Politics of Knowledge,* 17.

63 Howe, "Emergence of Scientific Philanthropy," 33.

64 CCNYR, International Grenfell Association, 1921–46, box 186, folio 8, Angell to Wilfred Grenfell, 31 May 1921.

65 PAD, IGA Collection, MG 63, box 86, file 63.1943, vol. 1, 28–9 March 1914 to 22 November 1932, meeting minutes, 21 May 1921.

66 PAD, IGA Collection, MG 63, box 86, file 63.1943, vol. 1, 28–9 March 1914 to 22 November 1932, meeting minutes, 3 December 1921.

67 CCNYR, International Grenfell Association, 1921–46, box 186, folio 8, Wilfred Grenfell to Angell, 17 December 1921. The attached list was not found in the collection, but a reference was found to the number of students in the Board of Directors minutes for 28 April 1922, Education Committee to the Board of Directors. See PAD, IGA Collection, MG 63, box 86, file 63.1943, vol. 1, 28–9 March 1914 to 22 November 1934, meeting minutes, 28 April 1922.

68 CCNYR, International Grenfell Association, 1921–46, box 186, folio 8, Angell to Wilfred Grenfell, 21 January 1922.

69 Grenfell, "Educational Fund," 46.

70 PAD, Wilfred Thomason Grenfell Collection, MG 327, reel 113, Huey Tetley, The Rectory, Curling, to Wilfred Grenfell, 7 August 1922.

71 PAD, IGA Collection, MG 63, box 86, file 63.1943, vol. 1, 28–9 March 1914 to 22 November 1934, Report from the Education Committee to the Board of Directors, meeting minutes, 28 April 1922.

72 PAD, Wilfred Thomason Grenfell Collection, MG 327, reel 114, Clara McLeod to Wilfred Grenfell, 2 September 1922.

73 CCNYR, International Grenfell Association, 1921–46, box 186, folio 8, Anne Grenfell to CCNY, 18 August 1922.

74 Charles Curtis, "It Should Be Told ... Part II," 56.

75 CCNYR, International Grenfell Association, 1921–46, box 186, folio 8, Anne Grenfell to CCNY, 27 August 1923.

76 PAD, IGA Collection, MG 63, box 86, file 63.1943, vol. 1, 28–9 March 1914 to 22 November 1932, meeting minutes, 26 April 1924.

77 McNeill, "Farewell."

78 CCNYR, International Grenfell Association, 1921–46, box 186, folio 8, Anne Grenfell to CCNY, 17 September 1927.

79 CCNYR, International Grenfell Association, 1921–46, box 186, folio 8, Anne Grenfell to CCNY, 17 September 1927.

80 Shannon Wilson, *Berea College*, 86. The Day Law of 1904 made interracial schools illegal in Kentucky. The college's appeal to the Supreme Court failed to overturn the law, so Berea provided funds to build the Lincoln Institute, a new Black school near Louisville.

81 "Dr Grenfell Visits Berea," *Berea Citizen*, 18 March 1920.

82 "Grenfell to Be Speaker," *Berea Citizen*, 21 May 1931.

83 Tallant, "Industrial Department and the People," 127.

84 Grenfell, "Berea College."

85 Louie, "Letter from Louie"; Pye, "Fond Are Our Memories."

86 Andersen, *Voyage to the Grand Banks*.

87 Laverty, *Silk Stocking Mats*, 103. More information on Dora Mesher can be found in MU-ASC, Rhoda Dawson Bickerdike, Coll-198.

88 Horace McNeill was appointed assistant superintendent of the IGA in 1959. He was educated at Berea College and studied co-operative management in Manchester, England. See "Horace W. McNeill." He is the son of Edgar ("Ted") McNeill, who is discussed in chapter 9 by Rafico Ruiz in this volume.

89 CCNYR, International Grenfell Association, 1921–46, box 186, folio 8, Anne Grenfell to Keppel, 11 July 1929.

90 PAD, IGA Collection, MG 63, box 86, file 63.1943, vol. 1, 28–9 March 1914 to 22 November 1934, IGA Board of Directors Minutes, 15 May 1929.

91 Lagemann, *Politics of Knowledge*, 62.

92 Lagemann, *Politics of Knowledge*, 108.

93 Some years later, Burke did receive the Order of the British Empire. See Stockwood, "Vincent Burke."

94 CCNYR, International Grenfell Association, 1921–46, box 186, folio 8, memorandum of interview – Memorial University College, Keppel, Burke, DAS, 15 November 1927.

95 CCNYR, International Grenfell Association, 1921–46, box 186, folio 8, memorandum of interview RML and Vincent P. Burke, 16 November 1927. Interoffice memoranda often used initials and usually refer to staff members at the CCNY. Robert M. Lester (RML) came to work at the CCNY offices in 1926.

96 CCNYR, International Grenfell Association, 1921–46, box 186, folio 8, RML to Vincent Burke, 17 February 1928.

97 MU-RA, Board of Trustees, box 1, John Paton to Vincent Burke, 18 September 1928.

98 MU-RA, Presidential Papers, box 1, Memorial University of Newfoundland, John Paton, "Report on Education in Labrador," 1929.

99 MU-RA, Presidential Papers, box 1, Memorial University of Newfoundland, John Paton, "Report on Education in Labrador," 1929, 8.

100 MU-RA, Presidential Papers, box 1, Memorial University of Newfoundland, John Paton, "Report on Education in Labrador," 1929, 8.

101 Michael Coleman, "Symbiotic Embrace," 6.

102 MU-RA, Presidential Papers, box 1, Memorial University of Newfoundland, John Paton, "Report on Education in Labrador," 1929.

103 MU-RA, Presidential Papers, box 1, Memorial University of Newfoundland, John Paton, "Report on Education in Labrador," 1929.

104 Telephone interview with Bonnie Waddell, Nova Scotia Agricultural College.

105 CCNYR, International Grenfell Association, 1921–46, box 186, folio 8, John Lewis Paton, Memorial University College to Keppel, 23 July 1929.

106 Loder, Daughter of Labrador; Loder, "Early School Days."

107 Loder, "Early School Days," 30.

108 Loder, "Early School Days," 41–2.

109 Loder, "Early School Days," 79.

110 Kerr, Wilfred Grenfell, 164.

111 Ronald Rompkey, Grenfell, 240.

CHAPTER NINE

1 Greene, "Opening of St Anthony Hospital," 100.

2 Ronald Rompkey, Grenfell, 284.

3 Cormier, "Writing the Tape-Recorded Life," 423.

4 Poednicks, "Introduction," 2.

5 Dorothy McNeill, interview.

6 Cosby, "New Hospital for St Anthony."

7 Demarest, "History of St Anthony Hospital," 103.

8 [International Grenfell Association], "Sixth Annual Report of the International Grenfell Association," 86.

9 Charles Curtis, "St Anthony Hospital," 26.

10 Hause, "Design and Installation of an Electric Lighting Plant."

11 Hause, "Design and Installation of an Electric Lighting Plant," 59–60.

12 "New St Anthony Hospital."

13 Grenfell, "New Hospital for St Anthony," ADSF 23 (October 1925): 102.

14 Grenfell, "New Hospital for St. Anthony," ADSF 23 (October 1925): 102.

15 Charles Curtis, "Year's Work at St Anthony Hospital," 148.

16 "Pleasant Commendation for the Hospital."

17 "Pleasant Commendation for the Hospital."

18 "Pleasant Commendation for the Hospital."

19 ADSF 25 (July 1927): [49].

20 Greene, "William Adams Delano."

21 Greene, "William Adams Delano."

22 "Men behind the Scenes," 66.

23 "Men behind the Scenes," 67.

24 "Men behind the Scenes," 67.

25 "Year at St Anthony Hospital."

26 Threlkeld-Edwards, "New Medical Era," 51.

27 Threlkeld-Edwards, "New Medical Era."

28 "Men behind the Scenes," 67.

29 Threlkeld-Edwards, "New Medical Era," 57.

30 Threlkeld-Edwards, "New Medical Era," 57.

31 Threlkeld-Edwards, "New Medical Era," 57.

32 Cited in Greene, "Opening of St Anthony Hospital," 101.

33 See *New English Hymnal*.

34 Greene, "Opening of St Anthony Hospital," 101.

35 Joel Howell refers to this broader trend, around the turn of the century, as the development of a "guidelines movement," in *Technology in the Hospital*, 245.

36 For example, Delano & Aldrich's Private Patients' Pavilion at the Flower Hospital in New York City, completed in 1914, was of Georgian influence, and "domestically scaled, reminiscent more of the firm's larger city houses and clubs"; Pennoyer and Walker, *Architecture of Delano & Aldrich*, 61.

37 Charles Curtis, "Activities at St Anthony in 1934," 3.

38 Adams, "Modernism and Medicine," 58.

39 Demarest, "History of St Anthony Hospital," 107.

40 Shields, "Knowing Space," 147.
41 Hornsby, "Trend of Modern Hospital Service," 98.
42 Cameron, de Leeuw, and Greenwood, "Indigeneity," 355.

CHAPTER TEN

The insights and contributions of Jennifer J. Connor are deeply
appreciated.
 1 J.T.H. Connor, "Putting the 'Grenfell Effect' in Its Place"; Coombs-
Thorne, "'Credit to All Concerned'"; Lawson and Noseworthy, "Newfoundland's Cottage Hospital System"; Lake, *Capturing an Era*;
Crellin, *Life of a Cottage Hospital*; Murphy, *Cottage Hospital Doctor*;
Bellamy, *Mustard Seed*; O'Brien, *Out of Mind, Out of Sight*; Candow,
"Signal Hill's Hospitals, 1870–1920."
      For other studies, see, for example, Martin, *Fluorspar Mines of New-
foundland*; Bishop-Stirling, "Negotiating Health Care"; Craig Palmer,
Sattenspiel, and Cassidy, "Boats, Trains, and Immunity"; House, *Light
at Last*; Neary, "Venereal Disease and Public Health Administration in
Newfoundland"; Crellin, *Home Medicine*; Nigel Rusted, *Medicine in
Newfoundland*.
 2 Connor, Connor et al., "Conceptualizing Health Care."
 3 Smith, "General Hospital." See also the editorial, "Healing the Sick,"
Daily Star (St John's), 2 December 1918, 4.
 4 Lodge, *Dictatorship in Newfoundland*, 227. Thomas Lodge, an English
civil servant, was commissioner for public utilities in Newfoundland
from 1934 to 1937.
 5 *First Interim Report of the Royal Commission on Health and Public
Charities, June 1930*, 10.
      On the Highland and Island Medical Service (HIMS), see McCrae,
National Health Service; Dupree, "Foreshadowing the Future." For the
connection between HIMS and Newfoundland, see MU-CNS, Kealey,
"From Mosdell to Medicare," typescript, 6; and Martin, *Leonard
Miller*, 38–48.
 6 Scrutator, "Hospitals Needed at Extern Points," *Daily Star* (St John's),
17 February 1919, 2; Wilfred T. Grenfell, "Bay Hospitals," *Daily Star*,
1 April 1919, 7–8; and Wilfred T. Grenfell, "Recent 'Flu' Epidemic
Shows Great Need of Bay Hospitals," *Daily Star*, 27 June 1919, 2.
 7 PAD, Commissioner for Public Health and Welfare, MG 38, S6-5-2,
file 14, "Of Enquiries concerning Public Matters," 11 June 1938, 21.
 8 MU-HSL, Neergaard, Agnew, and Craig, "Hospital Facilities in New-

foundland," typescript, 82. Most of these hospitals have since been demolished, but some have been "repurposed," in one case as a heritage centre (Bonne Bay Cottage Hospital Heritage Corporation, "Julia Ann Walsh Heritage Center"), and in another case, an organic winery that has preserved most of the original architecture and signage of the Markland Hospital (Rodrigues Winery, "About Us").

9 Kealey, "On the Edge of Empire"; Green, *Don't Have Your Baby in the Dory*. For comparison, see Giovannini, *Outport Nurse*. For details of one funding scheme for outport nurses, see House, *Way Out*. About midwives, see Piercey, *"True Tales of Rhoda Maude"*; and McNaughton, "Role of the Newfoundland Midwife"; Benoit, *Midwives in Passage*; and J.T.H. Connor, "Rural Medical Lives and Times."

10 [MacDermott], *MacDermott of Fortune Bay*, 267–8, 7–10.

11 [MacDermott], *MacDermott of Fortune Bay*, 281–7. A copy of his report for the almost three-month voyage is reproduced in Nigel Rusted, *It's Devil Deep Down There*, appendix 6. Rusted also notes that his father, Ernest E. Rusted, who settled in Newfoundland in 1903 as an Anglican minister, was taught about public health and emergency medicine as part of his training in England; he "often dispensed drugs … when a doctor could not be obtained": see 81.

12 Nigel Rusted, *It's Devil Deep Down There*; Jennifer Connor and Hyde, "Dr Nigel Rusted." The diaries of Robert Dove, who succeeded Rusted as medical officer on the *Lady Anderson*, remain unpublished but are under analysis; a preliminary study is Goudie, "Keeping Healthcare Afloat" (presentation at the annual conference of the History of Medicine Days). For details of Dove's career, see "Dr Robert Frederick Dove." Contemporary articles related to his work are "Report Medical, Hospital and Nursing Service S.W. Coast," *Evening Telegram* (St John's), 22 August 1938, 5–6; "Report of Medical Service South West Coast," *Daily News* (St John's), 22 August 1938, 44–5; "Health Services in Fortune and Hermitage Bays," *Daily News*, 23 August 1938, 4; and "The S.W. Coast Medical Service," *Daily News*, 23 August 1938, 4.

13 Several entries in the diary of Dr Robert Ecke relate to such events. See Ecke, *Snowshoe & Lancet*, 247–8, 252–3, 256, and 278. For details concerning medical aspects of the *Kyle*, see Jennifer Connor and Hyde, "Dr Nigel Rusted," 361; Hanrahan, *Alphabet Fleet*, 43–7; Brian Rusted, "Diary of a Medical Student on the ss *Kyle*"; Peters, "Doctor at $5.00 a Day"; Drover, "In Good Company"; and Hawkins, "A While on the Kyle." The ss *Kyle* was a 1,000-ton vessel built in 1913 in Newcastle and in service until 1967; see Hanrahan, *Alphabet Fleet*, 5–6, 199.

14 MU-HSL, Neergaard, Agnew, and Craig, "Hospital Facilities in New-
    foundland," 82.
15 [International Grenfell Association], *A Few Facts about the Grenfell
    Missions*. Clothing was always in demand (see "Clothing Emergency";
    and discussion in chapter 6 in this volume); so too were silk stockings
    sought to make the popular artistic Grenfell hooked rugs (ADSF 34
    [April 1936]: 35). Individuals might donate materials to equip a whole
    children's ward with beds, bedside tables, linen, blankets (ADSF 36 [Jan-
    uary 1939]: 165).
16 These figures and conclusions are derived from published IGA reports:
    [International Grenfell Association], "Staff and Volunteer Workers," 24
    (July 1926): 69–72; [International Grenfell Association], "Report of the
    Staff Selection Committee," ADSF 29 (July 1931): 80–3; "Report of the
    Staff Selection Committee," ADSF 34 (July 1936): 66–70; and "Report
    of the Staff Selection Committee," ADSF 37 (July 1939): 53–6. On Little
    and Curtis, see Ronald Rompkey, *Grenfell*.
17 "Two Loving Tributes to Dr Joseph A. Andrews"; Phinney, "'Eye Doc-
    tor'"; Charles Curtis, "Dr Frank Douglas Phinney." On Musson, see
    "In Memoriam: Emma E. Musson"; Musson, "Labrador."
18 Hospital admission records, St Anthony Hospital, International Gren-
    fell Association. The original restricted documents are housed at the
    Charles S. Curtis Memorial Hospital, Labrador-Grenfell Regional
    Health Authority, St Anthony, NL.
19 "The Hospital at St Anthony," *Daily News*, 9 September 1925, 4;
    "Pleasant Commendation for the Hospital"; Threlkeld-Edwards, "New
    Medical Era in St Anthony"; Greene, "Opening of St Anthony Hospi-
    tal"; Blackburn, "Informal Report of the Opening of the Hospital."
20 Greene, "William Adams Delano"; see also Pennoyer and Walker,
    Architecture of Delano & Aldrich.
21 For full details, see J.T.H. Connor, "'Medicine Is Here to Stay.'" For
    more about the construction of the Twillingate hospital, and that of
    the one in St Anthony, see Ruiz, "Sites of Communication," 403–89.
22 J.T.H. Connor, "'Medicine Is Here to Stay,'" 264n25; Olds, "Brief Ac-
    count of Medical Services in Notre Dame Bay," typescript, 27; see also
    Saunders, *Doctor Olds of Twillingate*. On the uptake of the ECG, see
    Joel Howell, *Technology in the Hospital*, 122–6; and Lawrence, "'Defi-
    nite and Material.'"
23 "Dr Charles E. Parsons"; Saunders, *Doctor Olds of Twillingate*; *Notre
    Dame Bay Memorial Hospital*; and Ecke, *Snowshoe & Lancet*.
24 "Professional Approval of St Anthony."

25 See J.T.H. Connor, "Notre Dame Bay Memorial Hospital, Twillingate, 1933," 307–8.
    In his 1923 tour of hospitals in America and Canada, A.E. Webb-Johnson, dean of the Medical School of the Middlesex Hospital, was much impressed with the clinical records at Johns Hopkins, as "many stenographers" kept them complete; similarly in Cleveland, Webb-Johnson believed that the hospital's record system there was "far better than ours." "I have no doubt in my mind," he noted further, "that we must give greater attention to this part of our hospital work, and take more interest in the filing of records of cases and following up the results, than in recording the proceedings of committees." See Webb-Johnson, *Notes on a Tour of the Principal Hospitals and Medical Schools*, 11, 15–16. For discussion of the rise of the efficient hospital record in American hospitals, see Joel Howell, *Technology in the Hospital*, 42–56; also Risse and Warner, "Reconstructing Clinical Activities."

26 On the role of the American College of Surgeons as the pioneering accreditor of hospitals in North America, see Neuhauser, *Coming of Age*, 39–41; and Agnew, *Canadian Hospitals*, 32–5, 251–2.

27 "Professional Approval of St Anthony."

28 Grenfell, *Forty Years for Labrador*, 279–80. For an account of the clinical activities specifically of Grenfell, see J.T.H. Connor, "Sir Wilfred Thomason Grenfell."

29 "St Anthony Hospital," *Daily News* (St John's), 17 February 1928, 4; "The Standardized Hospital," *Evening Telegram* (St John's), 20 February 1928, 6. See also the summary of these newspaper reports in the IGA magazine: "Comment from Newfoundland Papers."

30 J.T.H. Connor, "Notre Dame Bay Memorial Hospital, Twillingate, 1933."

31 Charles Curtis, "Hospital Stations," 73; Charles Curtis, "Year's Work at St. Anthony Hospital," 19; Charles Curtis, "St Anthony Hospital Report," ADSF 26 (April 1928): 26–7; Mount, "St Anthony Hospital Report," 24–5; Charles Curtis, "St Anthony Hospital Report: Jan. 1, 1929, to Dec. 31, 1929"; Charles Curtis, "St Anthony in 1930"; Charles Curtis, "St Anthony in 1931"; Charles Curtis, "St Anthony in 1932"; Charles Curtis, "St Anthony in 1933"; Charles Curtis, "Activities at St Anthony in 1934," 3–4; Charles Curtis, "St Anthony Hospital Statistics for 1935"; Charles Curtis, "St Anthony in 1936"; and Charles Curtis, "St Anthony in 1937."

32 In order to establish performance baselines for the St Anthony hospital, the following were consulted for comparison: Pinker, *English Hospital*

Statistics; Abel-Smith, *Hospitals*; Gagan and Gagan, *For Patients of Moderate Means*; and J.T.H. Connor, *Doing Good.*

33 Charles Curtis, "St Anthony in 1933," 13. Patients' place of origin had been identified for years earlier, as well; see, for example, *First Annual Report of the International Grenfell Association*, 10.

34 See, for example, "Here and There," *Evening Telegram* (St John's), 4 June 1910, 4; "Here and There," *Evening Telegram*, 11 December 1911, 8; "Sent to Hospital," *Evening Telegram*, 18 July 1911, 6; "Cured at St Anthony," *Evening Telegram*, 20 July 1912, 2; "Obituary," *Evening Telegram*, 12 December 1913, 9; George Ridout, "A Restored Patient," *Twillingate Sun*, 9 January 1909, 1; John Dawer, "Note of Thanks," *Evening Telegram*, 10 June 1909, 7; Wilfred T. Grenfell, "Eye Specialist," *Evening Telegram*, 16 May 1911, 7.

35 Another American influence of dubious distinction was eugenics and the sterilization of women deemed mentally unfit to bear children. See J.T.H. Connor, "'Human Subject,' 'Vulnerable Populations,' and Medical History."

36 Grenfell identifies a list of dentists who served from 1910 to 1926 in "Tribute to the Dental Volunteers." See also [International Grenfell Association], "Staff and Volunteer Workers," ADSF 24 (July 1926): 69–72; "Dentist's Report"; "Staff and Volunteer Workers," ADSF 22 (July 1924): 66–7.

37 Bellingham, "Humanitarian Service of Dentists in Grenfell's Sub-Arctic Labrador."

38 Grenfell, "Sir Wilfred's Log: Summer of 1930," 161; Grenfell, "Sir Wilfred's Letter," ADSF 30 (January 1933): 149; Grenfell, "Summer of 1933"; Grenfell, "Practice of Medicine in Labrador," 103. For more information related to radium, see Silverman, "Pittsburgh's Contribution to Radium Recovery"; and Hayter, *Element of Hope.*

39 J.T.H. Connor personal collection, St John's General Hospital General Register: August 1931–September 1936, entry #852 on 7 December 1935; and Hospital admission record #11173, St Anthony Hospital, International Grenfell Association. For details of radium use and related matters at Massachusetts General Hospital, see Suit and Loeffler, *Evolution of Radiation Oncology*, 19–20; concerning contemporary radioactive dosages, see Teperson, "Formulae for the Rapid Calculation of Millicuries of Radon."

40 "St Anthony Hospital," *Evening Telegram* (St John's), 18 February 1928, 6.

41 Stephan Curtis, "Introduction: Cores/Peripheries – Rural/Remote," 1–17.

42 Ecke, *Snowshoe & Lancet*, 225; see also J.T.H. Connor, "'Medicine Is Here to Stay,'" 150.

43 Johnson, *Doctor Regrets*, 125–6.

44 PAD, MG 38 S6-5-1, file 1a, "Of Enquiries concerning Public Matters," H.M. Mosdell to commissioner for public health and welfare, 24 February 1940, 8–10.

45 Vonderlehr and Heering, *Report of a Survey on Civil Health Services*, in Candow, "An American Report," 229. For context to this friendly invasion, see High, *Occupied St John's*; and Neary, "'Mortgaged Property.'"

46 Wheatley, *Politics of Philanthropy*, x. The mixed blessing of philanthropic support for organized medicine is explored by other scholars: E. Richard Brown, *Rockefeller Medicine Men*; Fedunkiw, *Rockefeller Foundation Funding and Medical Education*.

47 See Ward, Dreshman & Reinhardt, and its in-house online corporate history entitled "Voluntary Giving in a Free Land," 21.

CONCLUSION

We thank volume authors, who initially provided draft summaries of their chapters that appear here in revised form.

1 "Confederation."

2 Ashdown, "Changing Fields."

3 "In Memoriam: Cecil S. Ashdown"; and T.A.G., "Memorial Minute."

4 Center for Adventist Research, Adventist Digital Library, "Clippings Regarding John Harvey Kellogg, the Battle Creek Sanitarium, and Prominent Individuals from Battle Creek, Michigan, and the 1905 General Conference Session," "2 Famous Doctors Mark Birthdays: Future Still Challenges after 116 Years' Service" [*Battle Creek Enquirer and News*, 3 March 1940]; and "Sir Wilfred Grenfell Dies: Was Frequent Visitor Here," with photo titled "Death ends friendship," *Battle Creek Enquirer and News*, 10 October 1940, 210, 219.

5 "Battle Harbour Jottings," 23; Johnson, *Doctor Regrets*, 128.

6 That is, at least British physicians preached. See Curwen, *Labrador Odyssey*; on one occasion, for example, Curwen noted three services on one Sunday, with 130, 127, and 98 attendees (despite few hymn books), and an apparently separate service for the women (67). See also Johnson, *Doctor Regrets*, 149; [Wakefield], "Winter Work," 19; Wakefield, "St Anthony Items," 11; Wakefield, "Battle Harbour Hospital," 17.

7 Center for Adventist Research, Adventist Digital Library, Eric Hutton, "The One Weight-Control System That Works Every Time," *Maclean's*,

15 July 1961; reprinted in the American *Life and Health* 77 (June
1962): 8–9, 27, 29, 31, 34; see 31. Grenfell had visited this sanitarium
apparently annually from 1906 to 1909, but then remembered in the
notice of his death as visitor only three more recent times, twice with
his wife: in 1918, 1929, and 1931 ("Sir Wilfred Grenfell Dies").

 8 Greg Wood, quoted in Melanie Callahan, "Re-energizing Life on the
Tip of the Great Northern Peninsula," [MUN] *Gazette*, 11 December
2017, https://gazette.mun.ca/public-engagement/untapped-potential/. At
the same time, his name remained linked to the local co-operative store,
despite the history behind Grenfell's loose association with these commercial endeavours, and for the president of its board the closing of the
store in 2018 meant "seeing another of the Grenfell institutions that's
been around for 105 years in this community, that we weren't able to
rally around and save, that's distressing": see "After 105 Years, St
Anthony's Grenfell Co-op Closing," CBC News Newfoundland and
Labrador, 29 January 2018, https://www.cbc.ca/news/canada/new
foundland-labrador/st-anthony-grenfell-coop-closing-1.4508717.

 9 See Landmark Branding, "156 Fifth Avenue"; Miller, "Presbyterian
Building."

10 J.L.G., "Items from the Grenfell Association of America," 8.

11 John R. Matchim is working toward obtaining permissions to undertake research on the clinical records of the later ship, the *Strathcona III*,
which he plans to begin in the near future.

12 Ruiz, "Sites of Communication," 289–336.

13 Susan Flanagan, "Buttons or Berries," *Telegram* (St John's), 22 July
2017, http://www.pressreader.com/canada/the-telegram-st-johns/2017
0722/281689729872712.

14 Elisabeth Hamilton and Smith, "'All Offerings Gratefully Received.'"

15 Peirce, "Summer Volunteers in the United States, 1938." The wayside
stops were the Dog Team Tavern-by-the-River, Middlebury, VT; and the
Dog Team Tea House, Cheshire, CT. These volunteers were also identified under the "Industrial Department" section of "Report of the Staff
Selection Committee," ADSF 34 (July 1936): 69; and [International
Grenfell Association], "Report of the Staff Selection Committee," ADSF
35 (July 1937): 70. See also Anne Budgell, *Dear Everybody*. On the
stores, see "Industrial Shops."

16 Hamill, "Needlework Guild of America," 30.

17 See Laverty, *Silk Stocking Mats;* Luther, *Jessie Luther.*

18 Ruiz, "Media Infrastructure." Also, see IGA film footage examined by
Ruiz, "Moving Image."

19 Cards with Grenfell's drawings are still available in St Anthony. See
    Grenfell Historic Properties, Grenfell Handicrafts Store; and Labrador-
    Grenfell Health Regional Authority, Charles S. Curtis Hospital Auxil-
    iary, Grenfell Greeting Cards. For Grenfell's mat designs, see Laverty,
    Silk Stocking Mats, 15–16. His sketches appear in Kerr, *Wilfred Gren-
    fell*; Grenfell, *Yourself and Your Body*; Anne Grenfell and Spalding,
    Le Petit Nord. Monica Kidd noted his sketches in early clinical records
    in "'If We Can Make a Cure of Him'" (presented at Symposium on
    100 Years).

20 The collection of Newfoundland and Labrador materials of Rhoda
    Dawson (1897–1992), donated soon after her death based on her will
    under her later married name, is available for study at MU-ASC, Rhoda
    Dawson Bickerdike, Coll-198. See also Neary, "'Wry Comment.'"

21 "In Memoriam: Cecil S. Ashdown," 70.

22 See LeRoy Appleton's design on the cover of *ADSF* from 1943 until
    1981, and for which the editor initially sought comments about his
    "modernization" of the "traditional *Deep Sea Fishers* form," *ADSF* 41
    (October 1943): 66.

23 "Vassar Initiates Dramatic Workshop," *Vassar Miscellany News* 10,
    no. 38 (20 March 1926): 1; Hallie Flanagan, "Vassar Experimental
    Theatre," 161; Clothier, *She Canna Perish*, in *It's a Glorious Country*,
    202–26. Unlike *She Canna Perish*, *Right Machinery* appears not to
    have been published or performed; characters in this script appear as
    residents of White Bay in Clothier's letters. Thanks to Mark Graesser
    for information about *Right Machinery*.

24 These plays are all about royal pageants in the region. See MU-ASC,
    Rhoda Dawson Bickerdike, Coll-198, finding aid, at http://collections.
    mun.ca/cdm/ref/collection/ead/id/483.

25 [Wakefield], "Winter Work," 20. On Wakefield, see Jennifer Connor,
    "'Flits' of Medical Personnel on the Grenfell Labrador Mission" (pre-
    sented at the Health, Medicine and Mobility conference).

26 [White], "Items from the New England Grenfell Association," *ADSF* 8
    (October 1910): 7.

27 Berea College, "Berea College Early History."

28 Jennifer Connor, "'Dispensing Good Books and Literature.'"

29 Ronald Rompkey, *Grenfell*, 130–1, 136–8, 182; Treude, "Development
    of Reindeer Husbandry in Canada"; and Scotter, "Reindeer Ranching
    in Canada." The herder position would subsequently be held by an
    American, John J. Evans, from Philadelphia: see "International Grenfell
    Association."

30 Grenfell also served as a magistrate, and reflecting his belief in temper-
    ance, he is credited with suppressing the traffic of liquor by going after
    offenders. See Grenfell, *Forty Years for Labrador*, 139–40; Tanner,
    Outlines of the Geography, Life and Customs, 788.

31 "Tim Shannahan Gets There!," *Evening Telegram* (St John's), 27 Febru-
    ary 1912. At this time, Wakefield had undertaken separate public
    health work for a year at the request of Grenfell and the president of
    the Newfoundland Association for the Prevention of Consumption.

32 See also Connor, Connor et al., "Conceptualizing Health Care," 130.

33 See five oral histories in Kathleen Tucker, "Stories of the Grenfell
    Mission."

34 J.T.H. Connor, "'Human Subject,' 'Vulnerable Populations,' and Medi-
    cal History."

35 Rob Antle, "Work Underway to Cap St John's Dumpsite Abandoned by
    U.S. Military in 1960s," CBC News, 25 November 2017, https://www.
    cbc.ca/news/canada/newfoundland-labrador/us-military-dumpsite-
    work-white-hills-st-johns-1.4415785.

36 Jennifer Connor, "'Dispensing Good Books and Literature,'" 380.

37 Simon Macdonald, "Transnational History."

38 Conroy-Kutz, "'Engaged in the Same Glorious Cause,'" 24.

39 Porter, *Religion versus Empire?*, 299.

40 For example, Canadian University Students Overseas (CUSO), http://
    www.cusointernational.org/about/about; World University Service
    of Canada, and its "Students without Borders," http://uniterra.ca/
    en/volunteering/student-volunteering; Global Brigades, https://www.
    globalbrigades.org/about-us/vision-mission/. See Brouwer, "When
    Missions Became Development."

41 See, for example, *Yale Daily News* 56, 28 November 1949, 6; *Yale
    Daily News* 40, 3 November 1950, 8; *Yale Daily News* 62, 3 December
    1951, 4.

42 Toland, *Sort of Peace Corps*.

43 Brouwer, *Canada's Global Villagers*, 1.

Bibliography

Substantive primary sources that were published in two periodicals, *Among the Deep Sea Fishers* (ADSF) and *Them Days*, are identified in full in this bibliography by their author or title. All other primary source periodicals appear in the bibliography listed only by periodical or newspaper title consulted, with full citations to their articles provided in the endnotes.

ARCHIVAL SOURCES

Archives and Special Collections, Memorial University of Newfoundland, St John's, NL.
  Florence Miller Collection.
  Nathaniel Stuart Noel Correspondence.
  Newfoundland Outport Nursing and Industrial Association Collection.
  Rhoda Dawson Bickerdike Collection.
Bentley Historical Library, University of Michigan, Ann Arbor, MI.
  John Harvey Kellogg Papers.
Carnegie Corporation of New York Records, Rare Book and Manuscript Library Archives, Columbia University, New York.
  International Grenfell Association Correspondence.
Center for Adventist Research, Berrien Springs, MI.
  Adventist Digital Library. https://adventistdigitallibrary.org.
Centre for Newfoundland Studies, Memorial University of Newfoundland, St John's, NL.
  Linda Kealey. "From Mosdell to Medicare: Health Care in Newfoundland and Labrador." Typescript, 2004.

Charles S. Curtis Memorial Hospital, St Anthony, NL.
    International Grenfell Association, St Anthony Hospital Admission
    Records.
Concord Free Library, Concord, MA.
    Concord New England Branch of the International Grenfell Association,
    Meeting Minutes.
Faculty of Medicine Founders Archive, Memorial University of Newfound-
land, St John's, NL.
    Dr Cluny MacPherson Collection.
Folklore and Language Archives, Memorial University of Newfoundland, St
John's, NL.
    Ian McKinnon. "A Health and Medical Services Perspective of the
    Labrador Fishery from an Oral History Interview with Dr Nigel Rusted."
    Transcript, 26 March 1986, MS 86-120, FI3821C-12822C.
Grenfell Historic Properties Collection, St Anthony, NL.
    Florence F. Fuller Photograph Album.
Historical Collection, Health Sciences Library, Memorial University of New-
foundland, St John's, NL.
    Neergaard, Agnew, and Craig. "Hospital Facilities in Newfoundland: A
    Study Conducted for the Honourable J.R. Chalker, Minister of Health."
    Typescript, Toronto, 1952.
    Olds, John. "A Brief Account of Medical Services in Notre Dame Bay."
    Typescript, 1966.
Hutchins Library Special Collections and Archives, Berea College, Berea, KY.
    Newfoundland Student Registration Records.
J.T.H. Connor Personal Collection, Memorial University of Newfoundland,
St John's, NL.
    General Register, St John's General Hospital, August 1931–September
    1936.
Library and Archives Canada, Ottawa.
    William Lyon Mackenzie King Collection.
Manuscripts and Archives, Yale University, New Haven, CT.
    Elizabeth Page Harris Papers.
    Wilfred Thomason Grenfell Papers.
National Archives, London, UK.
    Records of the Colonial Office.
Provincial Archives Division, The Rooms, St John's, NL.
    Colonial Secretary's Office Fonds.
    Commissioner for Public Health and Welfare Fonds.
    Dorcas Society Fonds.

International Grenfell Association Collection.
Wilfred Thomason Grenfell Fonds.
Records Archives, Memorial University of Newfoundland, St John's, NL.
President's Office Records and Board of Governors' Records.
Royal National Mission to Deep Sea Fishermen, London, UK.
Grenfell Association Transfers Papers.
Sophia Smith Archive, Smith College, Northampton, MA.
Beatrice Farnsworth Powers Collection.
Carolyn Galbraith Correspondence.

UNPUBLISHED PAPERS AND INTERVIEWS

Bennett, Beverly. Provincial Archives Division, The Rooms, St John's, NL. Personal communication with Katherine Side, April 2016.
Connor, Jennifer J. "'Flits' of Medical Personnel on the Grenfell Labrador Mission before 1914." Paper presented at the Health, Medicine and Mobility: International Migrations in Historical Perspective conference, University of Prince Edward Island, Charlottetown, June 2016.
Didsbury, Kendell. "In the Shadow of the Clock Tower: One Hundred Years in the Life of Tilton School." Tilton, NH: Tilton School, 1967.
Goudie, Shaina. "Keeping Healthcare Afloat: Dr Dove and the *Lady Anderson*, 1936–38." Paper presented at the annual conference of the History of Medicine Days at the University of Calgary, 2010.
Jesseau, Ben. "A Most Interesting Game: The Introduction and Growth of Hockey in Newfoundland, 1894–1935." Unpublished.
Kidd, Monica. "'If We Can Make a Cure of Him': Lyrical Grenfell in the St Anthony Casebooks, 1906." Paper presented at "A Symposium on 100 Years of the International Grenfell Association and the Delivery of Health Care in Newfoundland and Labrador," St John's, NL, October 2014.
McNeill, Dorothy. Interview by Rafico Ruiz, St Anthony, NL, 22 November 2011.
Ruiz, Rafico. "Media Environments, Northern Natural Resources and Iceberg Economies for the 21st Century." Presentation at Memorial University of Newfoundland, St John's, NL, January 2016.
Scott, Shirley. "Cuffs, Vamps, Trigger Mitts and Drawers: The Knitted Heritage of Newfoundland and Labrador." Presentation at Newfoundland Historical Society, St John's, NL, February 2016. http://www.nlhistory.ca/pastLectures.html.
Waddell, Bonnie. Chief Librarian at MacRae Library, Nova Scotia Agricultural College. Telephone interview by Helen Woodrow, winter 2009.

Woodrow, Helen M. "'Serve the World': Learning and the Grenfell Mission in the 1920s." Master's report, Memorial University of Newfoundland, 2009.

PUBLISHED SOURCES

Mission, Church, College, and Oral History Periodicals

Among the Deep Sea Fishers. Toronto: [J. Greenshields], 1903–14; New York: Grenfell Association of America, 1914–81.
Canada Presbyterian
Good Health
Harvard Crimson
Medical Missionary
Missionary Outlook
P&S on the Labrador: An Account of the Work of the Columbia Unit of the Grenfell Mission at Spotted Islands, Labrador
Presbyterian Review
Them Days
Toilers of the Deep
Vassar Miscellany News
Yale Daily News

Newspapers and Media Sites

Allentown (PA) Leader
Berea Citizen (KY)
CBC News
CBC News Newfoundland and Labrador
Daily News (St John's)
Daily Star (St John's)
Evening Chronicle (St John's)
Evening Mercury (St John's)
Evening Star (Toronto)
Evening Telegram (St John's)
Evening Telegram (Toronto)
Globe (Toronto)
Huffington Post
Montreal Gazette
[MUN] *Gazette*

New York Herald
New York Sun
New York Times
Telegram (St John's)
Toronto Star
Twillingate Sun (NL)
Western Star (Corner Brook)

Government Documents

Annual Report of the Bureau of Education, 1927–1928. St John's, NF: Manning and Rabbitts, 1929.
Census of Newfoundland and Labrador, 1891. St John's, NF: J.W. Withers, Queen's Printer, 1893.
Census of Newfoundland and Labrador, 1901. St John's, NF: J.W. Withers, King's Printer, 1903.
Census of Newfoundland and Labrador, 1921. St John's, NF: 1923.
"Education Act 1903." *Acts of the General Assembly of Newfoundland.* St John's, NF: J.W. Withers, 1903.
First Interim Report of the Royal Commission on Health and Public Charities, June 1930. St John's, NF: King's Printer, 1930.
Journal of the House of Assembly of Newfoundland.
    An Act to Provide for the Better Accommodation of Female Passengers to and from Labrador. *JHA* 1882, 103–4, 116, 155, 176–7.
    "Medical Report of Dr Forbes, Labrador, 1885." *JHA* 1886, Appendix, 821–5.
    "Report of an Official Visit to the Coast of Labrador by the Governor of Newfoundland during the Month of August 1905." *JHA* 20 March 1907, 300–79.
    "Report of a Select Committee on Education." *JHA* 1891, 447–55.
    "Report of Dr Skelton on Medical Visit to Labrdor [*sic*], for the Year 1884." *JHA* 1885, Appendix, 505–13.
    Report of the Select Committee to Consider the Operation and Effectiveness of the Present Law in Respect to the Overcrowding of Vessels ... and the Employment of Female Labour Therein. *JHA* 1886, 55, 169–79.
    "Resolutions to Be submitted by Mr Murray to a Committee of the Whole House, May 8, 1890." *JHA* 1890, 147.
Report of the Public Schools of Newfoundland under Methodist Boards, 1920. St John's, NF, 1921.
"Report of the Public Schools of Newfoundland under Methodist Boards

for Year 1922–23." *Department of Education Report for 1922–1923.* St John's, NF, 1924.

Report of the Public Schools under Roman Catholic School Boards for the Year Ended December 31st 1917. St John's, NF, 1918.

United Kingdom Parliament. Commons Sitting, 14 December 1933, series 5, vol. 284, Orders of the Day, Newfoundland Bill. HC Deb 14 December 1933, vol. 284 cc. 565–701.

Articles, Books, Pamphlets, Reports, Theses, Websites

Aamodt, Terrie Dopp, Gary Land, and Ronald L. Numbers, eds. *Ellen Harmon White: American Prophet.* New York: Oxford University Press, 2014.

Abe, Ikuo. "Muscular Christianity in Japan: The Growth of a Hybrid." In *Muscular Christianity in Colonial and Post-Colonial Worlds,* ed. John MacAloon, 14–38. New York: Routledge, 2008.

Abel-Smith, Brian. *The Hospitals, 1800–1948: A Study of Social Administration in England and Wales.* Cambridge, MA: Harvard University Press, 1964.

Adams, Annmarie. "Modernism and Medicine: The Hospitals of Stevens and Lee, 1916–1932." *Journal of the Society of Architectural Historians* 58, no. 1 (1999): 42–61.

Agnew, G. Harvey. *Canadian Hospitals, 1920 to 1970: A Dramatic Half-Century.* Toronto: University of Toronto Press, 1974.

Alexander, David. "Newfoundland's Traditional Economy and Developments to 1934." In *Newfoundland in the Nineteenth and Twentieth Centuries: Essays in Interpretation,* ed. James Hiller and Peter Neary, 17–39. Toronto: University of Toronto Press, 1980.

Andersen, Raoul. *Voyage to the Grand Banks: The Saga of Captain Arch Thornhill.* St John's, NL: Creative, 1998.

Antikainen, Ari, and Katja Komonen. "Biography, Life Course, and the Sociology of Education." In *The International Handbook on the Sociology of Education: An International Assessment of New Research and Theory,* ed. Carlos Alberto Torres and Ari Antikainen, 143–59. Lanham, MD: Rowman & Littlefield, 2003.

Armour, James E. "Castles in the Air: The Life, Times and Influence of the Reverend Moses Harvey (1820–1901)." Master's thesis, Memorial University of Newfoundland, 2016.

Armstrong, Bess. "Summer Resort Industrial Sales: Labrador Visits New England." *ADSF* 28 (October 1930): 135–6.

Ashdown, Cecil S. "Changing Fields." *ADSF* 41 (October 1943): 68–9.

Avery, Donald. *"Dangerous Foreigners": European Immigrant Workers and Labour Radicalism in Canada, 1896–1932.* Toronto: McClelland and Stewart, 1979.

Badger, Theodore. "Wilfred Bertram Mesher." *ADSF* 70 (October 1973): 16–18.

Baehre, Rainer. "Whose Pine Clad Hills: Forest Rights and Access in Newfoundland and Labrador's History." *NQ* 103, no. 4 (2011): 42–7. https://www.mun.ca/harriscentre/reports/nlquarterly/MemPreNQ103-4.pdf.

"Balls." *Them Days* 7, no. 2 (1981): 44–7.

Barnes, Arthur. "The History of Education in Newfoundland." D.Ped. diss., New York University, 1917.

Battle Harbour. "Historic Trust." http://www.battleharbour.com/historic-trust.

– "History." http://www.battleharbour.com/history.

"Battle Harbour Jottings." *ADSF* 7 (January 1910): 16–24.

"Bell Island." *NQ* 1, no. 1 (July 1901): 2–3.

Bellamy, Kathrine E. *The Mustard Seed: The Story of St Clare's Mercy Hospital.* St John's, NL: Flanker, 2010.

Bellingham, Peter John. "The Humanitarian Service of Dentists in Grenfell's Sub-Arctic Labrador, 1910–1930." *Journal of the History of Dentistry* 54 (2006): 101–7.

Belvin, Cleophas. *The Forgotten Labrador: Kegashka to Blanc Sablon.* Montreal and Kingston: McGill-Queen's University Press, 2014.

Benoit, Cecilia M. *Midwives in Passage: The Modernization of Maternity Care.* St John's, NL: ISER Books, 1991.

Berea College. "Berea College Early History." 2018. https://www.berea.edu/about/history/.

Berthelsen, Karen. "Blue Denim." *ADSF* 30 (October 1932): 125–6.

Best, Ben. "School Days." *Them Days* 5, no. 3 (1980): 42–3.

Biddle, Pippa. "The Problem with Little White Girls, Boys and Voluntourism." *Huffington Post*, 23 February 2014. http://www.huffingtonpost.com/pippa-biddle/little-white-girls-voluntourism_b_4834574.html.

"Birthday Broadcasts." *ADSF* 34 (April 1936): 6–8.

Bishop-Stirling, Terry. "Negotiating Health Care: Epidemics, Public Health and Medical Care in Newfoundland and Labrador, 1918–1920." *NQ* 103, no. 2 (2010): 47–54.

Blackburn, Alice A. "An Informal Report of the Opening of the Hospital." *ADSF* 25 (October 1927): 106–8.

Blayney, Katharine L. "Nutrition Work in White Bay." *ADSF* 19 (January 1922): 123–5.

Bledsoe, Verda M. "Christmas-Tide at North West River." *ADSF* 54 (April 1956): 9–12.

Bonne Bay Cottage Hospital Heritage Corporation, Norris Point. "Julia Ann Walsh Heritage Center." 2017. http://www.norrispoint.ca/wp-content/up loads/2015/03/JuliaAnnWalshHeritageCenter.pdf.

Bourdieu, Pierre. *Distinction: A Social Critique of the Judgement of Taste.* London: Routledge and Kegan Paul, 1984.

Bourne, Grace E. "The School at Englee." *ADSF* 21 (April 1923): 27–8.

Brouwer, Ruth Compton. *Canada's Global Villagers: CUSO in Development, 1961–86.* Vancouver: UBC Press, 2013.

– "When Missions Became Development: Ironies of 'NGOization' in Mainstream Canadian Churches in the 1960s." *Canadian Historical Review* 91 (2010): 661–93.

Brower, Alice V. "A 'Tachie's' Retrospection." *ADSF* 23 (July 1925): 65–6.

Brown, E. Richard. *Rockefeller Medicine Men: Medicine and Capitalism in America.* Berkeley: University of California Press, 1979.

Brown, Lincoln, Horace McNeill, and Rachel Brown. *Inasmuch.* Winslow, ME: n.p., 1992.

Buckner, Phillip. "The Creation of the Dominion of Canada, 1860–1901." In *Canada and the British Empire,* ed. Phillip Buckner, 66–86. Oxford: Oxford University Press, 2008.

Budgell, Anne. *Dear Everybody: A Woman's Journey from Park Avenue to a Labrador Trapline.* Portugal Cove–St Philips, NL: Boulder, 2013.

Budgell, Nathan. "From a Newfoundland Agricultural Student." *ADSF* 26 (January 1929): 177.

– *A Newfoundland Son: Autobiography.* n.p.: 1st Books Library, 2001.

Bulgin, Iona. "Mapping the Self in the 'Utmost Purple Rim': Published Labrador Memoirs of Four Grenfell Nurses." PhD diss., Memorial University of Newfoundland, 2001.

Burstyn, Varda. *The Rites of Men: Manhood, Politics, and the Culture of Sport.* Toronto: University of Toronto Press, 1999.

Buxton, William J., and Charles R. Acland. *American Philanthropy and Canadian Libraries: The Politics of Knowledge and Information. Accompanied by Charles F. McCombs' "Report on Canadian Libraries" Submitted to the Rockefeller Foundation in 1941.* Montreal: Graduate School of Library and Information Studies and Centre for Research on Canadian Cultural Industries and Institutions, McGill University, 1998.

Byrne, Allan. "The Introduction of Moose to the Island of Newfoundland." September 2012. Newfoundland and Labrador Provincial Historic Commemorations Program, 2017. http://www.seethesites.ca/media/48059/introduction%20of%20moose.pdf.

– "Selling Simplicity: Lee Wulff, Stanley Truman Brooks, and the Newfoundland Tourist Development Board, 1925–1946." Master's report, Memorial University of Newfoundland, 2008.

Cadigan, Sean. "Battle Harbour in Transition: Merchants, Fishermen and the State in the Struggle for Relief in a Labrador Community during the 1930s." *Labour / Le Travail* 26 (1990): 125–50.

– *Newfoundland and Labrador: A History*. Toronto: University of Toronto Press, 2009.

Cameron, Emilie, Sarah de Leeuw, and Margo Greenwood. "Indigeneity." In *International Encyclopedia of Human Geography*, ed. Rob Kitchin and Nigel Thrift, 352–7. 5th ed. London: Elsevier, 2009.

Candow, James E. "An American Report on Newfoundland's Health Services in 1940." *NLS* 5 (1989): 221–39.

– *A History of the Labrador Fishery*. Microfiche report series 70. Ottawa: Parks Canada, 1983.

– "Signal Hill's Hospitals, 1870–1920." *Research Bulletin* no. 121. Ottawa: Parks Canada, 1980.

Card, Mary F. "Nutrition Work in White Bay, Newfoundland." *ADSF* 22 (April 1924): 26–7.

– "Nutrition Work in White Bay, Newfoundland: Summer of 1924." *ADSF* 22 (January 1925): 167–8.

Carleton, Fred P. "Notes on the Labrador Dialect." *ADSF* 21 (January 1924): 138–9.

Chadacre Agricultural Trust. "History." http://www.chadacre-trust.org.uk/history.html.

Chambers II, John Whiteclay. *The Tyranny of Change: America in the Progressive Era, 1890–1920*. 2nd ed. New Brunswick, NJ: Rutgers University Press, 2000.

Chaulk, Bertha. "Coombs Family History." *Them Days* 33, no. 1 (2009): 28–9.

Chaulk, Maud. "We Liked the Outdoor Life." *Them Days* 8, no. 1 (1982): 59–60.

Claudio, Luz. "Waste Couture: Environmental Impact of the Clothing Industry." *Environmental Health Perspectives* 115, no. 9 (2007): A448–A454.

Clothier, Florence. *It's a Glorious Country: Letters from Newfoundland, 1924–1925*. Edited by Mark Graesser. St John's, NL: DRC, 2015.

"The Clothing Emergency." *ADSF* 30 (April 1932): 38–9.

Coates, Laurie. "Item from Mud Lake Hospital." *ADSF* 11 (July 1913): 25–7.

Coleman, Daniel. *White Civility: The Literary Project of English Canada*. Toronto: University of Toronto Press, 2006.

Coleman, Michael. "The Symbiotic Embrace: American Indians, White
    Educators and the School, 1820s–1920s." *History of Education* 25,
    no. 1 (1996): 1–18.
"Comment from Newfoundland Papers." *ADSF* 26 (April 1928): 27.
"Confederation." *ADSF* 46 (October 1948): 67.
Congregationalist. "Patron Saint of Labrador." In *Grenfell Association of
    America* [New York: 1908], 14.
Connor, J.T.H. *Doing Good: The Life of Toronto's General Hospital.*
    Toronto: University of Toronto Press, 2000.
– "The 'Human Subject,' 'Vulnerable Populations,' and Medical History:
    The Problem of Presentism and the Discourse of Bioethics." *CBMH/BCHM*
    34 (2017): 496–520.
– "'Medicine Is Here to Stay': Rural Medical Practice, Frontier Life, and
    Modernization in 1930s Newfoundland." In *Medicine in the Remote and
    Rural North*, ed. J.T.H. Connor and Stephan Curtis, 129–51. London:
    Pickering & Chatto, 2011.
– "The Notre Dame Bay Memorial Hospital, Twillingate, 1933: An Institu-
    tional Profile in a Time of Transition." *NLS* 28 (2013): 293–330.
– "Putting the 'Grenfell Effect' in Its Place: Medical Tales and Autobiograph-
    ical Narratives in Twentieth-Century Newfoundland and Labrador."
    Papers of the Bibliographical Society of Canada 48, no. 1 (2010): 77–118.
– "Rural Medical Lives and Times." *NLS* 23 (2008): 231–43.
"Sir Wilfred Thomason Grenfell: Legendary Physician in Newfoundland
    and Labrador." *Hektoen International: A Journal of Medical Humanities*
    (Fall 2016). http://hekint.org/2017/01/29/sir-wilfred-thomason-grenfell-
    legendary-physician-in-newfoundland-and-labrador/.
Connor, J.T.H., Jennifer J. Connor, Monica G. Kidd, and Maria Mathews.
    "Conceptualizing Health Care in Rural and Remote Pre-Confederation
    Newfoundland as Ecosystem." *NLS* 30 (Spring 2015): 113–38.
Connor, Jennifer J. "'Dispensing Good Books and Literature' to Coastal
    Communities: The Role of the Grenfell Mission in Newfoundland and
    Labrador, 1890s–1940." *NLS* 32 (2017): 362–98.
– "Stalwart Giants: Medical Cosmopolitanism, Canadian Authorship, and
    American Publishers." *Book History* 12 (2009): 210–39.
Connor, Jennifer J., and Heidi Coombs-Thorne. "To the Rescue: Julia Green-
    shields for the Mission to Deep Sea Fishermen in Newfoundland and
    Labrador." *NQ* 107, no. 2 (Fall 2014): 32–6.
Connor, Jennifer J., and Angela J. Hyde. "Dr Nigel Rusted: A *CMAJ* Cente-
    nary Reader." *CMAJ* 183 (2011): 361–5.
Conroy-Kutz, Emily L. "'Engaged in the Same Glorious Cause': Anglo-

American Connections in the American Missionary Entrance into India, 1790–1815." *Journal of the Early Republic* 34 (Spring 2014): 21–44.

"Consumption from Fish: A New Source of Tuberculous Infection." *Good Health* 45 (1910): 103–5.

Cook, Harriet Huntington. "'Down' North with Dr Grenfell." ADSF 21 (April 1923): 25–7.

Cook, Ramsay. *The Regenerators: Social Criticism in Late Victorian English Canada*. Toronto: University of Toronto Press, 1985.

Coombs-Thorne, Heidi. "Conflict and Resistance to Paternalism: Nursing with the Grenfell Mission Stations in Newfoundland and Labrador, 1939– 1982." In *Caregiving on the Periphery: Historical Perspectives on Nursing and Midwifery in Canada*, ed. Myra Rutherdale, 210–42. Montreal and Kingston: McGill-Queen's University Press, 2010.

– "'A Credit to All Concerned': Community Involvement and the Bonne Bay Cottage Hospital." NQ 107, no. 2 (2014): 43–7.

– "'Mrs Tilley Had a *Very* Hasty Wedding!': The Class-Based Response to Marriages in the Grenfell Mission of Newfoundland and Labrador." CBMH/BCHM 27 (2010): 123–38.

– "Nursing with the Grenfell Mission in Northern Newfoundland and Labrador, 1939–81." PhD diss., University of New Brunswick, 2010.

– "A 'Radiating Center of Helpfulness': The Early Years of the King George V Seamen's Institute in St John's, 1912–18." NQ 109, no. 3 (2016–17): 39–47.

– "'Such a Many-Purpose Job': Nursing, Identity, and Place with the Grenfell Mission, 1939–1960." *Nursing History Review* 21 (2013): 89–96.

Cormier, Ken. "Writing the Tape-Recorded Life." *a/b: Auto/Biography Studies* 27, no. 2 (2012): 402–26.

Cosby, Arthur F. "A New Hospital for St Anthony." ADSF 23 (April 1925): 2–3.

Crane, Jean. "Across the River." *Them Days* 1, no. 4 (1976): 15–18.

Crellin, John K. *Home Medicine: The Newfoundland Experience*. Montreal and Kingston: McGill-Queen's University Press, 1994.

– *The Life of a Cottage Hospital: The Bonne Bay Experience*. St John's, NL: Flanker, 2007.

Cremin, Lawrence. *Popular Education and Its Discontents*. New York: Harper & Row, 1989.

– *Traditions of American Education*. New York: Basic Books, 1977.

Crimi, Elody, Diane Ney, and Ken Cobb. *Jewels of Light: The Stained Glass of Washington National Cathedral*. Washington, DC: Washington National Cathedral, 2004.

Criswell, Elizabeth. "Child Welfare Department Report, 1924." *ADSF* 22 (January 1925): 167–8.

– "Dental Work: Child Welfare." *ADSF* 23 (July 1925): 90–1.

– "Program of the Child Welfare Department." *ADSF* 22 (July 1924): 63–4.

– "School Health Work in Labrador." *Hygeia* (December 1933): 1088–9.

– "West Coast Travelling Health Unit." *ADSF* 21 (January 1924): 125–7.

Croci, Osvaldo. "(Association) Football and the Development of a National Identity in Newfoundland, 1870–1914." *Soccer and Society* 18 (September 2017): 1–18.

Crocker, Ruth. "From Gift to Foundation: The Philanthropic Lives of Mrs Russell Sage." In *Charity, Philanthropy, and Civility in American History*, ed. Lawrence Jacob Friedman and Mark D. McGarvie, 199–215. Cambridge: Cambridge University Press, 2003.

Cuerrier, Edith. "Newfoundland and Labrador Photographs from the George Eastman House Legacy Collection." Master's thesis, Ryerson University, 2009.

Cullen, Declan. "Race, Debt, and Empire: Racialising the Newfoundland Financial Crisis of 1933." *Transactions of the Institute of British Geographers*, 2018. https://doi.org/10.1111/tran.12229.

– "What to Do about Newfoundland?: Colonial Reconstruction and the Commission of Government, 1933–1941." PhD diss., Syracuse University, 2013.

Curtis, Charles S. "Activities at St Anthony in 1934." *ADSF* 33 (April 1935): 3–4.

– "Dr Frank Douglas Phinney." *ADSF* 36 (July 1938): 51.

– "The Hospital Stations: St Anthony Hospital Report, for Six Months Ending April 31 [*sic*], 1926." *ADSF* 24 (July 1926): 73.

– "It Should Be Told: The Grenfell Mission's Work for Education, Part I." *ADSF* 61 (April 1963): 5–9.

– "It Should Be Told: The Grenfell Mission's Work for Education, Part II." *ADSF* 61 (July 1963): 54–7.

– "Sixty Years Forward: Report of the Superintendent." *ADSF* 51 (April 1953): 4–9.

– "St Anthony Hospital." *ADSF* 23 (April 1925): 26.

– "St Anthony Hospital Report." *ADSF* 26 (April 1928): 26–7.

– "St Anthony Hospital Report: Jan. 1, 1929, to Dec. 31, 1929." *ADSF* 28 (April 1930): 32–3.

– "St Anthony Hospital Statistics for 1935." *ADSF* 34 (July 1936): 65–6.

– "St Anthony in 1930." *ADSF* 29 (April 1931): 11.

– "St Anthony in 1931." *ADSF* 30 (April 1932): 26.

– "St Anthony in 1932." *ADSF* 31 (April 1933): 3.

– "St Anthony in 1933: The Annual Report." *ADSF* 32 (April 1934): 12–13.

– "St Anthony in 1936." *ADSF* 35 (April 1937): 5.

– "St Anthony in 1937." *ADSF* 36 (April 1938): 5, 9.

– "Willingly to School." *ADSF* 56 (April 1958): 3–11.

"The Year's Work at St Anthony Hospital." *ADSF* 23 (January 1926): 147–9.

Curtis, Stephan. "Introduction: Cores/Peripheries – Rural/Remote: Medicine, Health-care Delivery and the North." In *Medicine in the Remote and Rural North*, ed. J.T.H. Connor and Stephan Curtis, 1–17. London: Pickering & Chatto, 2011.

Curwen, Eliot. *Labrador Odyssey: The Journal and Photographs of Eliot Curwen on the Second Voyage of Wilfred Grenfell, 1893.* Edited by Ronald Rompkey. Montreal and Kingston: McGill-Queen's University Press, 1996.

Cutter, Marian. "Pioneer Library Work in Labrador." *Library Journal* 41, no. 1 (February 1916): 102–3.

Davis, Harry. "Itinerant Teacher 1923–25." *Them Days* 3, no. 2 (1977): 22–5, 31.

Delatour, Beeckman J. "Reuben Henry Patey." *ADSF* 70 (April 1972): 18–19.

Demarest, Emma S. "History of St Anthony Hospital." *ADSF* 23 (October 1925): 103–7.

"The Dentist's Report." *ADSF* 15 (January 1918): 132–3.

Devens, Carol. "'If We Get the Girls, We Get the Race': Missionary Education of Native American Girls." *Journal of World History* 3, no. 2 (Fall 1992): 219–37.

"Directions for Making Mittens." *ADSF* 41 (October 1943): 91.

"Donations and Contributions." *ADSF* 1 (July 1903): 18–20.

Dove, Jas. "The Home Work." *Missionary Outlook* 12 (March 1892): 38–9.

"Dr Charles E. Parsons." *ADSF* 39 (April 1941): 30.

"Dr Robert Frederick Dove." *CMAJ* 104 (1971): 252.

Drover, W.H. "In Good Company [1935]." *Them Days* 9 (June 1984): 44–6.

Duley, Margot. "The Unquiet Knitters of Newfoundland: From Mothers of the Regiment to Mothers of the Nation." In *A Sisterhood of Suffering and Service: Women and Girls of Canada and Newfoundland during the First World War*, ed. Sarah Glassford and Amy Shaw, 51–74. Vancouver: UBC Press, 2012.

Duncan, Norman. *The Adventures of Billy Topsail.* New York: Fleming H. Revell, 1906.

– *Billy Topsail, MD: A Tale of Adventure with Doctor Luke of the Labrador.* New York: Fleming H. Revell, 1916.

– *Doctor Luke of the Labrador.* New York: Fleming H. Revell, 1904.
– *Dr Grenfell's Parish: The Deep Sea Fishermen.* New York: Fleming H. Revell, 1905.
Dupree, Marguerite. "Foreshadowing the Future: Health Services in Remote Areas, the National Health Service, and the Highlands and Islands of Scotland, 1948–74." In *Medicine in the Remote and Rural North, 1800–2000*, ed. J.T.H. Connor and Stephan Curtis, 75–90. London: Pickering & Chatto, 2011.
Earle, Karl Mcneil. "Cousins of a Kind: The Newfoundland and Labrador Relationship with the United States." *American Review of Canadian Studies* 28 (1998): 387–411.
Ecke, Robert S. *Snowshoe & Lancet: Memoirs of a Frontier Newfoundland Doctor, 1937–48.* Portsmouth, NH: Peter E. Randall, 2000.
Erdozain, Dominic. *The Problem of Pleasure: Sport, Recreation and the Crisis of Victorian Religion.* Woodbridge, UK: Boydell, 2013.
Etherington, Norman. "Education and Medicine." In *Missions and Empire*, ed. Norman Etherington, 261–84. Oxford: Oxford University Press, 2005.
Ewing, Kathleen. "The Educational Department: The School at Venison Tickle." *ADSF* 18 (July 1920): 53–5.
Faculty of Medicine, Memorial University of Newfoundland. http://www.med.mun.ca.
Fedunkiw, Marianne P. *Rockefeller Foundation Funding and Medical Education in Toronto, Montreal, and Halifax.* Montreal and Kingston: McGill-Queen's University Press, 2005.
Fingard, Judith. "College, Career, and Community: Dalhousie Coeds, 1881–1921." In *Youth, University and Canadian Society: Essays in the History of Higher Education*, ed. Paul Axelrod and John G. Reid, 26–50. Montreal and Kingston: McGill-Queen's University Press, 1989.
Fischer, Claude, and Michael Hout. *Century of Difference: How America Changed in the Last One Hundred Years.* New York: Russell Sage Foundation, 2006.
The Fishermen's Mission. "Our History." http://www.fishermensmission.org.uk/about-us/our-history/.
Fitzhugh, Lynn D. *The Labradorians: Voices from the Land of Cain.* St John's, NL: Breakwater, 1999.
Fitzpatrick, Ronald James. "Render unto Caesar?: The Roman Catholic Church and the Denominational Equipoise in the Newfoundland Civil Service, 1908–1934." Bachelor's Honours diss., Memorial University of Newfoundland, 1999.
Flanagan, Hallie. "The Vassar Experimental Theatre." *Vassar Quarterly* 13 (1 July 1928): 157–64.

Forsyth, C. Hogarth. "Sport on Labrador." *ADSF* 37 (October 1939): 96–7.
"Four Students Who Were at Berea College, Kentucky Last Winter." *ADSF* 21 (October 1923): 107.
Frankel, Miles. *I Want to Know If I Got to Get Married: A Doctor on the Grenfell Mission.* St John's, NL: Flanker, 2015.
Gagan, David, and Rosemary Gagan. *For Patients of Moderate Means: A Social History of the Voluntary Public General Hospital in Canada, 1890–1950.* Montreal and Kingston: McGill-Queen's University Press, 2002.
Garret, Helen. "From St John's to White Bay by Land." *ADSF* 22 (July 1924): 81–2.
Gathorne-Hardy, Robert. *Traveller's Trio.* London: Nelson, 1963.
Gerson, Carole. *Canadian Women in Print 1750–1918.* Waterloo, ON: Wilfrid Laurier University Press, 2010.
Giovannini, Margaret. *Outport Nurse.* Edited by Janet McNaughton. St John's, NL: Faculty of Medicine, Memorial University of Newfoundland, 1988.
Goldblatt, David. *The Ball Is Round: A Global History of Football.* New York: Riverhead Books, 2008.
Goodnow, Elinor. "Fisher Folk." *ADSF* 22 (January 1925): 158–9.
Gordon, Clara. *Labrador Teacher, 1919–1925: Clara Gordon's Journals.* Edited by Francis Buckle. Cartwright, NL: Anglican Parish of Cartwright, 2005.
Gordon, Henry. *The Labrador Parson: Journal of the Reverend Henry Gordon, 1915–1925.* Edited by F. Burnham Gill. St John's, NL: Provincial Archives, 1972.
Gorn, Elliot J., and Warren Goldstein. *A Brief History of American Sports.* Chicago: University of Illinois Press, 2004.
Gosden, P.H.J.H. *The Friendly Societies in England, 1815–1875.* Manchester: Manchester University Press, 1961.
Gosling, W.G. *Labrador: Its Discovery, Exploration, and Development.* Toronto: Musson, 1909.
Graham, Frank W. *Ready ... Set ... Go! A St John's Sports Pictorial.* St John's, NL: Creative, 1988.
Graves, Karen. *Girls' Schooling during the Progressive Era: From Female Scholar to Domesticated Citizen.* New York: Garland, 1998.
Green, H. Gordon. *Don't Have Your Baby in the Dory: A Biography of Myra Bennett.* Montreal: Harvest House, 1973.
Greene, Theodore A. "Items from St Barbe Islands." *ADSF* 10 (October 1912): 29–30.
– "The Opening of St Anthony Hospital." *ADSF* 25 (October 1927): 99–106.
– "William Adams Delano." *ADSF* 25 (July 1927): 64.

Greenleaf, Elisabeth Bristol. "Introduction." In *Ballads and Sea Songs of Newfoundland*, ed. Elisabeth Bristol Greenleaf and Grace Yarrow Mansfield. Cambridge, MA: Harvard University Press, 1933. Reprint, xix–xxxix. St John's, NL: Memorial University of Newfoundland, 2004.

Grenfell, Anne, and Katie Spalding. *Le Petit Nord or Annals of a Labrador Harbour.* Boston: Houghton Mifflin, 1920.

Grenfell Association of Great Britain and Ireland. *Medical Work in Labrador and Northern Newfoundland: Eleventh Annual Report for the Year Ending September 30th, 1937.* London: [1937].

– *Medical Work in Labrador and Northern Newfoundland: Sixth Annual Report for the Year Ending September 30th, 1932.* London, [1932].

Grenfell Historic Properties, St Anthony, NL. https://www.grenfell-properties.com/.

Grenfell Louie A. Hall Bed and Breakfast. "Our History." 2014. http://www.grenfellbandb.ca/home/6.

Grenfell, Michael. *Pierre Bourdieu: Education and Training.* New York: Continuum, 2007.

Grenfell, Wilfred T. *Adrift on an Icepan.* New York: Houghton Mifflin, 1909.

– *Adrift on an Icepan.* St John's, NL: Creative, 1992.

– *Adrift on an Icepan.* St John's, NL: Flanker, 2016.

– "American Jottings." *Toilers of the Deep* (1903): 150–1.

– "Battle Harbour." *ADSF* 18 (October 1920): 111–14.

– "Berea College." *ADSF* 21 (April 1923): 39.

– *The Challenge of Labrador.* London: Grenfell Association of Great Britain and Ireland, 1928.

– "The Dentist's Report." *ADSF* 15 (January 1918): 132–3.

– "Doctor Grenfell's Log." *ADSF* 10 (January 1913): 10–12.

– "Donation from the Philadelphia Nationals." *ADSF* 25 (July 1927): 95.

– *Down to the Sea: Yarns from the Labrador.* New York: Fleming H. Revell, 1910.

– "Dr Grenfell's American and Canadian Tour." *ADSF* 3 (July 1905): 12–35.

– "Dr Grenfell's American Tour." *ADSF* 3 (April 1905): 5–10.

– "Dr Grenfell's Log on Land." *ADSF* 16 (April 1918): 18–22.

– "The Educational Fund." *ADSF* 20 (July 1922): 45–7.

– *Forty Years for Labrador.* Boston: Houghton Mifflin, 1919. Reprint, Cambridge, MA: Riverside, 1932.

– *The Harvest of the Sea: A Tale of Both Sides of the Atlantic.* New York: Fleming H. Revell, 1905.

– "Labrador." In *The Newfoundland Guidebook, 1905*, ed. D.W. Prowse, 92–107. London: Bradbury, Agnew, 1905.

– *Labrador and North Newfoundland: An Outline History of the Work of the International Grenfell Association.* Boston: AEG [A.E. Gosling], 1928.
– *Labrador Days: Tales of the Sea Toilers.* Boston: Houghton Mifflin, 1919.
– *A Labrador Doctor: The Autobiography of Sir Wilfred Thomason Grenfell.* London: Hodder and Stoughton, 1929.
– *A Labrador Doctor: The Autobiography of Sir Wilfred Thomason Grenfell.* 13th ed. London: Hodder and Stoughton, 1941.
– *A Labrador Doctor: The Autobiography of Sir Wilfred Thomason Grenfell.* London: Hodder and Stoughton, 1948.
– *A Labrador Doctor: The Autobiography of Wilfred Thomason Grenfell.* Boston: Houghton Mifflin, 1919.
– "Leaves from Dr Grenfell's Diary." ADSF 23 (October 1925): 126–36.
– "The Log of the SS *Strathcona.*" ADSF 12 (January 1905): 11–19.
– "The Log of the *Strathcona* for 1927." ADSF 25 (October 1927): 114–26.
– "Medical Missions in Labrador." *Medical Missionary* 18 (5 May 1909): 344–59.
– "The Mission as Practical Religion." ADSF 26 (July 1928): 59–61.
– "The Missions." In Wilfred T. Grenfell and others, *Labrador: The Country and the People,* 226–250. New rev. ed. New York: Macmillan, 1922.
– "The New Hospital for St Anthony." ADSF 23 (July 1925): 51–2.
– "The New Hospital for St Anthony." ADSF 23 (October 1925): 99–103.
– *Off the Rocks: Stories of the Deep-Sea Fisherfolk of the Labrador.* Philadelphia: Sunday School Times, 1906.
– "The Practice of Medicine in Labrador." ADSF 34 (October 1936): 101–3.
– "Sir Wilfred's Log: Summer of 1930." ADSF 28 (January 1931): 161–75.
– "The Soul of Battle Creek: The Famous Institution Preaches a Gospel of Right Living – Food Only Part of the Creed." *Modern Hospital* 6 (April 1916): 277–80.
– "The Summer of 1933." ADSF 31 (October 1933): 109–11.
– *Tales of the Labrador.* Boston: Houghton Mifflin, 1916.
– "A Tribute to the Dental Volunteers." ADSF 25 (July 1927): 80–1.
– "An Urgent Call for Help." ADSF 3 (July 1905): 6–8.
– *Vikings of To-Day: Or Life and Medical Work among the Fishermen of Labrador.* London: Marshall Brothers, 1895.
– *What Life Means to Me.* Boston: Pilgrim, 1910.
– "Work among Labrador Fishermen." *Proceedings of the Canadian Club* 1904–5, 17 April 1905, 156–61.
– *Yourself and Your Body.* New York: Scribner's, 1924.
Grenfell, William T., and others. *Labrador: The Country and the People.* New rev. ed. New York: Macmillan, 1922.
Hallett, Vicki S. "A Class unto Itself: Phebe Florence Miller's Outport Literary

Salon." In *Creating This Place: Women, Family, and Class in St John's, 1900–1950*, ed. Linda Cullum and Marilyn Porter, 47–70. Montreal and Kingston: McGill-Queen's University Press, 2014.

Halverson, Anders. *An Entirely Synthetic Fish: How Rainbow Trout Beguiled America and Overran the World*. New Haven, CT: Yale University Press, 2010.

Hamill, Sarah C. "Needlework Guild of America." *ADSF* 25 (April 1927): 30–1.

Hamilton, Agnes E. "Football in Labrador." *ADSF* 21 (October 1923): 95.

Hamilton, Elisabeth L., and Shirley S. Smith. "'All Offerings Gratefully Received.'" *ADSF* 39 (April 1941): 14–15.

Hamilton, William B. "Society and Schools in Newfoundland." In *Canadian Education: A History*, ed. J. Donald Wilson, Robert M. Stamp, and Louis-Philippe Audet, 126–42. Toronto: Prentice-Hall, 1970.

Hanrahan, Maura. *The Alphabet Fleet: The Pride of the Newfoundland Coastal Service*. St John's, NL: Flanker, 2007.

Hardiman, David. "Introduction." In *Healing Bodies, Saving Souls: Medical Missions in Asia and Africa*. Wellcome Series in the History of Medicine: Clio Medica 80, ed. David Hardiman, 5–57. Amsterdam: Rodopi, 2006.

Harper, Richard H. "The Missionary Work of the Reformed (Dutch) Church in America in Oklahoma." *Chronicles of Oklahoma* 18, no. 3 (1940): 252–65. Electronic Publishing Center, Oklahoma Historical Society. https://cdm17279.contentdm.oclc.org/digital/collection/p17279coll4/id/10447/rec/3.

Harvard Crimson. http://www.thecrimson.com.

Hause, Frank E. "The Design and Installation of an Electric Lighting Plant for Dr W.T. Grenfell." In *Science and Technology Annual, Pratt Institute, 1908–1909*. New York: Pratt Institute, 1909.

Hawkins, David. "A While on the Kyle [1957]." *Them Days* 9 (June 1984): 65–76.

Hayter, Charles. *An Element of Hope: Radium and the Response to Cancer in Canada, 1900–1940*. Montreal and Kingston: McGill-Queen's University Press, 2005.

Heggie, Vanessa. "Sport (and Exercise) Medicine in Britain: Healthy Citizens and Abnormal Athletes." *CBMH/BCHM* 28, no. 2 (2011): 249–69.

Heidger-Osborne, Ruth. "Sports Day at Harrington." *ADSF* 25 (April 1927): 46.

Hickman, George Albert. "The History of Education in Newfoundland." Master's thesis, Acadia University, 1941.

Higginbotham, Peter. "Rowton Houses" in "The Workhouse: The Story of an Institution." 2018. http://www.workhouses.org.uk/Rowton.

Higgins, Jenny. "Grenfell Mission." Heritage Newfoundland and Labrador, 2018. http://www.heritage.nf.ca/articles/society/grenfell-mission.php.
– "The Truck System." Heritage Newfoundland and Labrador, 2018. http://www.heritage.nf.ca/articles/economy/truck-system.php.
Higgins, W.J. "Association Football, 1901." *NQ* 1 (December 1901): 10–11.
– "Football in Newfoundland." *NQ* 1 (July 1901): 4.
High, Steven. "From Outport to Outport Base: The American Occupation of Stephenville, 1940–1945." *NLS* 18 (2002): 84–113.
– *Occupied St John's: A Social History of a City at War, 1939–1946.* Montreal and Kingston: McGill-Queen's University Press, 2010.
– "Working for Uncle Sam: The 'Comings' and 'Goings' of Newfoundland Base Construction Labour, 1940–1945." *Acadiensis* 32, no. 2 (2003): 84–107.
Hiller, James K. "The Newfoundland Credit System: An Interpretation." In *Merchant Credit and Labour Strategies in Historical Perspective*, ed. Rosemary Ommer, 86–101. Fredericton, NB: Acadiensis, 1990.
– "The Nineteenth Century, 1815–1914." In Newfoundland Historical Society, *A Short History of Newfoundland and Labrador*, 77–102. Portugal Cove–St Philip's, NL: Boulder, 2008.
– "O'Brien, Sir John Terence Nicholls." *DCB* 13. 1994. http://www.biographi.ca/en/bio/o_brien_john_terence_nicholls_13E.html.
– "The Politics of Newsprint: The Newfoundland Pulp and Paper Industry, 1915–1939." *Acadiensis* 19, no. 2 (1990): 3–39.
– "Social Issues in Early 20th-Century Newfoundland: A Comparison of Wilfred Grenfell and William Coaker." *NQ* 89, no. 1 (1994): 27–31.
– "Status without Stature: Newfoundland, 1869–1949." In *Canada and the British Empire*, ed. Phillip Buckner, 127–39. Oxford: Oxford University Press, 2008.
Hobsbawm, Eric. *The Invention of Tradition.* Cambridge: Cambridge University Press, 2012.
Hollett, Calvin. *Beating against the Wind: Popular Opposition to Bishop Feild in Newfoundland and Labrador.* Montreal and Kingston: McGill-Queen's University Press, 2016.
Hopkins, Maud A. "Adventures in the Clothing Department." *ADSF* 23 (October 1925): 124–6.
Hopwood, F.J.S. "The Newfoundland Fisheries and Fishermen." *Toilers of the Deep* 7, no. 73 (1892): 34–44.
"Horace W. McNeill." *ADSF* 57 (April 1959): 4.
Hornsby, John A. "The Trend of Modern Hospital Service." *ADSF* 13 (October 1915): 97–9.

Horsman, Reginald. *Race and Manifest Destiny: The Origins of American Racial Anglo-Saxonism.* Cambridge, MA: Harvard University Press, 1981.

Houghteling, Harriet P. "The Educational Fund: Newfoundland Students in the United States." *ADSF* 22 (October 1924): 120.

House, Edgar. *Light at Last: Triumph over Tuberculosis in Newfoundland and Labrador, 1900–2005.* St John's, NL: Lung Association of Newfoundland and Labrador, 2005.

– *The Way Out: The Story of NONIA, 1920–1990.* St John's, NL: Creative, 1990.

Howe, Barbara. "The Emergence of Scientific Philanthropy, 1900–1920: Origins, Issues and Outcomes." In *Philanthropy and Cultural Imperialism: The Foundations at Home and Abroad,* ed. Robert Arnove, 26–54. Boston: G.K. Hall, 1980.

Howell, Colin, and Daryl Leeworthy. "Borderlands." In *Routledge Companion to Sports History,* ed. S.W. Pope and John Nauright, 71–84. New York: Routledge, 2010.

Howell, Colin D. *Blood, Sweat, Cheers: Sport and the Making of Modern Canada.* Toronto: University of Toronto Press, 2001.

Howell, Joel D. *Technology in the Hospital: Transforming Patient Care in the Early Twentieth Century.* Baltimore: Johns Hopkins University Press, 1995.

Hulan, Renee. "'A Brave Boy's Story for Brave Boys': Adventure Narrative Engendering." In *Echoing Silence: Essays on Arctic Narrative,* ed. John Moss, 183–190. Ottawa: Ottawa University Press, 1997.

Hustins, Donald. *Rivers of Dreams: The Evolution of Fly-Fishing and Conservation of Atlantic Salmon in Newfoundland and Labrador, 1700–1949.* St John's, NL: Tight Lines, 2010.

Hutchings, Corey. "Labrador-Inuit Games Report." April 2014. Newfoundland and Labrador Provincial Historic Commemorations Program. 2016. http://commemorations.ca/wp-content/uploads/2015/10/Labrador-Inuit-Games-Report-by-Corey-Hutchings-April-2014.pdf.

Imhoff, Sarah. "Manly Missions: Jews, Christians, and American Religious Masculinity, 1900–1920." *American Jewish History* 97, no. 2 (2013): 139–58.

"In Memoriam: Cecil S. Ashdown." *ADSF* 46 (October 1948): 68–70.

"In Memoriam: Emma E. Musson." *Iatrian* (February 1914): 3–10.

"The Industrial Shops." *ADSF* 28 (October 1930): 137–9.

"The International Grenfell Association." *ADSF* 12 (October 1914): 111.

International Grenfell Association. "Our History." 2018. http://www.grenfellassociation.org/who-we-are/history/.

[International Grenfell Association]. *A Few Facts about the Grenfell Missions of Newfoundland and Labrador.* [IGA, 1937.]

– *First Annual Report of the International Grenfell Association 1914.*

– "Report of the Staff Selection Committee." *ADSF* 27 (July 1929): 88–91; *ADSF* 28 (July 1930): 86–9; *ADSF* 29 (July 1931): 80–3; *ADSF* 30 (July 1932): 80–3; *ADSF* 31 (July 1933): 90–4; *ADSF* 32 (July 1934): 75–8; *ADSF* 33 (July 1935): 58–61; *ADSF* 34 (July 1936): 66–70; *ADSF* 35 (July 1937): 67–71; *ADSF* 36 (July 1938): 59–62; *ADSF* 37 (July 1939): 53–6.

– "Sixth Annual Report of the International Grenfell Association." *ADSF* 18 (July 1920): 76–96.

– "Staff and Volunteer Workers." *ADSF* 13 (July 1915): [83]–[4]; *ADSF* 14 (July 1916): 55–7; *ADSF* 15 (July 1917): 46–7; *ADSF* 16 (July 1918): 64–5; *ADSF* 17 (July 1919): 71–2; *ADSF* 18 (July 1920): 70–2; *ADSF* 20 (July 1922): 41–3; *ADSF* 21 (July 1923): 54–6; *ADSF* 22 (July 1924): 65–7; *ADSF* 23 (July 1925): 87–9; *ADSF* 24 (July 1926): 69–72; *ADSF* 25 (July 1927): 77–81; *ADSF* 26 (July 1928): 66–9.

– "The Summer Staff." *ADSF* 12 (July 1914): 79–80.

James, Cathy. "Reforming Reform: Toronto's Settlement House Movement, 1900–20." *Canadian Historical Review* 82 (2001): 55–90.

Jenish, D'Arcy. "Raising Steel." *Legion Magazine* (November–December 2009): 46–9.

J.L.G. "Items from the Grenfell Association of America." *ADSF* 8 (July 1910): 6–8.

Johnson, Donald Mc.I. *A Doctor Regrets: Being the First Part of "A Publisher Presents Himself."* London: Christopher Johnson, 1949.

Johnston, James. *Grenfell of Labrador.* London: S.W. Partridge, n.d.

Jones, Edgar. "Early Work of the Church of England in Labrador." *ADSF* 14 (October 1916): [91]–3.

Jones, Peter. "Clothing the Poor in Early-Nineteenth-Century England." *Textile History* 37, no. 1 (2006): 17–37.

"Jottings from the Grenfell Association of America." *ADSF* 6 (July 1908): 10.

Junek, O.W. *Isolated Communities: A Study of a Labrador Fishing Village.* New York: America Book, 1937.

Kealey, Linda. "On the Edge of Empire: The Working Life of Myra (Grimsley) Bennett." In *Caregiving on the Periphery: Historical Perspectives on Nursing and Midwifery in Canada,* ed. Myra Rutherdale, 84–105. Montreal and Kingston: McGill-Queen's University Press, 2010.

Keith, A. "Treves, Sir Frederick." Rev. by D.D. Gibbs. In *DNB* online ed., May 2006.

Kellogg, John Harvey. *The Crippled Colon.* Battle Creek, MI: Modern
  Medicine Publishing, 1931.
– *The Natural Diet of Man.* Battle Creek, MI: Modern Medicine Publishing,
  1923.
Kennedy, David. "Overview: The Progressive Era." *Historian* 37, no. 3 (May
  1975): 453–68.
Kennedy, John C. *Encounters: An Anthropological History of Southeastern
  Labrador.* Montreal and Kingston: McGill-Queen's University Press, 2015.
– "The Impact of the Grenfell Mission on Southeastern Labrador Communi-
  ties." *Polar Record* 24, no. 150 (1988): 199–206.
– *People of the Bays and Headlands: Anthropological History and the Fate
  of Communities in Unknown Labrador.* Toronto: University of Toronto
  Press, 1995.
Kerr, J. Lennox. *Wilfred Grenfell: His Life and Work.* Toronto: Ryerson,
  1959.
King, Stephen. "Reclothing the English Poor, 1750–1840." *Textile History*
  33, no. 1 (2002): 37–47.
Kinsey, Darin. "Seeding the Water as the Earth: The Epicentre and Periph-
  eries of a Western Aquacultural Revolution." *Environmental History* 11,
  no. 3 (2006): 527–66.
"Kirkina." *ADSF* 1 (January 1904): 22.
Korneski, Kurt. *Conflicted Colony: Critical Episodes in Nineteenth-Century
  Newfoundland and Labrador.* Montreal and Kingston: McGill-Queen's
  University Press, 2016.
Kverndal, Roald. *Seamen's Missions: Their Origin and Early Growth; A
  Contribution to the History of the Church Maritime.* Pasadena, CA:
  William Carey Library, 1986.
Labrador-Grenfell Regional Health Authority. "About Us." 2007. http://
  www.lghealth.ca/index.php?pageid=9.
– "2017 Grenfell Greeting Cards." http://www.lghealth.ca/index.php?page
  id=283.
– "Grenfell Foundation." 2007. http://www.lghealth.ca/index.php?page
  id=16.
"Labrador War Memorial." http://www.themdays.com/memorial/world_
  war_1.html.
Lagemann, Ellen Condliffe. *The Politics of Knowledge: The Carnegie Corporation, Philanthropy, and Public Policy.* Middletown, CT: Wesleyan University Press, 1989.
Lake, Edward F.J. *Capturing an Era: History of the Newfoundland Cottage
  Hospital System.* St John's, NL: Argentia Pilgrim, 2010.

Landmark Branding. "156 Fifth Avenue." 2014. http://landmarkbranding. com/154-158-fifth-avenue/.

Lane, Jeremy. *Pierre Bourdieu: A Critical Introduction*. London: Pluto, 2000.

Laverty, Paula. *Silk Stocking Mats: Hooked Mats of the Grenfell Mission*. Montreal and Kingston: McGill-Queen's University Press, 2005.

Lawrence, Christopher. "'Definite and Material': Coronary Thrombosis and Cardiologists in the 1920s." In *Framing Disease: Studies in Cultural History*, ed. Charles E. Rosenberg and Janet Golden, 50–82. New Brunswick, NJ: Rutgers University Press, 1992.

Lawson, Gordon S., and Andrew F. Noseworthy. "Newfoundland's Cottage Hospital System: 1920–1970." In *Making Medicare in Canada: New Perspectives on the History of Medicare in Canada*, ed. Gregory P. Marchildon, 229–48. Toronto: University of Toronto Press, 2012.

Lemare, Finley. "I Liked to Tease." *Them Days* 5, no. 1 (1979): 22–3.

"Letter from Louie [1924]." *Them Days* 3, no. 1 (1977): 18.

Loder, Millicent Blake. *Daughter of Labrador*. St John's, NL: Harry Cuff, 1989.

– "Early School Days." *Them Days* 5, no. 1 (1979): 36–40.

Lodge, T. *Dictatorship in Newfoundland*. London: Cassell, 1939.

Logan, Ann Stuart. "In the Land of the 'Chanty Punts.'" *ADSF* 21 (January 1924): 131–3.

Lombard, Rosalie. *Adventures of a Grenfell Nurse*. The Villages, FL: Xlibris, 2014.

Lougee, Willis E. "Items from the Grenfell Association of America." *ADSF* 7 (April 1909): 39–42.

Lush, Gail. "Nutrition, Health Education, and Dietary Reform: Gendering the 'New Science' in Northern Newfoundland and Labrador, 1893–1928." Master's thesis, Memorial University of Newfoundland, 2008.

Luther, Jessie. *Jessie Luther at the Grenfell Mission*. Edited by Ronald Rompkey. Montreal and Kingston: McGill-Queen's University Press, 2001.

– "Labrador Clothing and Routes." *ADSF* 10 (July 1912): 42–5.

[MacDermott, H.J.A.]. *MacDermott of Fortune Bay Told by Himself*. London: Houghton and Stoughton, 1938.

MacDonald, Robert H. *Sons of Empire: The Frontier and the Boy Scout Movement, 1890–1918*. Toronto: University of Toronto Press, 2000.

Macdonald, Simon. "Transnational History: A Review of Past and Present Scholarship." University College London, Centre for Transnational History. January 2013. https://www.ucl.ac.uk/centre-transnational-history/objectives/simon_macdonald_tns_review.

Mackay, R.A., with S.A. Saunders. "The Economy of Newfoundland." In *Newfoundland: Economic, Diplomatic, and Strategic Studies*, ed. R.A. Mackay, 39–242. Toronto: Oxford University Press, 1946.

Macklem, Elizabeth. "Report of the Labrador Needlework Guild of Canada." *ADSF* 6 (July 1908): 12.

Mangan, J.A. *Games Ethic and Imperialism: Aspects of the Diffusion of an Ideal.* New York: Viking, 1985.

Markel, Howard. *The Kelloggs: The Battling Brothers of Battle Creek.* New York: Pantheon Books, 2017.

Martin, John R. *The Fluorspar Mines of Newfoundland: Their History and the Epidemic of Radiation Lung Cancer.* Montreal and Kingston: McGill-Queen's University Press, 2012.

– *Leonard Miller: Public Servant.* Toronto: Fitzhenry and Whiteside, 1998.

"May Pardy." *Them Days* 1, no. 1 (1975): 36–8.

Mayou, Sister [Edith]. "Sketches of Dr Grenfell's Work on the Labrador and Northern Newfoundland." *ADSF* 6 (April 1908): 12–14.

McCann, Phillip. "Denominational Education in Twentieth-Century Newfoundland." In *The Vexed Question: Denominational Education in a Secular Age,* ed. William A. McKim, 60–79. St John's, NL: Breakwater, 1988.

– "The Politics of Denominational Education in the Nineteenth Century in Newfoundland." In *The Vexed Question: Denominational Education in a Secular Age,* ed. William A. McKim, 30–59. St John's, NL: Breakwater, 1988.

– *Schooling in a Fishing Society: Education and Economic Conditions in Newfoundland and Labrador, 1836–1986.* St John's, NL: ISER Books, 1994.

McCrae, Morrice. *The National Health Service in Scotland: Origins and Ideals, 1900–1950.* East Lothian, Scotland: Tuckwell, 2003.

McDevitt, Patrick F. *May the Best Man Win: Sport, Masculinity, and Nationalism in Great Britain and the Empire, 1880–1935.* Basingstoke, UK: Palgrave Macmillan, 2004.

McGrath, Judy. "Labrador Pastimes." *Them Days* 7, no. 2 (1981): 3–5.

McGrath, Robin. "Traditional Games of Newfoundland and Labrador." Newfoundland and Labrador Provincial Historic Commemorations Program. 2016. http://commemorations.ca/wp-content/uploads/2016/02/Traditional-Games-of-Newfoundland-and-Labrador-Commemoration-Paper-by-Robin-McGrath.pdf.

McLaren, Angus. *Our Own Master Race: Eugenics in Canada, 1885–1945.* Toronto: University of Toronto Press, 1990.

McNaughton, Janet. "The Role of the Newfoundland Midwife in Traditional Health Care, 1900 to 1970." PhD diss., Memorial University of Newfoundland, 1989.

McNeill, Horace. "Farewell." *ADSF* 49 (January 1952): 104–5.

"The Men behind the Scenes." *ADSF* 25 (July 1927): 66–7.

Mesher, Wilfred Bertram. Letter to the editor. *ADSF* 15 (July 1917): 45–6.

Miller, Tom. "The Presbyterian Building – 156 Fifth Avenue." 2011. http:// daytoninmanhattan.blogspot.ca/search?q=presbyterian+building.

Mitchell, Helen S. "Food Problems on the Labrador." *ADSF* 27 (October 1929): 99–103.

Moseley, Marion R. "The Third Year of Health Work." *ADSF* 20 (January 1923): 106–9.

Mount, Harry T. "St Anthony Hospital Report: Jan. 1, 1928, to Dec. 31, 1928." *ADSF* 27 (April 1929): 24–5.

Muir, Ethel. *The Ethical System of Adam Smith.* Halifax: J. Bowes, 1898.

Muir, Ethel Gordon. "The People on the Labrador and Their Needs." *ADSF* 8 (July 1910): 35–41.

– "A Summer School at Red Bay." *ADSF* 7 (January 1910): 31–4.

– "Summer Work at Eddies Cove." *ADSF* 11 (January 1914): 19–21.

Muir Family of Kirkcudbrightshire and Nova Scotia. Douglas J. Graham, comp. 2012. http://douglasjgraham.net/Muir.html.

Murphy, Noel. *Cottage Hospital Doctor: The Medical Life of Dr Noel Murphy, 1945–1954.* St John's, NL: Creative, 2003.

Musson, Emma E. "Labrador: Interesting Account of the Country, Its Interests, Hospitals, Etc." *Woman's Medical Journal* 20 (1910): 197–201.

Myers, Marcia. "Presbyterian Home Mission in Appalachia: A Feminine Enterprise." *American Presbyterians* 71, no. 4 (1993): 253–64.

Neary, Peter. "'A Mortgaged Property': The Impact of the United States on Newfoundland, 1940–49." In *Twentieth-Century Newfoundland: Explorations,* ed. James Hiller and Peter Neary, 179–93. St John's, NL: Breakwater, 1994.

– *Newfoundland in the North Atlantic World, 1929–1949.* Montreal and Kingston: McGill-Queen's University Press, 1988.

– "Venereal Disease and Public Health Administration in Newfoundland in the 1930s and 1940s." *CBMH/BCHM* 15 (1998): 129–51.

– "'Wry Comment': Rhoda Dawson's Cartoon of Newfoundland Society, 1936." *NLS* 8 (Spring 1992): 1–14.

Neuhauser, Duncan. *Coming of Age: A 50-Year History of the American College of Hospital Administrators and the Profession It Serves, 1933–1983.* Chicago: Pluribus, 1983.

"The New St Anthony Hospital." *ADSF* 23 (July 1925): 53.

New English Hymnal. Norwich, UK: Canterbury, 1986.

Newsome, David. *Godliness and Good Learning: Four Studies on a Victorian Ideal.* London: John Murray, 1961.

Nicholson, G.W.L. *The Fighting Newfoundlander: A History of the Royal Newfoundland Regiment*. Montreal and Kingston: McGill-Queen's University Press, 2006.

Noel, S.J.R. *Politics in Newfoundland*. Toronto: University of Toronto Press, 1971.

"Northern Pastimes: I – Fishing." *ADSF* 44 (July 1946): 47–50.

"North Wind: From New England." *ADSF* 37 (October 1939): 115–18

Notre Dame Bay Memorial Hospital: 50 Years in the Life of Our Hospital. n.p., [1974].

Numbers, Ronald L. *Prophetess of Health: A Study of Ellen G. White*. 3rd ed. Grand Rapids, MI: Wm B. Eerdmans, 2008.

– "Sex, Science, and Salvation: The Sexual Advice of Ellen G. White and John Harvey Kellogg." In *Right Living: An Anglo-American Tradition of Self-Help Medicine and Hygiene*, ed. Charles E. Rosenberg, 206–26. Baltimore, MD: Johns Hopkins University Press, 2003.

O. and M. "Strathcona's Secretary's Report." *ADSF* 12 (October 1914): 113–15.

O'Brien, Patricia. *The Grenfell Obsession: An Anthology*. St John's, NL: Creative, 1992.

– *Out of Mind, Out of Sight: A History of the Waterford Hospital*. St John's, NL: Breakwater, 1989.

O'Flaherty, Patrick. *Lost Country: The Rise and Fall of Newfoundland, 1843–1933*. St John's, NL: Long Beach, 2005.

– *The Rock Observed: Studies in the Literature of Newfoundland*. Toronto: University of Toronto Press, 1979.

O'Malley, Soren. "The Importance of the Bicycle to the Early Women's Liberation Movement." *Cranked Magazine* 4 (August 2006). https://cranked mag.wordpress.com/issues/issue-4/the-importance-of-the-bicycle-to-the-early-womens-liberation-movement/.

Overton, James. "Economic Crisis and the End of Democracy: Politics of Newfoundland during the Great Depression." *Labour / Le Travail* 26 (1990): 85–124.

– *Making a World of Difference: Essays on Tourism, Culture and Development in Newfoundland*. St John's, NL: ISER Books, 1996.

"Self-Help, Charity, and Individual Responsibility: The Political Economy of Social Policy in Newfoundland in the 1920s." In *Twentieth-Century Newfoundland: Explorations*, ed. James Hiller and Peter Neary, 79–122. St John's, NL: Breakwater Books, 1994.

P&S Club, Columbia University College of Physicians and Surgeons. "About P&S Club." http://psclub.columbia.edu/about.

Paddon, Harry. *The Labrador Memoir of Dr Harry Paddon, 1912–1938*. Edited by Ronald Rompkey. Montreal and Kingston: McGill-Queen's University Press, 2003.

Page, Elizabeth. "The Educational Department: White Bay, Newfoundland." *ADSF* 19 (January 1922): 129–34.

– "The Growth of the White Bay Work." *ADSF* 22 (April 1924): 24–6.

Palmer, Craig T., Lisa Sattenspiel, and Chris Cassidy. "Boats, Trains, and Immunity: The Spread of the Spanish Flu on the Island of Newfoundland." *NLS* 22 (2007): 473–504.

Palmer, H.M. "Hopwood, Francis John Stephens." Rev. by Mark Pottle, *DNB* online ed. January 2008.

Patey, Francis. *Veterans of the North*. St John's, NL: Creative, 2003.

Peirce, Margaret. "Summer Volunteers in the United States, 1938." *ADSF* 36 (July 1938): 62.

Pennoyer, Peter, and Anne Walker. *The Architecture of Delano & Aldrich*. New York: Norton, 2003.

Perry, Jill Samfya. "Nursing for the Grenfell Mission: Maternalism and Moral Reform in Northern Newfoundland and Labrador, 1894–1938." Master's thesis, Memorial University of Newfoundland, 1997.

Peters, E.S. "Doctor at $5.00 a Day [1933]." *Them Days* 9 (June 1984): 42–4.

Petrone, Penny, ed. *Northern Voices: Inuit Writing in English*. Toronto: University of Toronto Press, 1988.

Phillips, Clifton J. "Changing Attitudes in the Student Volunteer Movement of Great Britain and North America, 1886–1928." In *Missionary Ideologies in the Imperialist Era, 1880–1920*, ed. Torben Christen and William R. Hutchison, 131–45. Arhus, Denmark: Aros, 1982.

Phillips Brooks House Association. "Our History." 2015. http://pbha.org/about-us/our-history.

Phinney, Frank D. "'The Eye Doctor.'" *ADSF* 26 (January 1929): 152–4.

Picken, Mary Brooks. *The Language of Fashion: A Dictionary and Digest of Fabric, Sewing and Dress*. New York: Funk and Wagnalls, 1939.

Piercey, Rhoda Maude. *"True Tales of Rhoda Maude": Memoirs of an Outport Midwife*. Edited by Janet McNaughton. St John's, NL: Faculty of Medicine, Memorial University of Newfoundland, 1992.

Pinker, Robert. *English Hospital Statistics, 1861–1938*. London: Heinemann, 1966.

"Pleasant Commendation for the Hospital." *ADSF* 23 (January 1926): 192.

Pocius, Gerald L. "Tourists, Health Seekers and Sportsmen: Luring Americans to Newfoundland in the Early Twentieth Century." In *Twentieth-*

Century Newfoundland: Explorations, ed. James Hiller and Peter Neary, 47–77. St John's, NL: Breakwater, 1994.

Podnieks, Elizabeth. "Introduction: 'New Biography' for a New Millennium." *a/b: Auto/Biography Studies* 24, no. 1 (2009): 1–14.

Poppleton, M. Evelyn. "A Letter Concerning Flower's Cove." *ADSF* 30 (April 1932): 39.

Porter, Andrew. "Church History, History of Christianity, Religious History: Some Reflections on British Missionary Enterprise since the Late Eighteenth Century." *Church History* 71 (2002): 555–84.

– "Religion and Empire at Home and Abroad." Empire Online. 2018. www.empire.amdigital.co.uk/Essays/AndrewPorter.

– "Religion, Missionary Enthusiasm, and Empire." In *Oxford History of the British Empire*. Vol. 3, *The Nineteenth Century*, ed. Andrew Porter, 222–46. London: Oxford University Press, 2001.

– *Religion versus Empire?: British Protestant Missionaries and Overseas Expansion, 1700–1914*. Manchester: Manchester University Press, 2004.

Porterfield, Amanda. "Protestant Missionaries: Pioneers of American Philanthropy." In *Charity, Philanthropy and Civility in American History*, ed. Lawrence J. Friedman and Mark D. McGarvie, 49–69. Cambridge: Cambridge University Press, 2003 .

Powell, Ben. "Charlottetown." *Them Days* 9, no. 3 (1984): 56–62.

Power, Judith. *Hazel Compton-Hart: Angel from the North*. St John's, NL: Jesperson, 1995.

Pratt Institute, New York. "About Pratt Institute." https://www.pratt.edu/the-institute/history/.

– "Machine Construction Class of 1916." *Pratt Institute Annual 1916*. https://issuu.com/prattalumni/docs/1916prattannual.

"Prince Pomiuk's Friend." *ADSF* 16 (October 1918): 108–9.

"Professional Approval of St Anthony." *ADSF* 25 (January 1928): 180.

Putney, Clifford. *Muscular Christianity: Manhood and Sports in Protestant America, 1880–1920*. Cambridge, MA: Harvard University Press, 2001.

Pye, Gerald. "Fond Are Our Memories." *Them Days* 10 (1985): 49–50.

Rasenberger, Jim. *High Steel: The Daring Men Who Built the World's Greatest Skyline*. New York: HarperCollins, 2004.

Reeves, W.G. "Alexander's Conundrum Reconsidered: The American Dimension in Newfoundland Resource Development, 1898–1910." *NS* 5, no. 1 (1989): 1–37.

– "Aping the 'American Type': The Politics of Development in Newfoundland, 1900–1908." *NS* 10, no. 1 (1994): 44–72.

– "Newfoundlanders in the 'Boston States': A Study in Early Twentieth-Century Community and Counterpoint." *NS* 6, no. 1 (1990): 34–55.

Reynolds, George S. "The Mission Stations: Spotted Islands, 1920." *ADSF* 19 (April 1921): 10–16.

Reynolds, Katherine, and Susan Schram. *Separate Sisterhood: Women Who Shaped Southern Education in the Progressive Era*. New York: Peter Lang, 2002.

Rich, Phoebe. "Down Memory Lane." *Them Days* 4, no. 2 (1978): 59–61.

Richards, J.T. *Snapshots of Grenfell*. Edited by Irving Letto. Victoria, BC: Friesen, 2012.

Richmond, Vivienne. *Clothing the Poor in Nineteenth-Century England*. Cambridge: Cambridge University Press, 2013.

– "'Indiscriminate Liberality Subverts the Morals and Depraves the Habits of the Poor': A Contribution to the Debate on the Poor Law, Parish Clothing Relief and Clothing Societies in Early Nineteenth-Century England." *Textile History* 40, no. 1 (2009): 51–69.

Risse, Guenter B., and John Harley Warner. "Reconstructing Clinical Activities: Patient Records in Medical History." *Social History of Medicine* 5 (1992): 183–205.

Robbins, Cliff. "The Amalgamated Schools of Newfoundland." *NQ* 70, no. 1 (June 1973): 29–35.

Robbins, Sarah. "Woman's Work for Woman: Gendered Print Culture in American Mission Movement Narratives." In *Women in Print: Essays on the Print Culture of American Women from the Nineteenth and Twentieth Centuries*, ed. James P. Danky and Wayne A. Wiegand, 251–80. Madison: University of Wisconsin Press, 2006.

Robidoux, Michael A. *Stickhandling through the Margins: First Nations Hockey in Canada*. Toronto: University of Toronto Press, 2012.

Robinson, Barbara D. "Wilfred Thomason Grenfell and the Christ of Culture." Master's thesis, University of Manitoba, 1993.

Rochester, Maxine K. "Bringing Librarianship to Rural Canada in the 1930s: Demonstrations by the Carnegie Corporation of New York." *Libraries & Culture* 30 (1995): 366–90; reprinted in *Readings in Canadian Library History* 2, ed. Peter F. McNally, 241–63. Ottawa: Canadian Library Association, 1996.

Rodrigues Winery & Distillery, Whitbourne, NL. "About Us." http://rodrigues winery.com/aboutus.html.

Rollmann, Hans. "Hopedale: Gateway to the South and Moravian Settlement." *NLS* 28, no. 2 (2013): 153–92.

Rompkey, Ronald. *Grenfell of Labrador: A Biography*. Toronto: University
of Toronto Press, 1991; reprint ed. Montreal and Kingston: McGill-
Queen's University Press, 2009.
– "Grenfell, Sir Wilfred Thomason." DCB 16. 2011. http://www.biographi.ca
/en/bio/grenfell_wilfred_thomason_16E.html.
– "Heroic Biography and the Life of Sir Wilfred Grenfell." *Prose Studies* 12
(1989): 159–73.
– "Paddon, Henry Locke." DCB 16. 2013.
http://www.biographi.ca/en/bio/paddon_henry_locke_16E.html.
– "Sir Wilfred Thomason Grenfell: Spiritual Adventurer." *Touchstone* 25,
no. 3 (2007): 50–9.
Rompkey, William. *The Story of Labrador*. Montreal and Kingston: McGill-
Queen's University Press, 2005.
Rosenberg, Emily S. "Missions to the World: Philanthropy Abroad." In
Charity, Philanthropy and Civility in American History, ed. Lawrence J.
Friedman and Mark D. McGarvie, 241–57. Cambridge: Cambridge
University Press, 2003.
Rosenberg, Neil V., and Anna Kearney Guigné. "Foreword to the 2004
Reprint." In *Ballads and Sea Songs of Newfoundland*, ed. Elisabeth Bristol
Greenleaf and Grace Yarrow Mansfield. Cambridge, MA: Harvard Univer-
sity Press, 1933. Reprint ed., ix–xxv. St John's, NL: Memorial University of
Newfoundland, 2004.
Rowe, Frederick. *The Development of Education in Newfoundland*.
Toronto: Ryerson, 1964.
– *Education and Culture in Newfoundland*. Toronto: McGraw-Hill Ryerson,
1976.
Ruiz, Rafico. "Media Infrastructure: The Grenfell Mission of Newfoundland
and Labrador." *Continuum: Journal of Media & Cultural Studies* 29
(2015): 383–401.
– "The Moving Image on the North Atlantic, 1930–1950: The Case of the
Grenfell Mission." *Acadiensis* 44 (2015): 5–19.
– "Sites of Communication: The Grenfell Mission of Newfoundland and
Labrador." PhD diss., McGill University, 2014.
Rury, John L. *Education and Social Change: Themes in the History of Amer-
ican Schooling*. Mahwah, NJ: Lawrence Erlbaum, 2002.
Rusted, Brian. "Diary of a Medical Student on the SS *Kyle*, 1945: Ian E.L.
Rusted." NLS 26 (2011): 87–113.
Rusted, Nigel. *It's Devil Deep Down There: 50 Years Ago on the M.V.* Lady
Anderson, *a Mobile Clinic on the S.W. Coast of Newfoundland*. 2nd ed. St
John's, NL: Creative, 1987.

– , comp. *Medicine in Newfoundland c. 1497 to the Early 20th Century: The Physicians and Surgeons.* St John's, NL: Faculty of Medicine, Memorial University of Newfoundland, 1994.

Ryan, Betty. "Reaching for the Sky: The Newfoundland Ironworkers Leave Their Mark on Manhattan." *Newfoundland Lifestyle* 3 (August–September 1985): 8–12.

Ryan, Shannon. *The Ice Hunters: A History of Newfoundland Sealing to 1914.* St John's, NL: Breakwater, 1994.

Saunders, Gary L. *Doctor Olds of Twillingate: Portrait of an American Surgeon in Newfoundland.* St John's, NL: Breakwater, 1994.

Schoepflin, Rennie B. "The Mythic Mission Lands: Medical Missionary Literature, American Children, and Cultural Identity." In *Religion and the Culture of Print in Modern America*, ed. Charles L. Cohen and Paul S. Boyer, 72–104. Madison: University of Wisconsin Press, 2008.

Schumacher, Frank. "Anglo-Saxonism." In *Britain and the Americas ... A Multidisciplinary Encyclopedia*, ed. Will Kaufman and Heidi Slettedahl Macpherson. ABC Clio, 2005, 1:90–2.

Schwarz, Richard W. *John Harvey Kellogg, MD.* Nashville, TN: Southern Publishing Association, 1970.

Scott, John R. "Play at the Newfoundland Seal Fishery." *Culture and Tradition* 1 (1976): 63–71.

Scotter, George W. "Reindeer Ranching in Canada." *Journal of Range Management* 25, no. 3 (1972): 167–74.

Sealander, Judith. "Curing Evils at Their Source: The Arrival of Scientific Giving." In *Charity, Philanthropy and Civility in American History*, ed. Lawrence J. Friedman and Mark D. McGarvie, 217–39. Cambridge: Cambridge University Press, 2003.

Seidman, Steven. *Contested Knowledge: Social Theory Today.* Oxford: Blackwell, 2008.

Semple, Rhonda A. "Missionary Manhood: Professionalism, Belief and Masculinity in the Nineteenth-Century British Imperial Field." *Journal of Imperial and Commonwealth History* 36 (September 2008): 397–415.

Seton, David. *The College Y: Student Religion in the Era of Secularization.* New York: Palgrave Macmillan, 2007.

Sexty, Suzanne. "Dorcas Society: The Fruit of Her Hands." NQ 105, no. 4 (2013): 34–8.

Shackle, Samira. "The Rebirth of Women's Football: More Than a Century On, It's a Game Worth Watching." *New Statesman*, 17 October 2014. http://www.newstatesman.com/sport/2014/10/rebirth-women-s-football-more-century-it-s-game-worth-watching.

Shapiro, Henry. *Appalachia on Our Mind: The Southern Mountains and Mountaineers in the American Consciousness, 1870–1920*. Chapel Hill: University of North Carolina Press, 1978.

Sheard, A. "The Seamen's Institute." *ADSF* 12 (January 1915): 146.

Shields, Rob. "Knowing Space." *Theory, Culture & Society* 23, nos 2–3 (2006): 147–9.

Side, Katherine. "E. Mary Schwall: Traveller, Mission Volunteer, and Amateur Photographer." *NLS* 30 (Spring 2015): 53–88.

Silverman, Alexander. "Pittsburgh's Contribution to Radium Recovery." *Journal of Chemical Education* 27 (June 1950): 303–8.

Simms, Alvin, and Jamie Ward. *Regional Population Projections for Labrador and the Northern Peninsula 2016–2036: Report Prepared for the Harris Centre for Regional Development and Policy, Memorial University*. Population Project: Newfoundland and Labrador in Transition. St John's, NL: Memorial University of Newfoundland, 2016.

"Skating." *Them Days* 7, no. 2 (1981): 43.

Smith, Allan. *Canada: An American Nation? Essays on Continentalism, Identity, and the Canadian Frame of Mind*. Montreal and Kingston: McGill-Queen's University Press, 1994.

– *Doing the Continental: Conceptualizations of the Canadian-American Relationship in the Long Twentieth Century*. Canadian-American Public Policy Occasional Paper no. 44, December 2000. Orono, ME: Canadian-American Center, University of Maine, 2000.

Smith, Warwick. "The General Hospital." *Newfoundland Magazine* 2, no. 5 (1919): 2–3, 10–11.

Squarey, R.T. "The Newfoundland Government Inquiry into Charges against the Grenfell Mission." *ADSF* 15 (January 1918): 158–62.

"St Anthony Items." *ADSF* 10 (July 1912): 3–9.

"The St Anthony Mat Industry." *ADSF* 4 (January 1917): 137.

Stewart, Janet. "A Letter from Lockwood School." *ADSF* 31 (January 1934): 167–70.

Stirling, Gordon M. "Ice Hockey in Newfoundland." In *The Book of Newfoundland*, ed. Joseph R. Smallwood, 2:151–3. St John's, NL: Newfoundland Book Publishers, 1937.

Stockwood, Wayne. "Vincent Burke." In *ENL*, ed. Joseph R. Smallwood and Robert Pitt, 1:295–6. St John's, NL: Newfoundland Book Publishers, (1967) 1981.

Story, G.M., W.J. Kirwin, and J.D.A. Widdowson, eds. *Dictionary of Newfoundland English*. 2nd ed. Toronto: University of Toronto Press, 1990.

Heritage Newfoundland and Labrador. http://www.heritage.nf.ca/
dictionary/index.php.

Suit, Herman D., and Jay S. Loeffler. *Evolution of Radiation Oncology at Massachusetts General Hospital*. New York: Springer, 2011.

Sweeny, Robert. *Why Did We Choose to Industrialize? Montreal, 1819–1849*. Montreal and Kingston: McGill-Queen's University Press, 2015.

T.A.G. "A Memorial Minute to Cecil Spanton Ashdown." *ADSF* 47 (April 1949): 5.

Tallant, Edith. "The Industrial Department and the People." *ADSF* 27 (October 1929): 125–8.

– "An Itinerant Industrial Worker." *ADSF* 28 (October 1930): 124–8.

Tanner, V. *Outlines of the Geography, Life and Customs of Newfoundland-Labrador (The Eastern Part of the Labrador Peninsula)*. Helsinki, 1944.

Tatnall, Anna C. "An Effort for the Grenfell Mission." *ADSF* 39 (January 1942): 111.

– "Report of the American-Labrador Needlework Guild of America." *ADSF* 6 (July 1908): 11.

– "Seventh Annual Report of the Needlework Guild." *ADSF* 13 (July 1915): 60–1.

Taylor, Stephen, and Harold Horwood. *Beyond the Road: Portraits and Visions of Newfoundlanders*. Toronto: Van Nostrand Reinhold, 1976.

Teperson, Hyman I. "Formulae for the Rapid Calculation of Millicuries of Radon (Emanation) Destroyed and Dosage Delivered." *Radiology* 15 (1930): 129.

Thomas, G.W. "The International Grenfell Association: Its Role in Northern Newfoundland and Labrador. Part I: The Early Days." *CMAJ* 118 (1978): 308–10.

– "The International Grenfell Association. Part II: The Benefits of Newfoundland's Entry into Confederation." *CMAJ* 118 (1978): 446–9.

– *From Sled to Satellite: My Years with the Grenfell Mission*. Toronto: Irwin, 1987.

Threlkeld-Edwards, Herbert. "The New Medical Era in St Anthony." *ADSF* 25 (July 1927): 51–7.

Thurston, Harry. "The Fish Gang: Heaven-Storming Manhattan's Skyline with the Ironworkers of Newfoundland." *Equinox* 4 (September–October 1985): 54–63.

Toland, Harry G. *A Sort of Peace Corps: Wilfred Grenfell's Labrador Volunteers*. Bowie, MD: Heritage Books, 2001.

Treude, Erhard. "The Development of Reindeer Husbandry in Canada." *Polar Record* 14, no. 88 (1968): 15–19.

Tucker, Kathleen. "Stories of the Grenfell Mission: How the Grenfell Mission Changed People's Lives." St Anthony Basin Resources, Oral History Initiative, 2014. http://sabrinl.com/wp-content/uploads/2016/06/Grenfell-Mission.pdf.

Tucker, Leonard. "Hockey: A Story of the Creation of Hockey Teams on the Tip of the Great Northern Peninsula." St Anthony Basin Resources, Oral History Initiative, 2014. http://sabrinl.com/wp-content/uploads/2016/06/hockey.pdf.

"Two Loving Tributes to Dr Joseph A. Andrews." *ADSF* 26 (July 1928): 54–6.

Valen, Dustin. "Citizens, Protect Your Property: Perspectives on Public Health, Nationalism and Class in St John's Bowering Park, 1911–1930." *Journal of the Society for the Study of Architecture in Canada* 40, no. 2 (2015): 43–56.

Valverde, Mariana. *The Age of Light, Soap, and Water: Moral Reform in English Canada, 1885–1925.* Toronto: McClelland and Stewart, 1991.

Vanast, Walter. "Arctic Bodies, Frontier Souls: Missionaries and Medical Care in the Canadian North." PhD diss., University of Wisconsin at Madison, 1996.

Vassar Miscellany News. http://newspaperarchive.vassar.edu/.

Vaughn, Catherine. "Labrador Days in Florida: Grenfell Labrador Industries." *ADSF* 38 (April 1940): 32.

Vonderlehr, R.A., and R.E. Heering. *Report of a Survey on Civil Health Services as They Relate to the Health of Armed Forces in Newfoundland.* Washington, DC: United States Public Health Service, 1940.

Wakefield, A.W. "Battle Harbour Hospital." *ADSF* 11 (January 1914): 15–18.

– "St Anthony Items." *ADSF* 9 (July 1911): 8–12.

[Wakefield, A.W.]. "Winter Work at Cartwright." *ADSF* 8 (July 1910): 19–26.

Wall, R.R. "R.C.A.F. Station, Goose, Labrador." *ADSF* 45 (April 1947): 7–9.

Walls, Andrew. *The Missionary Movement in Christian History: Studies in the Transmission of Faith.* Edinburgh: T & T Clark, 1996.

Walls, Andrew F. "British Missions." In *Missionary Ideologies in the Imperialist Era: 1880–1920,* ed. Torben Christen and William R. Hutchison, 159–65. Arhus, Denmark: Aros, 1982.

Ward, Dreshman & Reinhardt. "Our Heritage." 2013. http://www.wdrincorp.com/our-heritage.

– "Voluntary Giving in a Free Land." 1955. http://www.wdrincorp.com/wp-content/uploads/2015/10/wdr-history.pdf.

Warren, Henry. "Winter Sports, St Anthony, 1920." *ADSF* 19 (July 1921): 47–9.

Webb, Jeff A. *Observing the Outports: Describing Newfoundland Culture, 1950–1980.* Toronto: University of Toronto Press, 2016.

Webb-Johnson, A.E. *Notes on a Tour of the Principal Hospitals and Medical Schools of the United States and Canada.* London, 1923; facsimile ed., Bibliolife, n.d.

Wheatley, Stephen C. *The Politics of Philanthropy: Abraham Flexner and Medical Education.* Madison: University of Wisconsin Press, 1988.

Whisnant, David. *All That Is Native and Fine: The Politics of Culture in an American Region.* Chapel Hill: University of North Carolina Press, 1983.

– "Second Level Appalachian History: Another Look at Some Fotched-On Women." *Appalachian Journal* 9, no. 2 (1982): 115–23.

[White, E.E.]. "Items from the New England Grenfell Association." ADSF 8 (October 1910): 5–8.

– "Items from the New England Grenfell Association." ADSF 10 (July 1912): 21–30.

– "Items from the New England Grenfell Association." ADSF 10 (October 1912): 24–8.

Whiteley, George. "The Story of Pomiuk." NQ 58, no. 2 (1959): 5, 41–2.

Wilson, Brian C. *Dr John Harvey Kellogg and the Religion of Biologic Living.* Bloomington: Indiana University Press, 2014.

Wilson, Shannon. *Berea College: An Illustrated History.* Lexington: University Press of Kentucky, 2006.

Withers, George. *Rock Harbour: A Chronicle of a Placentia Bay Community.* Portugal Cove–St Philip's, NL: White Rock, 2004.

Wong, Timothy Man-kong. "Local Voluntarism: The Medical Mission of the London Missionary Society in Hong Kong, 1842–1923." In *Healing Bodies, Saving Souls, Medical Missions in Asia and Africa.* Wellcome Series in the History of Medicine: Clio Medica 80, ed. David Hardiman, 87–113. Amsterdam: Rodopi, 2006.

Worth, Rachel. "Developing a Method for the Study of the Clothing of the 'Poor': Some Themes in the Visual Representation of Rural Working-Class Dress, 1850–1900." *Textile History* 40, no. 1 (2009): 70–96.

Wright, Donald. *The Professionalization of History in English Canada.* Toronto: University of Toronto Press, 2005.

Yale Daily News. "Yale Daily News Historical Archive." http://web. library.yale.edu/digital-collections/yale-daily-news-historical-archive.

"The Year at St Anthony Hospital." ADSF 25 (April 1927): 19.

Zecher, Ilsley. "Annual Sports on the Ice in St Anthony." ADSF 23 (October 1925): 121–3.

Zirin, Dave. *A People's History of Sport in the United States: 250 Years of Politics, Protest, People, and Play.* New York: New, 2008.

Zunz, Oliver. *Philanthropy in America: A History.* Princeton: Princeton University Press, 2011.

Contributors

JENNIFER J. CONNOR is professor of medical humanities in the Faculty of Medicine, cross-appointed to the Department of History, and affiliated with the Department of Gender Studies, Memorial University of Newfoundland. In 2015 she received both the Marie Tremaine Medal and the Watters-Morley Prize of the Bibliographical Society of Canada in recognition of her historical and bibliographical scholarship that focuses on medical book culture. Her essays have appeared in many books and journals, including *Science in Print* (University of Wisconsin Press, 2012), *Newfoundland and Labrador Studies*, CMAJ, *Victorian Periodicals Review*, and *Book History*.

J.T.H. CONNOR is John Clinch Professor of Medical Humanities and History of Medicine, Faculty of Medicine, Memorial University of Newfoundland; he also holds an appointment in the Department of History. A Fellow of the Royal Historical Society, he has published widely on the history of science, technology, and medicine in North America, as well as on aspects of medical museums. His most recent work has appeared in *Military Medicine, Journal of the History of Medicine and Allied Sciences, Canadian Bulletin of Medical History, Acadiensis*, and *Newfoundland and Labrador Studies*. He is also the author of *Doing Good: The Life of Toronto's General Hospital* (Toronto, 2000) and co-editor of *Medicine in the Remote and Rural North*, with Stephan Curtis (Pickering & Chatto, 2011).

HEIDI COOMBS-THORNE is a research associate with the Faculty of Medicine at Memorial University of Newfoundland. She has a PhD in history, specializing in nursing with the Grenfell mission in northern Newfoundland and Labrador, and she recently completed post-doctoral research on the negotiation of medical encounters between the Grenfell mission and the Southern Inuit of Labrador.

MARK GRAESSER was a member of the Department of Political Science, Memorial University of Newfoundland from 1970 to 2000, specializing in African and Newfoundland politics. Since retiring, he has divided his time between Newfoundland and New Zealand. He is the editor of *It's a Glorious Country* (DRC, 2015), letters by IGA volunteer Florence Clothier.

JAMES K. HILLER began PhD research on Wilfred Grenfell in the 1970s before moving on to another subject. However, he has maintained a strong interest in the history of Newfoundland and of Labrador, and was a member of the Department of History at Memorial University of Newfoundland until his retirement in 2008.

EMMA LANG is a graduate student in the Department of Folklore at Memorial University of Newfoundland. She holds a master's degree from George Washington University in museum studies. She designed and co-curated the bilingual, travelling exhibition, *Tangled Threads/Fils Entremêlés: Clothing and the Grenfell Mission 1880s–1920s*.

JOHN R. MATCHIM is a PhD candidate in the University of New Brunswick's Department of History. He earned a master of arts in history in 2010 and a master of philosophy in humanities in 2017, both from Memorial University of Newfoundland. His research has focused on maritime health and labour in the North Atlantic world, including medical care in the late-Victorian Royal Navy and Canada's east coast offshore oil industry and cod fishery. For several years he worked as research assistant on clinical records of the IGA, based in the Faculty of Medicine at Memorial University. His doctoral research will examine the marine operations of the IGA and its Strathcona line of hospital ships.

RONALD L. NUMBERS is Hilldale Professor Emeritus of the History of Science and Medicine and of Religion at the University of Wisconsin-Madison, where he taught for nearly four decades. He has written or edited more than two dozen books, including, most recently, *Galileo Goes to Jail and Other Myths about Science and Religion* (Harvard, 2009); *Biology and Ideology from Descartes to Dawkins* (Chicago, 2010), edited with Denis Alexander; *Science and Religion around the World* (Oxford, 2011), edited with John Hedley Brooke; *Wrestling with Nature: From Omens to Science* (Chicago, 2011), edited with Peter Harrison and Michael H. Shank; *Gods in America: Religious Pluralism in the United States* (Oxford, 2013), edited with Charles Cohen; *Ellen Harmon White: American Prophet* (Oxford, 2014), edited with Terrie Aamodt and Gary Land; and *Newton's Apple and Other Myths about Science*

(Harvard, 2015), with Kostas Kampourakis. He is a past president of the History of Science Society, the American Society of Church History, and the International Union of History and Philosophy of Science. He is currently writing a history of science in America and a biography of John Harvey Kellogg.

RAFICO RUIZ is a Social Sciences and Humanities Research Council of Canada Banting Post-doctoral Fellow in the Department of Sociology at the University of Alberta. From February to July 2018 he was the Fulbright Canada Research Chair in Arctic Studies at Dartmouth College, New Hampshire.

KATHERINE SIDE is professor, Department of Gender Studies, Memorial University of Newfoundland. Her research examines material artifacts, including photographs, associated with the Grenfell mission. She is principal researcher, grant holder, and co-curator of the bilingual, travelling exhibition *Tangled Threads/Fils Entremêlés: Clothing and the Grenfell Mission 1880s–1920s*, and author of *Patching Peace: Women's Civil Society Organizing in Northern Ireland* (ISER, 2015).

HELEN WOODROW is a historian, educator, and principal of Educational Planning and Design Associates and Harrish Press Publications. She is a scholar in the community whose publications and programs have supported the voices of various marginalized individuals and groups. She has edited collections of oral histories from fishers and plant workers, published memoirs from adults who returned to school, and prepared text on the important role of elders.

Index